Flavonoids and Anti-Aging

The nuclear factor erythroid 2-related factor 2 (Nrf2) was described as a master regulator of the cellular antioxidant response. Moreover, many critical biological functions linked to cell viability, metabolism, autophagy, inflammation, immunity, and differentiation have been attributed to Nrf2, which regulates over 600 genes. It is well known that oxidative stress, which Nrf2 can ameliorate, plays a key role in many pathologic processes such as aging, obesity, diabetes, cancer, and neurodegenerative diseases.

Flavonoids, on the other hand, through their ability to activate and upregulate Nrf2, can have anti-oxidative, anti-inflammatory, anti-mutagenic, and anti-carcinogenic properties. Flavonoids are an essential ingredient in nutraceuticals, functional foods, and pharmaceuticals. The present book *Flavonoids and Anti-Aging: The Role of Transcription Factor Nuclear Erythroid 2-Related Factor 2* focuses on the interaction between Nrf2 and flavonoids and their applications in various conditions such as aging, osteoporosis, cardiovascular diseases, and neurodegenerative disease and many other areas.

Key Features:

- Focuses on the mechanisms and use of flavonoids in activating Nrf2 as an anti-aging and "WELLNESS" molecule
- Provides a specific approach to flavonoid activation of Nrf2 and its implications in aging and various disease conditions and its applications as nutraceuticals
- Presents flavonoid-based functional foods
- Discusses the flavonoid nutraceuticals market and future trends

Written by experts in the field, this book provides a unique approach to understanding the flavonoid activation of the transcription factor Nrf2, which is responsible for many different disease conditions due to increased reactive oxidative species in the body caused by some physiological triggers.

Nutraceuticals: Basic Research and Clinical Applications
Series Editor: Yashwant Pathak, PhD

Nutraceuticals and Health: Review of Human Evidence
edited by Somdat Mahabir and Yashwant V. Pathak

Marine Nutraceuticals: Prospects and Perspectives
Se-Kwon Kim

Nutrigenomics and Nutraceuticals: Clinical Relevance and Disease Prevention
edited by Yashwant Pathak and Ali M. Ardekani

Food By-Product Based Functional Food Powders
edited by Özlem Tokuşoğlu

Flavors for Nutraceuticals and Functional Foods
M. Selvamuthukumaran and Yashwant Pathak

Antioxidant Nutraceuticals: Preventive and Healthcare Applications
Chuanhai Cao, Sarvadaman Pathak, and Kiran Patil

Advances in Nutraceutical Applications in Cancer: Recent Research Trends and Clinical Applications
edited by Sheeba Varghese Gupta and Yashwant Pathak

Flavor Development for Functional Foods and Nutraceuticals
M. Selvamuthukumaran and Yashwant Pathak

Nutraceuticals for Prenatal: Maternal and Offspring's Nutritional Health
Priyanka Bhatt, Maryam Sadat Miraghajani, Sarvadaman Pathak,
and Yashwant Pathak

Bioactive Peptides: Production: Bioavailability, Health Potential and Regulatory Issues
edited by John Oloche Onuh, M. Selvamuthukumaran, and Yashwant Pathak

Nutraceuticals for Aging and Anti-Aging: Basic Understanding and Clinical Evidence
edited by Jayant Lokhande and Yashwant Pathak

Marine-Based Bioactive Compounds: Applications in Nutraceuticals
edited by Stephen T. Grabacki, Yashwant Pathak, and Nilesh H. Joshi

Applications of Functional Foods and Nutraceuticals for Chronic Diseases
edited by Syam Mohan, Shima Abdollahi, and Yashwant Pathak

Flavonoids and Anti-Aging: The Role of Transcription Factor Nuclear Erythroid 2-Related Factor 2
edited by Karam F.A. Soliman and Yashwant V. Pathak

For more information about this series, please visit: https://www.crcpress.com/
Nutraceuticals/book-series/CRCNUTBASRES

Flavonoids and Anti-Aging
The Role of Transcription Factor Nuclear Erythroid 2-Related Factor 2

Edited by
Karam F.A. Soliman and
Yashwant V. Pathak

CRC Press
Taylor & Francis Group
Boca Raton London New York

CRC Press is an imprint of the
Taylor & Francis Group, an **informa** business

First edition published 2023
by CRC Press
6000 Broken Sound Parkway NW, Suite 300, Boca Raton, FL 33487-2742

and by CRC Press
4 Park Square, Milton Park, Abingdon, Oxon, OX14 4RN

CRC Press is an imprint of Taylor & Francis Group, LLC

Library of Congress Cataloging-in-Publication Data
Names: Soliman, Karam F. A., editor. | Pathak, Yashwant V., editor.
Title: Flavonoids and anti-aging : the role of transcription factor nuclear erythroid 2-related factor2 / edited by Karam F.A. Soliman and Yashwant V. Pathak.
Description: First edition. | Boca Raton : CRC Press, 2023. |
Series: Nutraceuticals: basic research/clinical applications |
Editor's name misspelled on title page; should read Karam F.A. Soliman. |
Includes bibliographical references and index.
Identifiers: LCCN 2022039544 (print) | LCCN 2022039545 (ebook) |
ISBN 9781032113739 (hardback) | ISBN 9781032125732 (paperback) |
ISBN 9781003225225 (ebook)
Subjects: LCSH: Aging–Nutritional aspects. | Flavonoids. |
Flavonoids–Therapeutic use. | Flavonoids–Physiological effect.
Classification: LCC RA776.75 .F537 2023 (print) | LCC RA776.75 (ebook) |
DDC 612.6/7–dc23/eng/20221202
LC record available at https://lccn.loc.gov/2022039544
LC ebook record available at https://lccn.loc.gov/2022039545

ISBN: 978-1-032-11373-9 (hbk)
ISBN: 978-1-032-12573-2 (pbk)
ISBN: 978-1-003-22522-5 (ebk)

DOI: 10.1201/9781003225225

Typeset in Times
by codeMantra

Dedication

This book is dedicated to my wife Samia, and my children John, Gina, Mark, and Mary for their love and endless support.

Karam F.A. Soliman

To the loving memories of my parents and Dr Keshav Baliram Hedgewar, who gave proper direction to my life, to my beloved wife Seema who gave positive meaning and my son Sarvadaman who gave a golden lining to my life.

I would like to dedicate this book to my brother Dr Pramod Pathak and sister Ms Charuta Pathak/Piplapure, who were my mentors from childhood, and I have learned a lot from them.

Yashwant V. Pathak

Contents

Preface

The primary objective of this book is to provide an overview of the anti-aging effects of the nuclear factor erythroid 2-related factor 2 (Nrf2) and the role of Nrf2 activators in delaying the aging process. In discussing this topic, we are emphasizing the use of flavonoids (potent Nrf2 activators) as commonly available nutraceuticals.

One of the hallmarks of aging is the reduced capacity of cellular homeostatic mechanisms that protect the body against various oxidative, toxicological, and pathological insults. The decline in endogenous antioxidant (EAO) levels leaves the cell susceptible to several internal and environmental stresses. Due to the central role of EAO in cellular protective mechanisms, the induction of enzymes required for its synthesis represents a critical adaptive response to oxidative injury. In aging, however, when basal levels of oxidative stress become elevated, EAO and the enzymes from which it is synthesized do not concomitantly increase but decline in many tissues. This lack of cellular compensatory response to loss in EAO and the existence of a prooxidant state in aging cells lead to many pathological manifestations.

One of the most important factors in the body to reduce oxidative stress is (Nrf2), which controls the basal and induced expression of an array of antioxidant response element–dependent genes to regulate the physiological and pathophysiological outcomes of oxidative stress. The release of Nrf2, the principal transcription factor, regulates antioxidant response element (ARE)-mediated gene transcription to enhance cellular defense systems. By regulating an extensive cytoprotective network of genes, Nrf2 activation is critical for the body's ability to cope with internal and external stressors, including inflammatory, oxidative, and environmental. It is also essential for mitochondrial homeostasis and structural integrity.

Activation of Nrf2 creates a downstream production of proteins and antioxidant enzymes, which provide benefits beyond direct-acting antioxidants. These products are not fully consumed in redox reactions; they can restore EAO. Additionally, they have a long duration of action, so they do not need to be continuously produced. The ability of Nrf2 to induce phase 2 liver enzymes also makes it a powerful detoxification agent. While oxidative stress activates Nrf2, researchers have looked for other ways to induce this protein for human benefit. Interestingly, there are many Nrf2 activators in foods, and many of these activators are available in the market as nutraceuticals. As we will see in this book, many of these nutraceuticals are used to delay or prevent many chronic diseases associated with aging. These diseases, as discussed in this book, include neurodegeneration, obesity, cardiovascular diseases, liver diseases, bone diseases, ocular diseases, and hearing loss.

We are extremely thankful to Mr Steve Zollo and Ms Laura Piedrahita and the staff of CRC Press and CodeMantra who helped us a lot to get this book out in the market.

Karam F.A. Soliman, PhD, Distinguished Professor of Pharmaceutical Sciences, Associate Dean for Research and Graduate Studies, College of Pharmacy and Pharmaceutical, Florida A&M University (FAMU), Tallahassee, FL 32307, USA

and

Yashwant V. Pathak, MPharm, Executive MBA, MSCM, PhD, FAAAS
Professor and Associate Dean for Faculty Affairs, USF Health Taneja College of Pharmacy, University of South Florida, 12901 Bruce B Downs Blvd, MDC 030, Tampa, FL 33612, USA
Tel: 01-813-974-1026, Email: ypathak1@usf.edu

Editors

Dr Karam F.A. Soliman is the Associate Dean for Research and Graduate Studies and Distinguished Professor of Pharmaceutical Sciences at the College of Pharmacy and Pharmaceutical Sciences Institute of Public Health of Florida A&M University (FAMU). Dr Soliman received his MS and PhD degrees in Physiology from the University of Georgia in 1971 and 1972, respectively. He started his professional career in 1972 as an Assistant Professor of Physiology at the School of Veterinary Medicine of Tuskegee Institute. He moved to FAMU in 1975, where he was involved with the Research Center in Minority Institution (RCMI) program for 36 years since its inception in 1985. Also, his record includes the training of 30 PhDs in Pharmacology/Toxicology. He has published extensively in national and international refereed journals (203). His record includes one book, five book chapters, and four US patents. His research has been supported by NIH, NASA, Office of Naval Research, and Department of Energy grants. During his tenure at FAMU, he was awarded federal grants totaling over $96 million. Dr Soliman's research interests in cancer have been focused on cancer cell pH as a crucial factor in the biological functions of cancer cell proliferation, invasion, metastasis, drug resistance, and apoptosis. Also, he contributed significantly to the area of the involvement of Nrf2 in aging, COVID-19, neurodegeneration, and cancer. Dr Soliman is a member of the Society for Neuroscience, American Society of Pharmacology and Experimental Therapeutics, American Physiological Society, American Society for Investigative Pathology, Endocrine Society, Society of Experimental Biology and Medicine, and the American Association of Cancer Society.

Dr Yashwant V. Pathak completed PhD in Pharmaceutical Technology from Nagpur University, India and EMBA and MS in Conflict Management from Sullivan University. He is Professor and Associate Dean for Faculty Affairs at College of Pharmacy, University of South Florida, Tampa, Florida. With extensive experience in academia as well as industry, he has more than 300 research publications, including research papers, chapters and reviews, and three US patents approved. Dr Pathak has over 62 edited books published in nanotechnology, nutraceuticals, and drug delivery systems. He has several edited books in cultural studies and conflict management. He has received several national and international awards including two Fulbright awards. Dr Pathak was selected as fellow of American Association for the Advancement of Sciences (FAAAS) in 2021. He is also an Adjunct Professor at Faculty of Pharmacy, Airlangga University, Surabaya, Indonesia.

Contributors

Getinet M. Adinew
Division of Pharmaceutical Sciences
College of Pharmacy and Pharmaceutical
  Sciences, Institute of Public Health
Florida A&M University
Tallahassee, Florida

Emmanuel Boadi Amoafo
Department of Pharmaceutical Sciences
North Dakota State University
Fargo, North Dakota

Seth Kwabena Amponsah
Department of Medical Pharmacology
University of Ghana Medical School
Accra, Ghana

Aparoop Das
Department of Pharmaceutical Sciences
Dibrugarh University
Assam, India

Madhavi Gangapuram
College of Pharmacy and Pharmaceutical
  Sciences, Institute of Public Health
Florida A&M University
Tallahassee, Florida

Urvashee Gogoi
Department of Pharmaceutical Sciences
Dibrugarh University
Assam, India

Aaron L. Hilliard
Division of Pharmaceutical Sciences
College of Pharmacy and Pharmaceutical
  Sciences
Florida A&M University
Tallahassee, Florida

Archita Jha
College of Arts and Sciences
University of South Florida
Tampa, Florida

Charles A. Lewis
College of Pharmacy and Pharmaceutical
  Sciences, Institute of Public Health
Florida A&M University
Tallahassee, Florida

Elizabeth Mazzio
Division of Pharmaceutical Sciences
College of Pharmacy and Pharmaceutical
  Sciences, Institute of Public Health
Florida A&M University
Tallahassee, Florida

Patricia Mendonca
Division of Pharmaceutical Sciences
College of Pharmacy and Pharmaceutical
  Sciences, Institute of Public Health
Florida A&M University
Tallahassee, Florida

Samia Messeha
Division of Pharmaceutical Sciences
College of Pharmacy and Pharmaceutical
    Sciences, Institute of Public Health
Florida A&M University
Tallahassee, Florida

Augustine T. Nkembo
Department of Pharmaceutical Sciences
Taneja College of Pharmacy
University of South Florida
Tampa, Florida

Emmanuel Kwaku Ofori
Department of Chemical Pathology
University of Ghana Medical School
Accra, Ghana

Kalyani Pathak
Department of Pharmaceutical Sciences
Dibrugarh University
Assam, India

Manash Pratim Pathak
Faculty of Pharmaceutical Sciences
Assam Down Town University
Assam, India

Yashwant V. Pathak
Taneja College of Pharmacy
University of South Florida
Tampa, Florida

Kinfe K. Redda
College of Pharmacy and Pharmaceutical
    Sciences, Institute of Public Health
Florida A&M University
Tallahassee, Florida

Tanya D. Russell
Center for Advanced Professional
    Excellence
University of Colorado Anschutz
Aurora, Colorado

Riya Saikia
Department of Pharmaceutical Sciences
Dibrugarh University
Assam, India

Karam F.A. Soliman
Division of Pharmaceutical Sciences
College of Pharmacy and Pharmaceutical
    Sciences, Institute of Public Health
Florida A&M University
Tallahassee, Florida

Equar Taka
Division of Pharmaceutical Sciences
College of Pharmacy and Pharmaceutical
    Sciences, Institute of Public Health
Florida A&M University
Tallahassee, Florida

Flavonoids

Sources, Chemical Classification, and Pharmacological Activities

1

Madhavi Gangapuram and Kinfe K. Redda
Florida A&M University

Contents

DOI: 10.1201/9781003225225-1

INTRODUCTION

Flavonoids are a large class of polyphenolic compounds present in all vascular plants having a structure of benzo-γ-pyrone. More than 10,000 different classes of flavonoids are reported within the literature and appear to exhibit a wide range of biological activities. Flavonoids are secondary metabolites accountable for many health benefits [1–3]. The basic structure of flavonoids has a 15-carbon atom skeleton with two A and B aromatic rings linked by a heterocyclic C-ring [4]. Their chemical structure and oxidation properties, the B-ring attached with the C-ring, flavonoids will be characterized into various subgroups like flavones, flavanones, flavonols, isoflavonoids, neoflavonoids, anthocyanins, and chalcones [5–8].

Flavonols

Flavonols and flavones have an identical structure except for the hydroxyl group on the third position of the C-ring, which can even be glycosylated [2]. O-glycoside forms of flavonols are the most common and most significant subgroup of flavonoids. About 900 O-glycosides of flavonols are present in plants and form the glycoside bond at 3, 7, 3′, and 4′ [9]. Flavonols are found abundantly in various fruits and vegetables, including apples, berries, grapes, tomatoes, onions, lettuce, celery, and parsley; the most studied flavonols are quercetin, kaempferol, and myricetin (Figure 1.1, Table 1.1). Cranberries, lingonberries, and elderberries are the rich source of quercetin and other kaempferol. Myricetin is found in berries and currants in high concentrations and peaches and pears in low concentrations [10,11].

Flavanones

Flavanones, also called dihydroflavones, are the intermediate precursor and end products in the flavonoid biosynthetic pathway. Flavanones and flavonols are structurally similar, except that flavanones have a chiral center at the second position and absence of a double bond between the second and third positions in the C-ring. Flavanones are most commonly found in citrus fruits like oranges, lemons, and grapefruits. Hesperidin

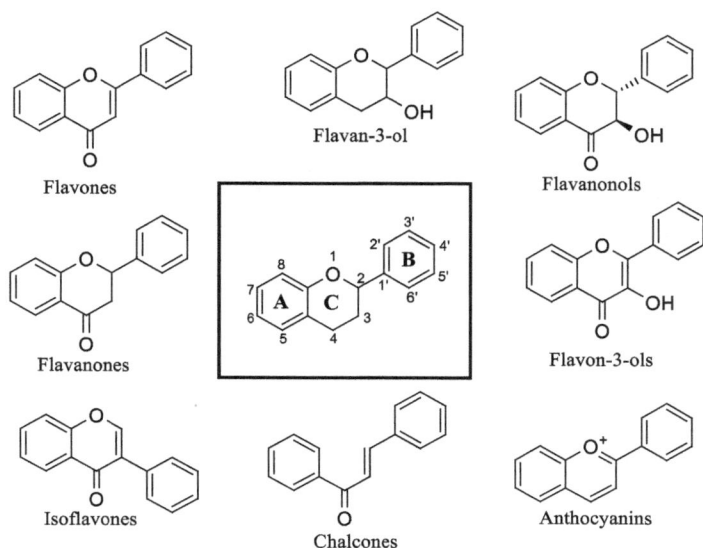

FIGURE 1.1   Flavonoids' chemical structures and classification [6].

and naringin are examples of this class (Figure 1.1, Table 1.1). Due to their free-radical scavenging properties, these compounds show engaging pharmacological activities as antioxidant, anti-inflammatory, and cholesterol-lowering agents [12,13].

Flavanonols: Flavanonols are 3-hydroxy derivatives of flavanones and are also called dihydroflavanonols. Taxifolin is a well-known example of this class and is abundant in citrus fruits [14].

Isoflavonoids

In isoflavonoids, the chromone ring (A&C) is attached to a B-ring at the third position rather than the second position in other flavonoids. Genistein and daidzein are examples of isoflavonoids and less disturbed in plants. Available sources of these compounds are the Chinese medicinal herbs Genista tinctoria, soybeans, beans, other leguminous plants, and microbes [13]. In some animal models, these compounds show estrogenic activities and are considered phytoestrogens [15–17]. Isoflavones can be stored in vacuoles by O-glycoxidation modification to form β-glucosides and 6-O-manlonylgucosides [18]. Isoflavones in the form of aglycones are more biologically active than the glycoside forms. In soybean seeds, 90% of isoflavone is in glycoside form and is more water-soluble and suitable for vacuole storage [19].

Flavanols

Flavanols are also referred to as catechins or flavan-3-ols because the hydroxyl group is bound to the third position of the C-ring. Flavanols do not have the double bond between

TABLE 1.1 Flavonoid's structure, natural source, and health benefits [4,6]

FLAVONOID CLASS	FLAVONOID STRUCTURE	DIETARY SOURCE	HEALTH BENEFITS
Flavonols	Quercetin Myricetin Kaempferol Isorhamnetin	Onions, broccoli, tea, apple, blueberries, spinach, dark chocolate, nuts	Antioxidant, anticoagulant, anti-inflammatory activities, control the blood pressure, glycemic levels
Flavones	Apigenin Luteolin Chyrysin	Celery, parsley, chamomile tea, fenugreek, onion, citrus fruits, garlic, pepper, some herbs	Anticancer, antimicrobial, antioxidant activities, anti-edematogenic activity, and controls blood glucose level

(Continued)

TABLE 1.1 (Continued) Flavonoid's structure, natural source, and health benefits [4,6]

FLAVONOID CLASS	FLAVONOID STRUCTURE	DIETARY SOURCE	HEALTH BENEFITS
Flavanones	Naringenin Hesperetin Eriodictyol	Citrus fruits, mint, tomatoes	Antiulcer activity, antioxidant activity
Flavanols	(+)-Catechin (+)-Epicatechin	Apricots, cocoa, chocolates, red grapes, red wine, green tea, cereals, milk, reduced fat	Antiulcerogenic, anti-inflammatory, antioxidant activities, lowering the risk of heart attack and antimicrobial activity, antibacterial activity

(Continued)

TABLE 1.1 (Continued)   Flavonoid's structure, natural source, and health benefits [4,6]

FLAVONOID CLASS	FLAVONOID STRUCTURE	DIETARY SOURCE	HEALTH BENEFITS
Anthocyanidins	Cyanidin, Delphindin, Malvidin, Petunidin	Berries, red wine, red cabbage, cherries, currants, rice, beans, onions	Anti-inflammatory, antimicrobial, anticarcinogenic, neuroprotective activities, prevention of LDL oxidation, antifungal activity
Isoflavones	Genistein, Daidzein, Glycitein	Soybeans, dairy products, leguminous plants, eggs, soy-based products, and meat	Lowering the LDL cholesterol, balancing hormone levels, antifibrosis, anti-atherosclerosis, anticancer, and antioxidant activities

(Continued)

TABLE 1.1 (Continued) Flavonoid's structure, natural source, and health benefits [4,6]

FLAVONOID CLASS	FLAVONOID STRUCTURE	DIETARY SOURCE	HEALTH BENEFITS
Chalcones	Arbutin, Phloretin, Phloridzin, Chalconaringenin	Apples, tomatoes, pears, strawberries, and wheat products	Antineoplastic, anti-inflammatory, and antioxidant activities

C-2 and C-3, and also the keto group at the fourth position of the C-ring. Flavanols have two chiral centers on the second and third places in the molecules that generate four diastereoisomers: (+)-catechin, (−)-catechin, (+)-epicatechin, and (−)-epicatechin [14]. Esterification of flavanols with gallate groups can form gallic acid conjugates epicatechin gallate, epigallocatechin, and epigallocatechin gallate [2]. Flavanols can create polymers called proanthocyanidins or condensed tannins. Proanthocyanidins generally contain 2–60 units of flavanol monomers. Flavanols are abundant in bananas, apples, blueberries, and green tea (Figure 1.1 and Table 1.1).

Flavones

Flavones have a double bond between the second and third positions and a keto group at the fourth position of the C-ring. Most vegetables and fruits containing flavones have the hydroxyl group at the fifth position of ring A. According to the taxonomic classification of fruits and vegetables, hydroxylation occurs at the seventh position of the A-ring and 3′ and 4′ of the B-ring [10]. O-glycosidation occurs mainly at the fifth and seventh positions and methylation and acylation at 3′ and 4′ of the B-ring. Apigenin, chrysin, luteolin, and tangeritin are well-known compounds in the flavone subgroup. They are usually present in celery parsley, red pepper, chamomile, mint, and *Ginkgo biloba* peels of citrus fruits [20–23].

Neoflavonoids

The less-studied flavonoids were neoflavonoids. Neoflavonoids have a B-ring attached to the C-ring at the fourth position. The first neoflavone was isolated from calophyllodlide from *Calophyllum inophyllum* seeds and was found in the Sri Lankan *Mesua thwaitesii* plant [10,11,24,25].

Anthocyanidin

The structure of anthocyanidin is different from other flavonoid subgroups. Anthocyanidins lack a keto group at the fourth position on the C-ring and have a positive charge on the oxygen atom, also referred to as flavylium cations; due to this, these compounds are unstable and not found in plants. Anthocyanidins have existed as chloride salts. Anthocyanins are the glycosylated form of anthocyanidins and are water-soluble. Anthocyanins are the pigments that give color to plants, flowers, and fruits, which depend upon the pH and methylation or acylation at the hydroxyl group on the A- & B-ring. The most commonly available anthocyanins are cyanidin, delphinidin, malvidin, pelargonidin, peonidin, and petunidin. These compounds are present in berry, red cabbage, red grape, currant, barley, banana, chocolate, tea, wine, onion, mango, and lentil [26–28].

Chalcones

Chalcones are among the leading subclass of flavonoids and are also called open-chain flavonoids or benzyl acetophenone [29]. Phloridzin, arbutin, phloretin, and chalconarin-genin are significant examples. Nutritional sources for chalcones are apples, tomatoes, pears, strawberries, and certain wheat products [10,30,31].

FLAVONOID SOURCES

Recent data analysis by the U.S. Department of Agriculture (USDA) and the National Health and Nutrition Examination Survey (NHANES) estimated that the median intake of flavonoids in adults was 344.83 ± 9.13 mg/day. The three major individual flavonoids were catechin, epicatechin, and polymers. The most important sources of total flavonoid intake in U.S. adults were tea, wine, beer, citrus fruits, and apples [32–35]. In plants, flavonoids are found in free-state aglycones and O- or C-glycoside-bound forms. The common hydroxylated position of flavonoids is at 2, 3, 5, 7, 3', 4', and 5'. In nature, glyco-sylation of flavonoids occurs at the third or seventh position; therefore, the carbohydrates are often D-glucose, L-rhamnose, D-galactose, D-xylose, and L-arabinose [2,36–38].

SYNTHESIS OF FLAVONOIDS

Naturally found flavonoids show promising biological and pharmacological activities. Therefore, flavonoid synthesis has widespread application in organic chemistry [39]. Several synthetic methods were developed to get flavonoids [40–42]. Flavonoids were conventionally synthesized by the Baker–Venkatraman rearrangement and the Claisen–Schmidt condensation. The condensation of 2-hydroxy acetophenone with benzalde-hydes under basic conditions leads to chalcones. Intramolecular cyclization of chalcones under acidic conditions furnishes various flavonoid analogs (Figure 1.2).

THE PHARMACOLOGICAL ACTIVITIES OF FLAVONOIDS

Recent research has focused on the flavonoid-rich food diet and its health benefits, including disease prevention [37]. Flavonoids are the plant's secondary metabolites hav-ing a polyphenolic compound with different biological activities in various signaling

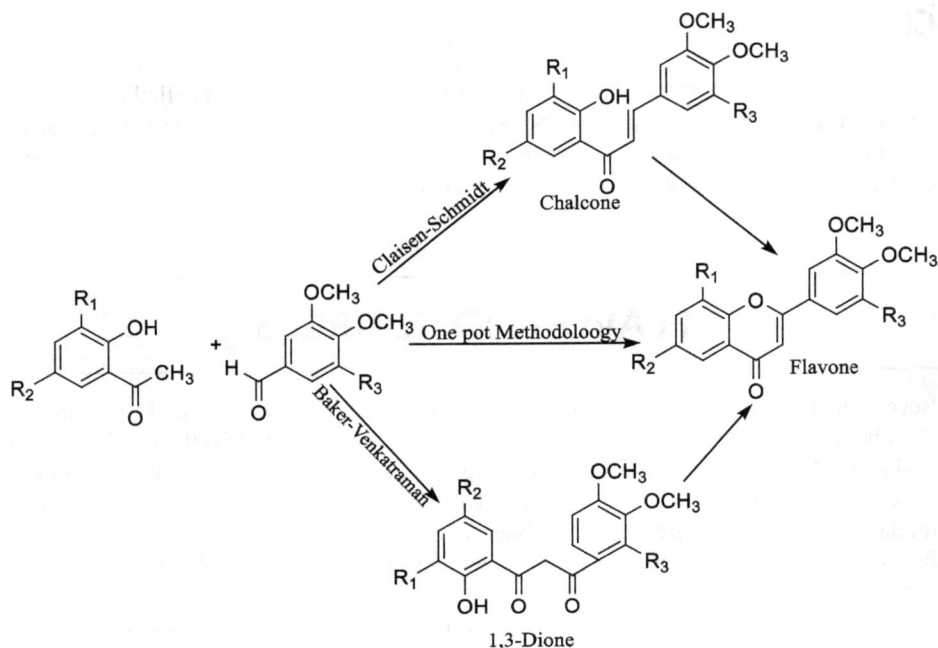

FIGURE 1.2   Basic reaction scheme for the synthesis of flavonoids [40,41].

pathways associated with chronic diseases like protecting cardiovascular disease (CVD) [43], anti-inflammatory [44], antioxidant [45], antibacterial, antiviral [46–49], and anticancer activities [50,51].

Antioxidant Activity

Flavonoids protect against reactive oxygen species (ROS) formation, which plays an essential role in cellular redox reactions, immune response, and normal cell functioning. The increased ROS level ends up imbalanced in the antioxidant defense mechanism. It will result in oxidative stress, which can cause chronic and pathological conditions, including diabetes, hepatocellular damage, atherosclerosis, and cancers [52,53]. Flavonoids are also called free-radical scavengers and act as antioxidants. The antioxidant properties of flavonoids rely upon the functional groups' arrangement, configuration, and the total number of hydroxyl groups [54,55]. The presence of hydroxyl groups in flavonoids can stabilize the free radicals, scavenge the ROS, and chelate the metal ions. However, substituting hydroxyl groups on rings A and C has little or no superoxide scavenging effect. The antioxidant activity of flavonoids usually increases with the increase in hydroxyl groups and decreases with O-methylation or glycosylation of the hydroxyl groups [56]. Flavonoids protect the lipids against peroxidation by various mechanisms like suppressing ROS formation either by enzyme inhibition or by metal chelating involved in a free-radical generation [4]. In vitro studies show that quercetin, epicatechin, and rutin are potent inhibitors of lipid peroxidation. In flavan-3-ols, hydroxyl groups on the B-ring form the hydrogen bond with 3-OH, aligning the B-ring with the C and A rings reveals the antioxidant activity. In the case of flavonols, intramolecular hydrogen bonding between 3-OH and 3', 4'-catechol will elucidate the antioxidant activity [57]. Procyanidins' antioxidant activity or scavenging of reactive species increases with increasing polymerization. Procyanidin dimers and trimers are more effective than monomers in scavenging superoxide anions. Similarly, procyanidin tetramers are more effective than trimers against peroxynitrite- and superoxide-mediated oxidation.

Anti-Inflammatory Activity

Inflammation is a normal biological process in response to the invasion of the pathogen, tissue injury, and removal of necrotic and damaged cells [58]. If the inflammation persists for an extended time, it causes various chronic diseases [59]. The anti-inflammatory activities of hesperidin, apigenin, luteolin, anthocyanin, and quercetin were reported [60]. In literature, it has been reported that flavonoids' anti-inflammatory activity is arbitrated through several mechanisms, such as inhibition of cyclooxygenase-2 (COX-2), lipoxygenase, and iNOS (nitric oxide synthase). Flavonoids also inhibit NF-κB and phosphodiesters involved in cell activation [61,62]. Higher concentrations of flavonoids like apigenin, quercetin, and luteolin inhibit COX-2 and NOS production [63]. Proanthocyanidins extracted from the grape seed are shown to control the inflammatory immune system and induce the production of prostaglandin E2 and nitric oxide production [64].

Anticancer Activity

Cancer is the second leading cause of death worldwide after heart attack. Oxidative stress, genetic mutation, pollution, smoking, and radiation develop cancer [65]. In vitro animal studies have shown that flavonoids can act as antioxidants in normal conditions and pro-oxidants in cancer cells triggering the apoptotic pathways [66,67]. Pro-oxidant activity of flavonoids could suppress the proliferation of cancer cells by inhibiting epidermal growth factor receptor/mitogen-activated protein kinase (EGFR/MAPK), phosphatidylinositide 3-kinase (PI3K), protein kinase B (Akt), and nuclear factor kappa-light-chain-enhancer of activated B cells (NF-κB) [26,68]. Quercetin, belonging to the flavonol group, was the first tyrosine kinase inhibitor tested in the human phase I trial and exhibited antiproliferative, antimetastatic, anti-angiogenic, apoptotic, and chemo-sensitizing effects [4]. Isoflavone, genistein, has phytoestrogen properties and might act as an estrogen antagonist that targets multiple cellular signal transduction pathways and arrests cell cycle at the G2/M phase. Hydroxylated flavonoids possess more potent inhibitory activity than their methoxylated counterparts on neoplastic cell lines. Hydroxylation on the third position of ring C will improve the biological activity. Apigenin antiproliferative activity is lower when compared to kaempferol because of the

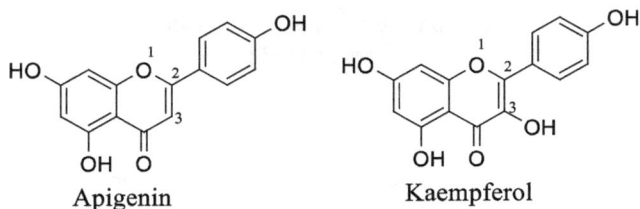

FIGURE 1.3 Apigenin and kaempferol structures.

lack of a 3-OH group on the C-ring (Figure 1.3). According to literature studies, flavonoids like quercetin, kaempferol, myricetin, luteolin, and apigenin exhibited anticancer activity against lung cancer, gastric cancer, colon cancer, glioma cancer, and liver cancer and antitumor activity [6,69,70].

Antimicrobial Activity

The flavonoids extracted from plants have a considerable effect against microbial infection. In vitro studies show that flavonoids have antimicrobial activity against many microorganisms. Quercetin, apigenin, isoflavone, flavone, and flavanone are the most potent antibacterial active compounds [71,72]. The two mechanisms were involved with the interaction of flavonoids and lipid bilayers. The most common molecular actions are that flavonoids form a complex with protein or phospholipids through non-specific forces such as hydrogen bonding, covalent bonding, and hydrophobic effect. Their antibacterial mode of action can be associated with their ability to deactivate microbial adhesion cell envelope, enzymes, and proteins [4]. The lipophilic nature of flavonoids may disrupt microbial membranes [73]. In vitro antibacterial effect of catechins against *Vibrio cholerae*, *Shigella*, *Streptococcus mutans*, and other bacteria are studied, and catechin showed a more potent action to inactivate cholera toxin in *V. cholerae* and also inhibited glucosyltransferase in *S. mutans* [4]. Hydroxyl groups on the B-ring of flavonoids may form hydrogen bonding with the nucleic acid bases and further result in DNA-RNA synthesis inhibition in bacteria. The antimicrobial activity of other flavonoids, naringenin, and sophoraflavanone G was also found effective against methicillin-resistant *Staphylococcus aureus* . This effect of flavonoids might be due to the reduction of membrane fluid in hydrophobic and hydrophilic regions and outer and inner membrane layers. The connection between antibacterial activity and membrane interference supports the concept that flavonoids can reduce the membrane fluidity of bacteria and exhibit antibacterial activity. Flavonoids having a hydroxyl group at the seventh, fifth, and sixth positions on the A-ring are essential for their antibacterial activity [74,75].

Antifungal Activity

Fungal infections are increased constantly in the current decade, mainly in immunocompromised people. Among all the fungal infections, *Candida*, *Aspergillus*, *Pneumocystis*,

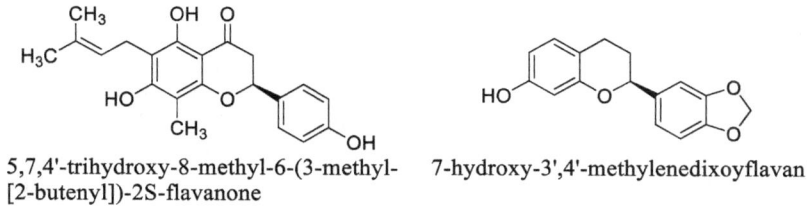

5,7,4'-trihydroxy-8-methyl-6-(3-methyl-
[2-butenyl])-2S-flavanone

7-hydroxy-3',4'-methylenedixoyflavan

FIGURE 1.4 Chemical structure of *Eysenhardria texana* and *Termanalia bellerica* extracts.

and *Cryptococcus* are the main aggressive agents worldwide due to severe and higher incidences of the diseases [76,77]. The flavonoids such as nobiletin, langeritin, and hesperidin have been extracted from the tangerine orange peels and tested their activity against *Deuterophoma tracheiphila*, showing suitable antifungal activities [78]. The flavonoids, 5, 7,4'-trihydroxy-8-methyl-6-(3-methyl-[2-butenyl])-2S-flavanone and 7-hydroxy-3', 4'-methylene dioxy flavan extracted from *Eysenhardtia texana* and *Terminalia bellerica* (Figure 1.4) exhibit potential antifungal activity against *A. flavus* [79]. The flavonoids such as kaempferol, rutin, quercetin, myricetin, baicalein, and apigenin have antifungal properties [80]. Flavonoids' inhibitory activity of fungal growth depends on various mechanisms such as plasma membrane disruption, induction of mitochondrial dysfunction, and inhibition of cell wall formation, cell division, RNA and protein synthesis, and efflux-mediated pumping system [26,77,81]. Flavonoids extracted from medicinal plants have been explored. Their antifungal activities can be promising, cost-effective agents for inhibiting fungal growth.

Cardioprotective Effects

CVDs are the leading cause of death globally. It is predicted that 44% of the U.S. population will have CVD by 2030 [82]. In recent years, it has been reported that the imbalance between the formation of ROS and ROS-degrading antioxidant systems causes endothelium damage and develops CVDs [83]. Research studies suggest that the daily consumption of flavonoid-rich food may reduce approximately 10% of the CVD risk [43]. In vitro, in vivo, and clinical studies found that the antioxidant activity of flavonoids may reduce the adverse side effects of anticancer drug doxorubicin and reported their cardioprotective properties through various mechanisms, including the inhibition of ROS generation, mitochondrial dysfunction, apoptosis, NF-κB, p53, and DNA damage. Flavonols (kaempferol, isorhamnetin) and flavones (rutin, luteolin) showed activity against doxorubicin-induced cardiotoxicity without affecting the doxorubicin antitumor activity [84,85]. In another study, the presence of thymoquinone in *Nigella sativa* showed a cardioprotective effect by reducing lipoprotein, cholesterol, and triglycerides [86]. Based on animal studies, black and red rice grains, fruits, and vegetables rich in flavonoids, like anthocyanins, proanthocyanidins, and apigenin, exhibited significant improvement in the myocardial antioxidant status during the administration of anticancer drugs and chemical-induced cardiac dysfunction. The chance of ischemic stroke and CVD can be lowered with a higher intake of flavonoids [27,87,88].

Antiviral Activity

Many natural phenolic compounds are an essential source for developing antiviral drugs because of their availability and having fewer side effects. Naturally occurring flavonoids have been recognized for antiviral activity since 1940, and many scientific reports have revealed their antiviral activity. There is an urgent need to develop an efficient drug against the human immunodeficiency virus (HIV). The effect of the antiviral activity of flavonoids depends on the inhibition of various enzymes linked with the life cycle of those viruses. Flavan-3-ol was more effective in inhibiting HIV-1 and 2 than flavones and flavanones [4,89,90]. The flavonoid compound. Baicalin isolated from *Scutellaria baiclensis* was more effective against HIV-1 infection and replication inhibition. Flavonoids, including quercetin, naringin, hesperetin, and catechin, have more potent antiviral activity, affecting specific DNA and RNA viruses [91]. The antiviral activity of flavonoids is expounded to the non-glycosidic compounds and hydroxylation at the third position. The antiviral mechanism of action includes inhibiting viral polymerase and binding of viral nucleic acid or viral capsid protein [92].

Hepatoprotective Activity

The organ liver plays an essential role in the physiological processes in the body like secretion, storage, metabolism, detoxification, and biochemical processes. The liver metabolizes fats and carbohydrates by the secretion of bile and storing vitamins. The significant factors for liver damage are autoimmune disorders, biological factors, and chemicals found in antituberculosis drugs and CCl_4 [93]. Flavonoids such as catechin, apigenin, naringenin, rutin, quercetin, and venoruton also possess hepatoprotective activities [94]. Grapefruit is a good source of the naringin flavonoid, which is metabolized as naringenin in the body. Lee et al. [95] reported that in rats, the hepatoprotective activity of naringenin was found, and the hepatic damage was induced by dimethylnitrosamine (DMN). Silymarin is a flavonoid with three structural components, silydianin, silychristine, and silibinin, extracted from the seeds and fruits of mild thistle *Silybum marianum* (Compositae, Figure 1.5).

In damaged livers, *Silymarin* stimulates the enzymatic activity of DNA-dependent RNA polymerase-1 and subsequent biosynthesis of RNA and protein, resulting in the cell proliferation and biosynthesis of DNA, resulting in liver regeneration [95]. It also involves regulating cell membrane permeability and integrity, ROS scavenging, inhibition of leukotriene, and collagen production [4]. Apigenin hepatic activity mode of action downregulates Nrf2-signaling and upregulates BCL-2 apoptotic pathway; this can improve hepatic health conditions during severe liver disease [96]. Flavonoids extracted from *Laggera alata* showed hepatoprotective activity against carbon tetrachloride (CCl_4)-induced liver damage in rats. Histopathological and in vivo studies showed that 50, 100, and 200 mg/kg of flavone administration reduced the aspartate transaminase (AST), alanine transaminase (ALT), total protein levels, and hydroxyproline and sialic acid levels in the liver. Several clinical studies also revealed the effect of flavonoids in treating hepatobiliary dysfunction, including nausea, abdominal pain, feeling of bloating, and less appetite [4].

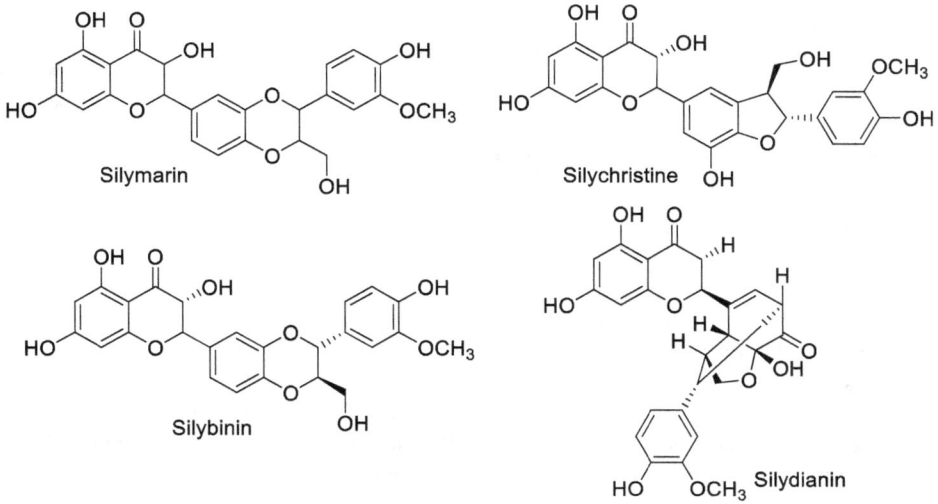

FIGURE 1.5 Sulymarin and structural components.

Antidiabetic Effects

Diabetes mellitus, commonly referred to as diabetes, is one of the widespread metabolic disorders characterized by hyperglycemia, negative nitrogen balance, hyperlipidemia, glycosuria, and ketonemia [97]. Numerous in vitro animal and in vivo cell studies support the hyperglycemic activity of flavonoids [98]. Several studies indicate that consuming a flavonoid-rich diet controls carbohydrate digestion and insulin secretion by regulating different intracellular pathways. Flavonols, quercetin, and kaempferol have antidiabetic effects on streptozotocin (STZ)-induced diabetic mice, reduce hyperglycemia, increase glucose uptake, and decrease the hyperglycemia-stimulating gluconeogenesis. O-methylated flavonol, isorhamnetin, extracted from *Ginkgo biloba*, *Hippophae rhamnoides*, and *Oenanthe javantica* also reduces the hypoglycemia and oxidative stress in STZ-induced diabetic mice [99]. Glycosylate quercetin, also known as rutin, rutoside, and sophorin, isolated from buckwheat, oranges, grapes, and citrus fruits has antidiabetic activity and reduces the fasting blood sugar levels. In diabetic rats, studies showed that rutin could protect against and improve myocardial dysfunction apoptosis, inflammation, and oxidative stress in the heart of rats [100]. Naringin and hesperidin also lower blood glucose levels by upregulating the PPARγ (peroxisome proliferator-activated receptor), hepatic glucokinase, and adipocyte GLUT4 [101]. The most common mechanism of flavonoids' antidiabetic activity is reducing glucose absorption. In another mechanism, flavonoids can inhibit the activity of α-glucosidase in the small intestine [37]. Anthocyanins extracted from bilberries studied their antidiabetic effect on mice with type-II non-insulin-dependent diabetes. The bilberries extract has improved hyperglycemia and insulin sensitivity by targeting AMPK (adenosine monophosphate-activated protein kinase) and GLUT4 (insulin-regulated glucose transporter type 4). Non-obese diabetic mice model studies show that daidzein or genistein in the diet at a dose of 0.2% can inhibit diabetes and increase glucose homeostasis through the function of pancreatic β-cell stabilization [98].

Antiatheroscleroitc Effects

Atherosclerosis is a chronic disease in which inflammation occurs in large arteries and forms plaque in the arteries. It is one of the significant factors contributing to the incidence of stroke myocardial infarction and leads to significant mortality in western countries. The primary risk factor for atherosclerosis development is the increased levels of lipoproteins and cholesterol in plasma. Other risk factors for developing atherosclerosis are age, diabetes, obesity, hypertension, diet, and smoking. Several studies have been conducted to evaluate the beneficial effects of flavonoids against atherosclerosis [102]. A high intake of a flavonoid-rich diet can reduce the risk factors that develop atherosclerosis, including high tolerance to glucose, lowering blood pressure, and maintaining a good body mass index. Pomegranate juice is rich in proanthocyanidins and anthocyanidins. A apoE-deficient mice model study shows the effects of pomegranate juice such as reduction of lipid peroxides and accumulation of macrophage CE without affecting the cholesterol level in plasma [103]. In the same mice model study, supplementation of polyphenolic compound resveratrol containing chow diet for 4 months reduced the total plasma cholesterol level and LDL-C and increased HDL cholesterol [104]. Another animal model study indicates that chronic administration of polyphenols has a positive effect on apolipoprotein B, plasma triglycerides, and cholesterol levels [105]. It has been observed that moderate consumption of red wine during meals significantly reduces the incidence of atherosclerotic disease by decreasing lipoproteins oxidation and endothelial toxicity instigated by oxidized LDL molecules. Administration of flavonoids in rabbits with hypercholesterolemia reduces the lipid accumulation in the iliac artery. Naringenin plays a significant role in overcoming the metabolic disturbances linked to insulin resistance and dyslipidemia and preventing the development of atherosclerosis in mice fed a high-fat diet [104].

Antiulcer Activity

An ulcer is characterized as a rupture of the protective barrier by acid and pepsin secretion in the gastrointestinal tract. It can probably exist due to the imbalance between the protective and aggressive agents of the gastric mucosa. The mucosal protective or defense factors include prostaglandins, mucus, bicarbonate, nitric oxide, bile, and the endogenous oxidative system. The aggressive agents include pepsin, acid secretion, bile reflux, and *Helicobacter pylori* infection [106]. Flavonoids' antiulcer effect consists of the functions like anti-acid secretion, inhibition of pepsin activity and level, and increasing gastric mucus and bicarbonate secretion. In animal studies, quercetin shows antiulcer activity by inhibiting the enzyme histidine decarboxylate and reducing histamine formation in the gastric mucosa. Hesperidin and neohesperidine were found in citrus fruits, and their antiulcer activity is due to their antioxidant and mucoprotective effects. Free radicals play a vital role in the formation of stomach ulcers. Oxidative stress model studies of rats reported that hesperidin prevents oxidative cell damage by increasing the levels of certain enzymes (superoxide dismutase (SOD), gastric glutathione (GHS), catalase (CAT), and mucin) in the gastric mucosa and decreasing the levels of lipid peroxidation and inflammatory marker [37,107].

CONCLUSION

Flavonoids are the polyphenolic compounds present in plants. The dietary sources of flavonoids are vegetables, fruits, tea, and wine. Flavonoids have different biological activities in various signaling pathways related to chronic diseases, such as protection against CVD and anti-inflammatory, antioxidant, antibacterial, antiviral, and anticancer activities with no or minimal side effects.

REFERENCES

1. Nabavi, S.M., Šamec, D., Tomczyk, M., Milella, L., Russo, D., Habtemariam, S., Suntar, I., Rastrelli, L., Daglia, M., Xiao, J., Giampieri, F., Battino, M., Sobarzo-Sanchez, E., Nabavi, S.F., Yousefi, B., Jeandet, P., Xu, S., & Shirooie, S. (2020). Flavonoid biosynthetic pathways in plants: Versatile targets for metabolic engineering. *Biotechnology Advances*, 38, 107316.
2. Kopustinskiene, D.M., Jakstas, V., Savickas, A., & Bernatoniene, J. (2020). Flavonoids as anticancer agents. *Nutrients*, 12(2), 457.
3. Sangeetha, K.S.S., Umamaheswari, S., Reddy, C.U.M., & Kalkura, S.N. (2016). Flavonoids: Therapeutic potential of natural pharmacological agents. *International Journal of Pharmaceutical Sciences and Research*, 7(10), 3924–3930.
4. Kumar, S., & Pandey, A.K. (2013). Chemistry and biological activities of flavonoids: An overview. *The Scientific World Journal*, 2013, 1–16.
5. Khan, J., Deb, P.K., Priya, S., Medina, K.D., Devi, R., Walode, S.G., & Rudrapal, M. (2021). Dietary flavonoids: Cardioprotective potential with antioxidant effects and their pharmacokinetic, toxicological and therapeutic concerns. *Molecules (Basel, Switzerland)*, 26(13), 4021.
6. Ekalu, A., & Habila, J.D. (2020). Flavonoids: Isolation, characterization, and health benefits. *Beni-Suef Univ Journal of Basic Applied Science*, 9(1), 1–14.
7. Sülsen, V.P., Lizarraga, E., Mamadalieva, N.Z., & Lago, J. (2017). Potential of terpenoids and flavonoids from asteraceae as anti-inflammatory, antitumor, and antiparasitic agents. *Evidence-Based Complementary and Alternative Medicine: ECAM*, 2017, 6196198.
8. Karak, P. (2019). Biological activities of flavonoids: An overview. *International Journal of Pharmaceutical Sciences and Research*, 10(4), 1567–1574.
9. Zhang, Q., Zhao, X., & Qiu, H. (2013). Flavones and flavonols: Phytochemistry and biochemistry. In *Natural Products: Phytochemistry, Botany and Metabolism of Alkaloids, Phenolics and Terpenes*. Heidelberg, Germany: Springer, 1821–1847.
10. Panche, A.N., Diwan, A.D., & Chandra, S.R. (2016). Flavonoids: An overview. *Journal of Nutritional Science*, 5, e47.
11. Iwashina, T. (2013). Flavonoid properties of five families newly incorporated into the order caryophyllales (review). *Bulletin of the National Museum of Nature and Science, Series B*, 39(1), 25–51.

12. Jung, U.J., Lee, M.K., Park, Y.B., Kang, M.A., & Choi, M.S. (2006). Effect of citrus flavonoids on lipid metabolism and glucose-regulating enzyme mRNA levels in type-2 diabetic mice. *The International Journal of Biochemistry & Cell Biology*, 38(7), 1134–1145.
13. Matthies, A., Clavel, T., Gütschow, M., Engst, W., Haller, D., Blaut, M., & Braune, A. (2008). Conversion of daidzein and genistein by an anaerobic bacterium newly isolated from the mouse intestine. *Applied and Environmental Microbiology*, 74(15), 4847–4852.
14. Tsao, R. (2010). Chemistry and biochemistry of dietary polyphenols. *Nutrients*, 2(12), 1231–1246.
15. Aoki, T., Akashi, T., & Ayabe, S. (2000). Flavonoids of leguminous plants: Structure, biological activity, and biosynthesis. *Journal of Plant Research*, 113(4), 475–488.
16. Dixon, R.A., & Ferreira, D. (2002). Genistein. *Phytochemistry*, 60(3), 205–211.
17. Veitch, N.C. (2013). Isoflavonoids of the leguminosae. *Natural Product Reports*, 30(7), 988–1027.
18. Ahmad, M.Z., Li, P., Wang, J., Rehman, N.U., & Zhao, J. (2017). Isoflavone malonyltransferases GmIMaT1 and GmIMaT3 differently modify isoflavone glucosides in soybean (Glycine max) under various stresses. *Frontiers in Plant Science*, 8, 735.
19. Zaheer, K., & Humayoun Akhtar, M. (2017). An updated review of dietary isoflavones: Nutrition, processing, bioavailability and impacts on human health. *Critical Reviews in Food Science and Nutrition*, 57(6), 1280–1293.
20. Braicu, C., Ladomery, M.R., Chedea, V.S., Irimie, A., & Berindan-Neagoe, I. (2013). The relationship between the structure and biological actions of green tea catechins. *Food Chemistry*, 141(3), 3282–3289.
21. Rosen, T. (2012). Green tea catechins: Biologic properties, proposed mechanisms of action, and clinical implications. *Journal of Drugs in Dermatology: JDD*, 11(11), e55–e60.
22. Babu, P.V., & Liu, D. (2008). Green tea catechins and cardiovascular health: An update. *Current Medicinal Chemistry*, 15(18), 1840–1850.
23. Manach, C., Scalbert, A., Morand, C., Rémésy, C., & Jiménez, L. (2004). Polyphenols: Food sources and bioavailability. *The American Journal of Clinical Nutrition*, 79(5), 727–747.
24. Nishimura, S., Taki, M., Takaishi, S., Iijima, Y., & Akiyama, T. (2000). Structures of 4-aryl-coumarin (neoflavone) dimers isolated from Pistacia chinensis BUNGE and their estrogen-like activity. *Chemical & Pharmaceutical Bulletin*, 48(4), 505–508.
25. Garazd, M.M., Garazd, Y.L., & Khilya, V.P. (2003). Neoflavones. 1. Natural distribution and spectral and biological properties. *Chemistry of Natural Compounds*, 39, 54–121.
26. Abotaleb, M., Samuel, S.M., Varghese, E., Varghese, S., Kubatka, P., Liskova, A., & Büsselberg, D. (2018). Flavonoids in cancer and apoptosis. *Cancers*, 11(1), 28.
27. Maria, J.K., Davies, N., Myburgh, K.H., & Lecour, S. (2014). Proanthocyanidins, anthocyanins and cardiovascular diseases. *Food Research International*, 59, 41–52.
28. Giusti, M., & Wrolstad, R. (2003). Acylated anthocyanins from edible sources and their applications in food systems. *Biochemical Engineering Journal*, 14(3), 217–225.
29. Abbas, A., Naseer, M.M., Hasan, A., & Hadda, T.B. (2014). Synthesis and cytotoxicity studies of 4-alkoxychalcones as new anti-tumor agents. *Journal of Materials and Environmental Science*, 5(1), 281–292.
30. Tomás-Barberán, F.A., & Clifford, M.N. (2000). Flavanones, chalcones, and dihydrochalcones—nature, occurrence, and dietary burden. *Journal of the Science of Food and Agriculture*, 80, 1073–1080.
31. Salehi, B., Quispe, C., Chamkhi, I., El Omari, N., Balahbib, A., Sharifi-Rad, J., Bouyahya, A., Akram, M., Iqbal, M., Docea, A.O., Caruntu, C., Leyva-Gómez, G., Dey, A., Martorell, M., Calina, D., López, V., & Les, F. (2021). Pharmacological properties of chalcones: A review of preclinical including molecular mechanisms and clinical evidence. *Frontiers in Pharmacology*, 11, 592654.
32. Bhagwat, S., & Haytowitz, D.B. (2015). USDA Database for the Flavonoid Content of Selected Foods, Release 3.2. U.S. Department of Agriculture, Agricultural Research Service. Nutrient Data Laboratory Home Page: Http://www.ars.usda.gov/nutrientdata/flav.

33. Chun, O.K., Chung, S.J., & Song, W.O. (2007). Estimated dietary flavonoid intake and major food sources of U.S. adults. *The Journal of Nutrition*, 137(5), 1244–1252.
34. Harnly, J.M., Doherty, R.F., Beecher, G.R., Holden, J.M., Haytowitz, D.B., Bhagwat, S., & Gebhardt, S. (2006). Flavonoid content of U.S. fruits, vegetables, and nuts. *Journal of Agricultural and Food Chemistry*, 54(26), 9966–9977.
35. U.S. Department of Agriculture. (May 2014). USDA Database for the Flavonoid Content of Selected Foods, Release 3.1. Available at: Http://www.ars.usda.gov/SP2UserFiles/Place/80400525/Data/Flav/Flav_R03-1.pdf. Accessed 8/25/15.
36. Teles, Y., Souza, M., & Souza, M. (2018). Sulphated flavonoids: Biosynthesis, structures, and biological activities. *Molecules (Basel, Switzerland)*, 23(2), 480.
37. Rana, A.C., & Gulliya, B. (2019). Chemistry, and pharmacology of flavonoids: A review. *Indian Journal of Pharmaceutical Education and Research*, 53, 8–20.
38. Rauter, A.P., Lopes, R.G., & Martins, A. (2007). C-Glycosylflavonoids: Identification, bioactivity, and synthesis. *Natural Product Communication*, 2, 1175–1196.
39. Seijas, J.A., Vázquez-Tato, M.P., & Carballido-Reboredo, R. (2005). Solvent-free synthesis of functionalized flavones under microwave irradiation. *The Journal of Organic Chemistry*, 70(7), 2855–2858.
40. Kshatriya, R., Yaseen, I.S., & Gulam, M.N. (2013). Synthesis of flavone skeleton by different methods. *Oriental Journal of Chemistry*, 29, 1475–1487.
41. Mills, C.J., Mateeva, N.N., & Redda, K.K. (2006). Synthesis of novel substituted flavonoids. *Journal of Heterocyclic Chemistry*, 43, 59–64.
42. Sarbu, L.G., Bahrin, L.G., Babii, C., Stefan, M., & Birsa, M.L. (2019). Synthetic flavonoids with antimicrobial activity: A review. *Journal of Applied Microbiology*, 127(5), 1282–1290.
43. Kozłowska, A., & Szostak-Wegierek, D. (2014). Flavonoids – Food sources and health benefits. *Roczniki Panstwowego Zakladu Higieny*, 65(2), 79–85.
44. Vrhovsek, U., Rigo, A., Tonon, D., & Mattivi, F. (2004). Quantitation of polyphenols in different apple varieties. *Journal of Agricultural and Food Chemistry*, 52(21), 6532–6538.
45. Saul, R.C., Saraí, C.H., Karen L.H.R., Luis A. Cira-Chávez, M.I., Estrada-Alvarado, L.E., Gassos, O., Jesús O.P., & Marco, A.L.M. (August 23, 2017). Flavonoids: Important biocompounds in food, flavonoids – From biosynthesis to human health, goncalo C. *Justino, Intechopen*, 354–369.
46. Procházková, D., Boušová, I., & Wilhelmová, N. (2011). Antioxidant and prooxidant properties of flavonoids. *Fitoterapia*, 82(4), 513–523.
47. Naik, K.K., Thangavel, S., Alam, A., & Kumar, S. (2017). Flavone analogues as antimicrobial agents. *Recent Patents on Inflammation & Allergy Drug Discovery*, 11(1), 53–63.
48. Li, A.N., Li, S., Zhang, Y.J., Xu, X.R., Chen, Y.M., & Li, H.B. (2014). Resources and biological activities of natural polyphenols. *Nutrients*, 6(12), 6020–6047.
49. Rodríguez-García, C., Sánchez-Quesada, C., & J Gaforio, J. (2019). Dietary flavonoids as cancer chemopreventive agents: An updated review of human studies. *Antioxidants (Basel, Switzerland)*, 8(5), 137.
50. Yahfoufi, N., Alsadi, N., Jambi, M., & Matar, C. (2018). The immunomodulatory and antiinflammatory role of polyphenols. *Nutrients*, 10(11), 1618.
51. Valko, M., Rhodes, C.J., Moncol, J., Izakovic, M., & Mazur, M. (2006). Free radicals, metals, and antioxidants in oxidative stress-induced cancer. *Chemico-Biological Interactions*, 160(1), 1–40.
52. Pham-Huy, L.A., He, H., & Pham-Huy, C. (2008). Free radicals, antioxidants in disease and health. *International Journal of Biomedical Science: IJBS*, 4(2), 89–96.
53. Ku, Y.S., Ng, M.S., Cheng, S.S., Lo, A.W., Xiao, Z., Shin, T.S., Chung, G., & Lam, H.M. (2020). Understanding the composition, biosynthesis, accumulation, and transport of flavonoids in crops for the promotion of crops as healthy sources of flavonoids for human consumption. *Nutrients*, 12(6), 1717.
54. Mondal, S., & Rahaman, S.T. (2020). Flavonoids: A vital resource in healthcare and medicine. *Pharm Pharmacol International Journal*, 8(2), 91–104.

55. Liu, K., Luo, M., & Wei, S. (2019). The bioprotective effects of polyphenols on metabolic syndrome against oxidative stress: Evidence and perspectives. *Oxidative Medicine and Cellular Longevity*, 2019, 6713194.

56. Rice-Evans, C.A., Miller, N.J., & Paganga, G. (1996). Structure-antioxidant activity relationships of flavonoids and phenolic acids. *Free Radical Biology & Medicine*, 20(7), 933–956.

57. Tiwari, C.S., Husain, N. (2017). Biological activities and role of flavonoids in human health – A review. *Indian Journal of Scientific Research*, 12(2), 193–196.

58. Pan, M.H., Lai, C.S., & Ho, C.T. (2010). Anti-inflammatory activity of natural dietary flavonoids. *Food & Function*, 1(1), 15–31.

59. Ozcan, T., Delikanli, B., Yilmaz-Ersan, L., Akpinar-Bayizit, A. (2014). Phenolics in human health. *International Journal of Chemical Engineering and Application*. 5(5), 393–396.

60. Cho, J.Y., Kim, P.S., Park, J., Yoo, E.S., Baik, K.U., Kim, Y.K., & Park, M.H. (2000). Inhibitor of tumor necrosis factor-alpha production in lipopolysaccharide-stimulated RAW264.7 cells from Amorpha fruticosa. *Journal of Ethnopharmacology*, 70(2), 127–133.

61. Ueda, H., Yamazaki, C., & Yamazaki, M. (2004). A hydroxyl group of flavonoids affects oral anti-inflammatory activity and inhibition of systemic tumor necrosis factor-alpha production. *Bioscience, Biotechnology, and Biochemistry*, 68(1), 119–125.

62. Tripathi, K.D. (2013). Insulin, oral hypoglycemic drugs and glucagon. In *Essentials of Medical Pharmacology*, 7th ed. New Delhi: J.P. Medical Ltd., 258.

63. Terra, X., Valls, J., Vitrac, X., Mérrillon, J.M., Arola, L., Ardèvol, A., Bladé, C., Fernandez-Larrea, J., Pujadas, G., Salvadó, J., & Blay, M. (2007). Grapeseed procyanidins act as anti-inflammatory agents in endotoxin-stimulated RAW 264.7 macrophages by inhibiting NFkB signaling pathway. *Journal of Agricultural and Food Chemistry*, 55(11), 4357–4365.

64. Blackadar C.B. (2016). Historical review of the causes of cancer. *World Journal of Clinical Oncology*, 7(1), 54–86.

65. Hadi, S.M., Asad, S.F., Singh, S., & Ahmad, A. (2000). Putative mechanism for anticancer and apoptosis-inducing properties of plant-derived polyphenolic compounds. *Iubmb Life*, 50(3), 167–171.

66. Link, A., Balaguer, F., & Goel, A. (2010). Cancer chemoprevention by dietary polyphenols: Promising role for epigenetics. *Biochemical Pharmacology*, 80(12), 1771–1792.

67. Neagu, M., Constantin, C., Popescu, I.D., Zipeto, D., Tzanakakis, G., Nikitovic, D., Fenga, C., Stratakis, C.A., Spandidos, D.A., & Tsatsakis, A.M. (2019). Inflammation and metabolism in cancer cell-mitochondria key player. *Frontiers in Oncology*, 9, 348.

68. Wang, T.Y., Li, Q., & Bi, K.S. (2018). Bioactive flavonoids in medicinal plants: Structure, activity, and biological fate. *Asian Journal of Pharmaceutical Sciences*, 13(1), 12–23.

69. Bhattacharya, T., Dutta, S., Akter, R., Rahman, M.H., Karthika, C., Nagaswarupa, H.P., Murthy, H., Fratila, O., Brata, R., & Bungau, S. (2021). Role of phytonutrients in nutrigenetics and nutrigenomics perspective in curing breast cancer. *Biomolecules*, 11(8), 1176.

70. Chandra, H., Bishnoi, P., Yadav, A., Patni, B., Mishra, A.P., & Nautiyal, A.R. (2017). Antimicrobial resistance and the alternative resources with special emphasis on plant-based antimicrobials – A review. *Plants (Basel, Switzerland)*, 6(2), 16.

71. Cushnie, T.P., & Lamb, A.J. (2005). Antimicrobial activity of flavonoids. *International Journal of Antimicrobial Agents*, 26(5), 343–356.

72. Mishra, A.K., Mishra, A., Kehri, H.K., Sharma, B., & Pandey, A.K. (2009). Inhibitory activity of Indian spice plant Cinnamomum zeylanicum extracts against Alternaria solani and Curvularia lunata, the pathogenic dematiaceous moulds. *Annals of Clinical Microbiology and Antimicrobials*, 8, 9.

73. Alcaráz, L.E., Blanco, S.E., Puig, O.N., Tomás, F., & Ferretti, F.H. (2000). Antibacterial activity of flavonoids against methicillin-resistant Staphylococcus aureus strains. *Journal of Theoretical Biology*, 205(2), 231–240.

74. Tsuchiya, H., & Iinuma, M. (2000). Reduction of membrane fluidity by antibacterial sopho-raflavanone G isolated from Sophora exigua. *Phytomedicine: International Journal of Phytotherapy and Phytopharmacology*, 7(2), 161–165.

75. Xie, Y., Yang, W., Tang, F., Chen, X., & Ren, L. (2015). Antibacterial activities of flavo-noids: Structure-activity relationship and mechanism. *Current Medicinal Chemistry*, 22(1), 132–149.

76. Lu, M., Li, T., Wan, J., Li, X., Yuan, L., & Sun, S. (2017). Antifungal effects of phyto-compounds on Candida species alone and in combination with fluconazole. *International Journal of Antimicrobial Agents*, 49(2), 125–136.

77. Aboody, M., & Mickymaray, S. (2020). Antifungal efficacy and mechanisms of flavonoids. *Antibiotics (Basel, Switzerland)*, 9(2), 45.

78. Taleb-Contini S.H., Salvador, M.J., Watanabe, E., Ito, I.Y., & Oliveira, D.C.R. (2003). Antimicrobial activity of flavonoids and steroids isolated from two Chromolaena species. *Revista Brasileira De Ciências Farmacêuticas*. 39(4), 403–408.

79. Wächter, G.A., Hoffmann, J.J., Furbacher, T., Blake, M.E., & Timmermann, B.N. (1999). Antibacterial and antifungal flavanones from Eysenhardtia texana. *Phytochemistry*, 52(8), 1469–1471.

80. Bestia, M., Leonte, A., & Oancea, I. (1984). Phenolic compounds with biological activity. *Bull. Univ. Galati Faso.* 6, 23–27.

81. Jin Y.S. (2019). Recent advances in natural antifungal flavonoids and their derivatives. *Bioorganic & Medicinal Chemistry Letters*, 29(19), 126589.

82. Benjamin, E.J., Muntner, P., Alonso, A., et al. American Heart Association Council on Epidemiology and Prevention Statistics Committee and Stroke Statistics Subcommittee. (2019). Heart disease and stroke statistics-2019 update: A report from the american heart association. *Circulation*, 139(10), e56–e528.

83. Wenzel, P., Kossmann, S., Münzel, T., & Daiber, A. (2017). Redox regulation of cardio-vascular inflammation – Immunomodulatory function of mitochondrial and nox-derived reactive oxygen and nitrogen species. *Free Radical Biology & Medicine*, 109, 48–60.

84. Han, X.Z., Gao, S., Cheng, Y.N., Sun, Y.Z., Liu, W., Tang, L.L., & Ren, D.M. (2012). Protective effect of naringenin-7-O-glucoside against oxidative stress induced by doxoru-bicin in H9c2 cardiomyocytes. *Bioscience Trends*, 6(1), 19–25.

85. Tungmunnithum, D., Thongboonyou, A., Pholboon, A., & Yangsabai, A. (2018). Flavonoids and other phenolic compounds from medicinal plants for pharmaceutical and medical aspects: An overview. *Medicines (Basel, Switzerland)*, 5(3), 93.

86. Shafiq, H., Ahmad, A., Masud, T., & Kaleem, M. (2014). Cardio-protective and anticancer ther-apeutic potential of Nigella sativa. *Iranian Journal of Basic Medical Sciences*, 17(12), 967–979.

87. Waheed Janabi, A.H., Kamboh, A.A., Saeed, M., et al. (2020). Flavonoid-rich foods (FRF): A promising nutraceutical approach against lifespan-shortening diseases. *Iranian Journal of Basic Medical Sciences*, 23(2), 140–153.

88. Mérillon, J.M., & Ramawat, K.G. (2019). *Bioactive Molecules in Food*, 1st ed. Cham, Switzerland: Springer Nature, 230–256.

89. Gerdin, B., & Svensjö, E. (1983). Inhibitory effect of the flavonoid O-(beta-hydroxyethyl)-rutoside on increased microvascular permeability induced by various agents in rat skin. *International Journal of Microcirculation, Clinical and Experimental*, 2(1), 39–46.

90. Mateeva, N., Eyunni, S., Redda, K.K., et al. (2017). Functional evaluation of synthetic flavonoids and chalcones for potential antiviral and anticancer properties. *Bioorganic & Medicinal Chemistry Letters*, 27(11), 2350–2356.

91. Lalani, S., & Poh, C.L. (2020). Flavonoids as antiviral agents for enterovirus A71 (EV-A71). *Viruses*, 12(2), 184.

92. Zandi, K., Teoh, B.T., Sam, S.S., Wong, P.F., Mustafa, M.R., & Abubakar, S. (2011). Antiviral activity of four types of bioflavonoid against dengue virus type 2. *Virology Journal*, 8, 560.

93. Adewusi, E., & Afolayan, A. (2010). A review of natural products with hepatoprotective activity. *Journal of Medicinal Plants Research*. 4(13), 1318–1334.

94. Tapas, A., Sakarkar, D.M., & Kakde, R. (2008). Flavonoids as nutraceuticals: A review. *Tropical Journal of Pharmaceutical Research*. 7(3), 1089–1099.
95. Lee, M.H., Yoon, S., & Moon, J.O. (2004). The flavonoid naringenin inhibits dimethylnitrosamine-induced liver damage in rats. *Biological & Pharmaceutical Bulletin*. 27(1), 72–76.
96. He, Q., Kim, J., & Sharma, R.P. (2004). Silymarin protects against liver damage in BALB/c mice exposed to fumonisin B1 despite increasing accumulation of free sphingoid bases. *Toxicological Sciences: An Official Journal of the Society of Toxicology*, 80(2), 335–342.
97. Brahmachari, G. (2011). Bioflavonoids with promising antidiabetic potentials: A critical survey. In: Tiwari, V.K., Mishra, B.B., editors. *Opportunity, challenge, and scope of natural products in medicinal chemistry*. Trivandrum: Research Signpost, 2, 187–212.
98. Kawser Hossain, M., Abdal Dayem, A., Han, J., Yin, Y., Kim, K., Kumar Saha, S., Yang, G.M., Choi, H.Y., & Cho, S.G. (2016). Molecular mechanisms of the anti-obesity and anti-diabetic properties of flavonoids. *International Journal of Molecular Sciences*, 17(4), 569.
99. Lee, Y.S., Lee, S., Lee, H.S., Kim, B.K., Ohuchi, K., & Shin, K.H. (2005). Inhibitory effects of isorhamnetin-3-O-beta-D-glucoside from Salicornia herbacea on rat lens aldose reductase and sorbitol accumulation in streptozotocin-induced diabetic rat tissues. *Biological & Pharmaceutical Bulletin*, 28(5), 916–918.
100. Wang, Y.B., Ge, Z.M., Kang, W.Q., Lian, Z.X., Yao, J., & Zhou, C.Y. (2015). Rutin alleviates diabetic cardiomyopathy in a rat model of type 2 diabetes. *Experimental and Therapeutic Medicine*, 9(2), 451–455.
101. Agrawal, Y.O., Sharma, P.K., Shrivastava, B., et al. (2014). Hesperidin produces cardioprotective activity via PPAR-γ pathway in ischemic heart disease model in diabetic rats. *PLoS One*, 9(11), e111212.
102. Hackam, D.G., & Anand, S.S. (2003). Emerging risk factors for atherosclerotic vascular disease: A critical review of the evidence. *JAMA*, 290(7), 932–940.
103. Aviram, M., Volkova, N., Coleman, R., et al. (2008). Pomegranate phenolics from the peels, arils, and flowers are antiatherogenic: Studies in vivo in atherosclerotic apolipoprotein e-deficient (E 0) mice and in vitro in cultured macrophages and lipoproteins. *Journal of Agricultural and Food Chemistry*, 56(3), 1148–1157.
104. Mulvihill, E.E., & Huff, M.W. (2010). Antiatherogenic properties of flavonoids: Implications for cardiovascular health. *The Canadian Journal of Cardiology*, 26 Suppl A, 17A–21A.
105. Ciumărnean, L., Milaciu, M.V., Runcan, O., et al. (2020). The effects of flavonoids in cardiovascular diseases. *Molecules (Basel, Switzerland)*, 25(18), 4320.
106. Zhang, W., Lian, Y., Li, Q., et al. (2020). Preventative and therapeutic potential of flavonoids in peptic ulcers. *Molecules (Basel, Switzerland)*, 25(20), 4626.
107. Serafim, C., Araruna, M.E., Júnior, E.A., Diniz, M., Hiruma-Lima, C., & Batista, L. (2020). A review of the role of flavonoids in peptic ulcer (2010–2020). *Molecules (Basel, Switzerland)*, 25(22), 5431.

Flavonoids' Classification and Their Applications as Nutraceuticals

2

Augustine T. Nkembo
University of South Florida

Contents

DOI: 10.1201/9781003225225-2

INTRODUCTION

Flavonoids are a group of natural compounds classified in the class of plants-derived secondary metabolites with benzo-γ-pyrone polyphenolic structure. Flavonoids are ubiquitously distributed in plants, typically abundant in the nucleus of mesophyll cells. They possess a lot of antioxidant properties and are widely found in certain beverages, fruits, and vegetables. Several studies show that flavonoids possess mitigating effects on atherosclerosis, cancer, Alzheimer's disease (AD), and antifungal and antibacterial activities [1,2]. Over 4,000 varieties of flavonoids have been identified and classified into different classes, including flavones (e.g., chrysin, luteolin, and apigenin); flavonols (e.g., quercetin, kaempferol, myricetin, and galangin); flavanones (e.g., hesperetin and naringenin); flavanonol (e.g., taxifolin); isoflavones (e.g., genistein and daidzein); and flavan-3-ols (e.g., catechin and epicatechin) [3]. The different classes of flavonoids occur as aglycones, glycosides, or methylated derivatives, with aglycone being the basic structure for the flavonoids [4]. In the aglycone structure, a common benzo-γ-pyrone polyphenolic structure based on a 15-carbon skeleton consisting of two benzene rings (A and B) is linked via a heterocyclic pyrane ring (C), as shown in Figure 2.1 [4]. The classes differ from one another by the level of oxidation and pattern of substitution on the C ring, while compounds in the same class differ by the pattern of substitution on the A and B rings [3]. Flavonoids have numerous protective biological activities, and several have been reported. Some of the biological effects of flavonoids reported so far include anti-inflammatory, antiallergic, antihemorrhagic, antimutagenic, antineoplastic, and antihepatoprotective [5–8]. Epidemiological studies of dietary components of flavonoids suggest a protective role against coronary heart disease [9–11]. The pharmacological and biochemical activities of flavonoids would result from their antioxidant activity and inhibition of certain enzymes in mammalian systems [5]. Flavonoids are increasingly gaining interest as critical dietary components and potential therapeutics against several different diseases. Flavonoids are major dietary components in nutraceuticals which are food or parts of food that provide medical or health benefits. Nutraceuticals may include isolated nutrients, dietary supplements, genetically engineered designer food, herbal products, and processed products such as soups, cereals, and beverages. Flavonoids constitute a large portion of human diets as they are ubiquitously distributed

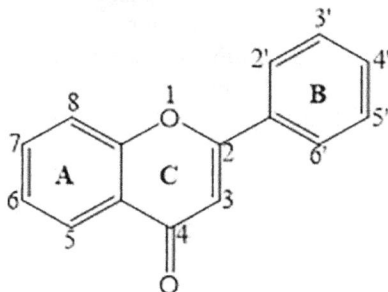

FIGURE 2.1 Basic structure of flavonoids.

in plants. Significant amounts of flavonoids are consumed daily, especially as the toxicity is extremely low in animals. Toxic LD_{50} doses of 2–10 g of flavonoids have been reported in rats, which is unrealistic in humans. However, as a precaution, a dose of less than 1 mg per day for adults is recommended for human consumption [12].

CLASSIFICATION AND STRUCTURE OF FLAVONOIDS

Flavonoids is a collective noun for plant pigments that are mostly derived from benzo-γ-pyrone, which is synonymous with chromone [13]. For a long time, flavonoids have been the subject of considerable study due to their nutritional and therapeutic properties. This class of compounds is ubiquitously distributed in green plant cells and, as such, should be expected to have a role in plant photosynthesis. However, there is no evidence of direct involvement of flavonoids in photosynthesis [7]. Some studies have revealed the mutagenic activity of flavonoids, and this is of particular interest to botanical taxonomists and hence a red flag to health professionals and nutritionists as it shows the potential dangers of the consumption of natural products [14]. Nutritionists estimate that an average safe intake of flavonoids by human beings on a normal diet is 1–2 g per day [7,14]. This safe, high daily intake dose recommendation continues to exponentially attract a lot of interest in research and in the fields of nutrition and medicine. There is a great zeal to better understand, discover, and analyze the different classes and/or groups of flavonoids and study their nutritional and health benefit in humans. This is because of the wide safety window upon exposure and consumption of flavonoids by a human. A compendium of research and development has reported a comprehensive description of the isolation processes, structures, and laboratory synthesis of flavonoids. It has also unveiled an avalanche of nutritive and therapeutic benefits to man [7].

It is worth noting that flavonoids are one of the largest groups of natural products known in terms of quality and quantity. Nearly all flavonoids are pigments, and undoubtedly, their colors are associated with some of their nutritive and therapeutic properties. It is thought to be the reason flavonoids might be ubiquitously distributed in plants and available in all geographical zones of herbal growth. Biochemical and structural analyses also reveal that all the colors of the light spectrum, including the UV region, are represented in the spectra of flavonoids, and their electronic properties include not only energy capture and transfer but also biological selectivity [7]. This has led to the great variability of the flavonoids, which arises from (a) differences in the ring structure of the aglycone and its state of oxidation/reduction; (b) differences in the extent of hydroxylation of the aglycone and the positions of the hydroxyl groups; and (c) differences in the derivatization of the hydroxyl groups, for example, with methyl groups, carbohydrates, or isoprenoids [7].

Currently, over 4,000 different flavonoids have been identified, and the number is growing fast. Computational permutation calculation based on the variability of the flavonoids reveals an estimated theoretical number of other structural members of flavonoids to be about 2 million [3,7]. Interestingly, members of each class of flavonoids are related structurally and, in their property, especially in their swiftness to decompose [15]. However, due to their relatively high molecular weight and complicated structure, in vitro identification and chemical synthesis of flavonoids represent a challenge to plant and synthetic chemists [7] (Table 2.1).

TABLE 2.1   Flavonoid classes, subclasses, and natural sources

FLAVONOID CLASSES	FLAVONOID SUBCLASSES	NATURAL SOURCES
 Anthocyanins	*Cyanidin *Malvidin *Delphinidin *Peonidin	-Fruits -Vegetables -Nuts and dry fruits -Medicinal plants and other
 Chalcones	*Phloretin *Arbutin *Phlioridzin *Chalconaringenin *Butein	-Fruits -Vegetables -Medicinal plants and other
 Flavanones	*Hesperitin *Naringin *Naringenin *Eriodictyol *Hesperidin	-Fruits -Medicinal plants and other
 Flavones	*Apigenin *Tangeretin *Baicalein *Rpoifolin *Luteolin	-Fruits -Medicinal plants and other
 Flavonols	*Quercetin *Myricetin *Rutin *Morin *Kaempferol	-Fruits -Vegetables -Medicinal plants and other

(Continued)

TABLE 2.1 (*Continued*)   Flavonoid classes, subclasses, and natural sources

FLAVONOID CLASSES	FLAVONOID SUBCLASSES	NATURAL SOURCES
Isoflavonoids	*Genistin *Genistein *Daidzein *Glycitein *Daidzin	-Legumes -Medicinal plants

Source: Aadapted from [7,16]

NUTRACEUTICALS

The word "nutraceutical" was coined from nutrition+pharmaceutical in 1989 by Stephen De Felice. Stephen is the founder and chair of the Foundation for Innovation in Medicine (FIM), an American organization that encourages medical health, based in Cranford, NJ, USA [18,19]. What Felice meant is that nutraceutical is any substance that can be defined as food or part of a food that provides health or medical benefits including but not limited to the prevention or treatment of diseases. It is also worth noting that health Canada defines nutraceuticals as "a product that is prepared from food but sold in the form of pills, or powder or other medicinal forms not usually associated with food but have demonstrated to have a physiological benefit, including benefit against chronic disease" [20]. Nutraceutical products range from isolated nutrients, dietary supplements, and specific diets to genetically engineered designer foods and herbal products [18]. These products emerge from the food industry, pharmaceutical industry, herbal and dietary supplement markets, and the recently merged pharmaceutical/agribusiness/nutrition conglomerates [20] (Figure 2.2).

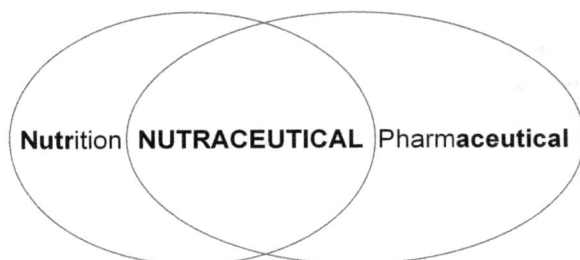

FIGURE 2.2   Nutraceutical was coined from nutrition and pharmaceutical.

BRIDGING THE GAP BETWEEN FOOD AND MEDICINE

Nutraceuticals are sometimes confused with functional foods. However, there is a slight difference between the two. Functional food is a food that is cooked or prepared using scientific knowledge with or without knowledge of how or why it is being used. Functional foods are expected to provide the body with macromolecules, including proteins, carbohydrates, fats, and vitamins. On the other hand, nutraceuticals are functional foods that help in the prevention and/or treatment of disease or disorders, excluding anemia. Examples include fortified dairy products such as milk and citrus juices.

Dietary Supplement Health and Education Act (DSHEA) of 1994 defines a dietary supplement in the following different ways: (a) a product (other than tobacco) that is intended to supplement the diet that bears or contains one or more of the following dietary ingredients: vitamins, minerals, herbs, or other botanicals, amino acids or dietary substance for use by humans to supplement the diets by increasing the total daily intake or concentrate, constituent, extract, metabolite, or a combination of these ingredients, (b) a product intended for ingestion in pills, capsules, tablets, or liquid form, (c) a product not represented for use as a conventional food or as the sole item of meal or diet, and (d) is labeled as a "dietary supplement."

From the consumer point of view, the benefits of nutraceuticals and functional food may include increased health value of diets, help man to live longer, help to avoid specific medical health conditions, physiological benefits by doing something positive to one's health, perceived to be more "natural" than conventional medicine and less likely to produce unpleasant side effects, and may present food for populations with special needs such as nutrient-dense foods for the elderly. A nutraceutical can be viewed as a nontoxic food extract supplement that has been shown scientifically to possess health benefits for both the prevention and treatment of certain diseases [21] (Figure 2.3).

CLASSIFICATION OF NUTRACEUTICALS

Nutraceuticals are consumable products with essential nutrients to improve human health/life that can be derived from the animal, plant, or fungi kingdom. Phytochemicals, on the other hand, are non-nutrients derived solely from the plant kingdom [23]. Nutraceuticals can be grouped or classified based on the application for easier understanding. Nevertheless, this classification is mainly for the purpose of academic instruction, clinical trial study, functional food development, and/or dietary recommendations. As such, we have [20] the following:

1. Dietary fiber
2. Probiotics

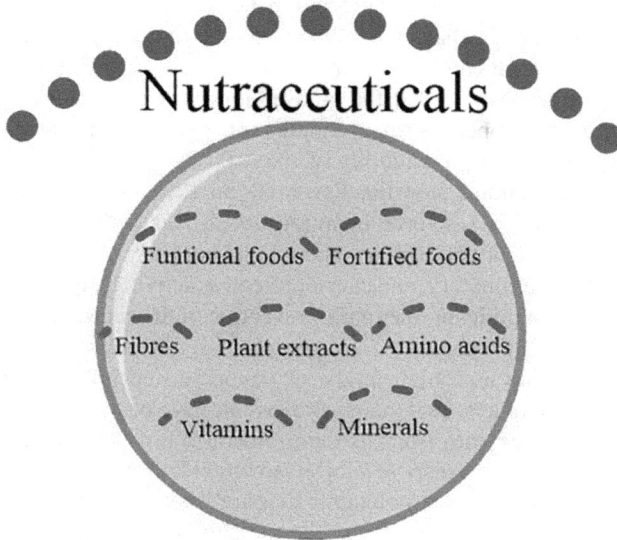

FIGURE 2.3 Different types of products described as "nutraceutical" (adapted from Williamson et al. [22]).

3. Prebiotics
4. Polyunsaturated fatty acids
5. Antioxidant vitamins
6. Spices
7. Polyphenols

Some common criteria used for the classification of nutraceuticals are based on food sources, chemical nature and structure, and mechanism of action. More broadly, nutraceuticals can be classified into two categories: potential nutraceuticals (one that holds a promise of specific health or medical benefit) and established nutraceuticals. Potential nutraceuticals become established nutraceuticals once sufficient clinical data of health and medical benefit have been established. Nevertheless, most nutraceutical products are still in the potential category [20].

The dietary polyphenolic flavonoid-rich compounds are currently the most common active ingredients in nutraceuticals. The simple reason behind this most sorted category of compounds is that flavonoids possess antioxidant, antimicrobial, anti-inflammatory, and cardioprotective activities and play a role in the prevention of neurodegenerative diseases and diabetes mellitus [24]. These categories of compounds are also of great interest because they have been shown in vitro to have substantial effects on numerous molecular processes in the cell, including gene expression, apoptosis, platelet aggregation, and intercellular signaling that can have anticarcinogenic and anti-atherogenic implications [25]. More rigorous research on polyphenols has revealed that flavonoids modulate the expression of an important rate-limiting enzyme involved in glutathione synthesis called γ-glutamylcysteine synthetase. It should be noted that glutathione is important in redox regulation of transcription factors and enzymes for signal transduction. The polyphenol-mediated regulation of glutathione significantly alters cellular effects, such as detoxification of xenobiotics and glutathionylation of proteins [26]. It is equally important to note that the bioavailability of polyphenols depends on the polyphenols' chemical properties, their conjugation and re-conjugation in the intestine, intestinal absorption, and the availability of enzymes for metabolism [27].

Several analytical studies show that flavonoids are the major active component of the polyphenols from plants that are used in nutraceuticals. Like other phenolic compounds, they play the role of potent antioxidants and metal chelators, in addition to their known antimicrobial, anti-inflammatory, and cardioprotective activities. Numerous indicate that flavonoids also play a significant role in the prevention of neurodegenerative diseases and diabetes mellitus [24,28]. Despite the armamentarium of health benefits of flavonoids, quantity or dose matters as a high intake of flavonoid-rich polyphenols from dietary sources could result in toxicity in humans. Flavonoids have been reported to induce MLL gene cleavage, inhibit enzymes (such as topoisomerase) involved in DNA structure and replication, and hence may predispose subjects to infant leukemia [27]. Even though most flavonoids possess reduced redox potentials that are lower than those of the superoxide and peroxyl radicals, the effectiveness of the radicals in generating lipid peroxidation, DNA adducts, and mutations may still be significant in disease development, and as such flavonoid-rich nutraceuticals must be consumed with prudence [20].

THE HEALTH BENEFITS OF FLAVONOID-RICH NUTRACEUTICALS

According to the Merriam-Webster Dictionary, the term "nutraceutical" is defined as "a foodstuff (as a fortified food or dietary supplement) that provides health benefits in addition to its basic nutritional value." As more studies and recommendations for the benefits of flavonoids are continuously made public, high-value flavonoid-rich nutraceutical products, including juice, wine, jelly, raisins, and jam obtained from flavonoid-rich sources, are on the rise. Byproducts such as pomace, seeds, skins, and seed oil from grapes processing are also being commercialized in various forms of different granulates and concentrated or dried powders that can be used for different types of nutraceuticals. Flavonoid-rich nutraceuticals have been reported to improve brain function, obesity and diabetes, cancer prevention, cardiovascular diseases (CVDs), and enhanced hepatoprotective activity [29]. Although our focus herein is on flavonoid-rich nutraceuticals, it is worth noting that the nutraceutical industry currently earns more than $200 billion per year, which, therefore, underscores the importance of nutraceuticals to the pharmaceutical industry and the exponential rise in the dietary supplement industry. The dietary supplement industry defines nutraceutical as "any nontoxic food component that has scientifically proven health benefits, including treatment and prevention, according to the original definition of nutraceutical and the FDA definition. It would be normal to extrapolate a generalized and simplified definition of nutraceutical from the definitions for nutraceuticals proposed or discussed here as follows: a substance that is cultivated/produced/extracted or synthesized under optimal and reproducible conditions and, when consumed, would provide the nutrient(s) required for bringing altered body structure and function back to normal, thus improving the health and well-being of the patients. Some specific health benefits that would be gained from the consumption of flavonoid-rich nutraceuticals include the following.

FLAVONOID-RICH NUTRACEUTICALS AS ANTIOXIDANTS

Antioxidant molecules help to reduce the accumulation of free radicals such as reactive oxygen species (ROS) in the body. The accumulation of free radicals usually leads to oxidative stress (OS). This occurs when ROS accumulate in the cell, from either excessive production or insufficient neutralization, causing damage to DNA, proteins, and lipids. Flavonoids possess the ideal structure for chelating and scavenging free radicals' activity, making them potent antioxidants. In fact, numerous in vitro research analyses showed that they are more effective antioxidants than the well-documented tocopherols and ascorbates. Each class or group of flavonoids has been well documented for their peculiarity to function as antioxidants. The ability of flavonoids to chelate the transition metals (particularly iron and copper) makes them unavailable to interact with other compounds to initiate damaging biological reactions [17]. This includes the inhibition of lipid peroxidation, oxidation of linoleic acid, and ferrous ion (Fe^{2+}), catalyzed by the oxidation of glutamine synthase through free radical scavenging and removal of metal ions from catalytic sites via scavenging [2,30]. Flavonoids also possess reducing power, which appears to contribute to the termination of lipid peroxidation chain reaction with their electron and hydrogen (H^+) donating capability. Like other classical and well-documented antioxidants, α-tocopherol and vitamin C, flavonoids can function as both antioxidant and pro-oxidant, that is, acting as pro-oxidant in the absence of free radicals [17]. Green tea, which is rich in catechins, is an example of catechin-rich flavonoid nutraceuticals that possess the antioxidative and pro-oxidative characteristics of Cu^{2+}-induced low-density lipoprotein (LDL) oxidation. In the initiation phase, LDL oxidation is inhibited by the action of catechins, but in the propagation phase of LDL oxidation, it serves as an accelerator of oxidation [31–34].

Oxygen is very vital for life. However, about 5% of the oxygen inhaled from the atmosphere is converted to ROS. On exposure to sunlight, ozone, X-rays, tobacco smoke, automobile exhaust, and environmental pollutants, ROS is also produced. The presence of the unpaired electron in the outer orbits of atoms enables ROS to be highly reactive to macromolecules such as proteins, nucleic acids, carbohydrates, and lipids, with dire consequences on the immune functions resulting in degenerative diseases [35–37]. OS is the consequence of the production of free radicals in the human body at a rate that overwhelms the body's antioxidant defense system. The OS is imposed on cells due to an increase in oxidant generation, a decrease in antioxidant protection, and failure in the repair of oxidative damage. It is also worth noting that exposure to pathogens, inappropriate lifestyle, excessive exercise, and byproducts of normal metabolisms are also contributing factors to OS [38,39]. OS deregulates the cellular mechanisms leading to neurodegenerative diseases, gastro-duodenal pathogenesis, cancer, cataracts, premature aging, inflammation, and cardiovascular and metabolic dysfunction [40,41].

Antioxidation is known to mitigate the effects of free radicals, hence reducing the risk of OS and associated disorders. Antioxidants inactivate the ROS or delay OS processes by interrupting the radical chain reaction of lipid peroxidation at the cellular levels [28,42]. Phytochemicals, including polyphenols, are powerful natural antioxidants found in food substances such as fruits, vegetables, and whole grains. The health benefits from the consumption of these food substances lead to protection against oxidative deterioration, which results in a reduced risk of chronic diseases associated with OS [41,43–45]. Catechins and flavonols are the most powerful flavonoids for protecting the body against ROS [46]. Cells and tissues of the human body are continuously threatened by damages caused by ROS and free radicals, which are produced during normal oxygen metabolism or are induced by exogenous damage [5,47]. A lot of medical and clinical conditions are associated with ROS and free radicals, as pictorially summarized by the illustration below:

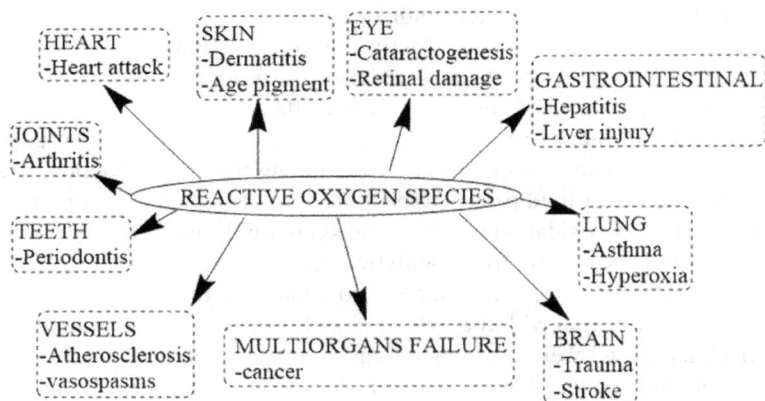

HEART
-Heart attack

SKIN
-Dermatitis
-Age pigment

EYE
-Cataractogenesis
-Retinal damage

GASTROINTESTINAL
-Hepatitis
-Liver injury

JOINTS
-Arthritis

REACTIVE OXYGEN SPECIES

TEETH
-Periodontis

LUNG
-Asthma
-Hyperoxia

VESSELS
-Atherosclerosis
-vasospasms

MULTIORGANS FAILURE
-cancer

BRAIN
-Trauma
-Stroke

In addition to scavenging the free radicals, flavonoids are also powerful metal chelators [48]. They function as a potent chain-breaking antioxidant and possess vitamin C stabilizing activity as they increase its absorption [17]. The arrangement of functional groups on the structure determines the activity of flavonoids [40]. Flavonoids possess antineoplastic effects as they interact with cellular pathways that control the cell cycle, differentiation, and apoptosis. Flavonoid-rich nutraceuticals have been shown to have therapeutic benefits in gastrointestinal hemorrhages, radiation reactions, erythroblastosis, menorrhagia, bleeding cystitis, tuberculosis, hemoptysis, periodontal disease, epitasis, and ophthalmic disorders [49,50]. The activity of some enzymes, including protein kinase C, protein tyrosine kinase, aldose reductase, myeloperoxidase, NADPH oxidase, xanthine oxidase, lipoxygenase, and cyclooxygenase are modified. Some of these enzymes have a crucial role in immune functions, cellular transformation, tumor growth, and metastasis [17,51,52].

FLAVONOIDS-RICH NUTRACEUTICALS AND ANTI-INFLAMMATION

Inflammation is a protective physiologic response mechanism by the body to eliminate damaged and necrotic cells as a result of several stress factors, including cell injury, pathogen invasion, and irritation [53,54]. Acute inflammation would eliminate unwanted effects on injured cells or tissues. However, chronic inflammation could promote or accelerate the development or the onset of chronic diseases such as neurodegenerative disease, CVD, diabetes, arthritis, AD, and autoimmune and pulmonary diseases [53,55,56]. Several flavonoid-rich nutraceuticals produced from grapes have been shown to be effective in reducing ROS levels and deregulating and/or modulating inflammatory pathways. Similarly, freeze-dried extract of wine from Jacquez grapes that contains flavonoids and anthocyanins also showed higher anti-inflammatory activity compared with the activity of indomethacin, a commercial non-steroidal anti-inflammatory drug [29,57]. This evidence, thus, further enhances the preference and demand for flavonoid-rich nutraceuticals for holistic treatment of chronic diseases such as arthritis, diabetes, cardiovascular and respiratory disorders, neurodegenerative diseases, and cancer.

FLAVONOID-RICH NUTRACEUTICALS AND BRAIN FUNCTION

The consumption of nutraceuticals has been shown to improve general health and delay the aging process by supporting the structure and function of the body, thus contributing to an increase in life expectancy. Numerous studies have been published demonstrating the beneficial effects of consumption of flavonoid-rich grapes on brain function and the central nervous system [58]. Krikorian et al. reported findings that concord grape juice supplement and polyphenol compounds found in berry fruits, in particular flavonoids, have been associated with health benefits, including improvement in cognition and neuronal function with aging [59,60]. Also, a 12-week clinical study by Krikorian et al. revealed that supplementation of diet with concord grape (*Vitis labrusca*) juice might improve memory functions in mild/moderate memory declined older adults. Anthocyanin flavonoid-rich grape has also been shown to have positive results in preventing neurodegenerative diseases both by reducing OS and inhibiting neuroinflammation [29,61]. Catechins and epicatechins, natural polyphenolic flavonoid compounds, are in the category of flavan-3-ols (or flavanols). These polyphenol-rich flavonoids from grape seed extract have been shown to have significant capability to disrupt and disintegrate the ultrastructure of native paired helical filaments, which is a key neuropathological feature in AD [62].

Several in vitro studies using flavonoids quercetin which is abundant in several common foods such as apples and capers, on C6 glioma and SH-SY5Y neuroblastoma cells showed its ability to alleviate OS induced by hydrogen peroxide or interleukin-1β and protect against Parkinson's disease (PD) toxin 6-OHDA, respectively [63,64]. Several in vivo studies also demonstrate that quercetin could be developed as a novel therapeutic for neurodegeneration since it has been shown to improve memory and hippocampal synaptic plasticity in models of impairment induced by chronic lead exposure [65]. Quercetin also provides neuroprotection against colchicine administration, which similarly causes cognitive impairments [66]. It decreases the size of the ischemic lesion and suppresses hippocampal neuronal death in the rat ischemia model using middle cerebral artery occlusion [67] and also improves motor function after administration of quercetin post-injury in the model of acute spinal cord injury [68].

Epigallocatechin 3-gallate (EGCG) is another flavonoid-rich polyphenol phytochemical that is abundant in green tea. Numerous in vitro and in vivo studies on neuronal cells system showed that EGCG induced an effective neuroprotective effect against many oxidative insults and improved cell functions; hence could be a viable therapeutic candidate for chronic neurodegenerative diseases such as AD, PD, ALS, or Huntington's disease [69]. Some of the studies included using cerebellar granule neuron (CGN) model rats, and results indicated that EGCG selectively protects cultured rat CGNs from OS, as CGNs were incubated with the Bcl-2 inhibitor, HA14-1 (ethyl 2-amino-6-bromo-4-(1-cyano-2-ethoxy-2-oxoethyl)-4H-chromene-3-carboxylate) to undergo mitochondrial OS and intrinsic apoptosis [70,71]. Oral administration of EGCG nutraceutical antioxidant to several models of neurodegeneration also showed its ability to preserve neuronal survival and function. In one of the studies, oral administrations of EGCG protected mice from the dopaminergic toxicity caused by the Parkinson's neurotoxin, 1-methyl-4-phenyl-1,2,3,6-tetrahydropyridine (MPTP). EGCG treatment prevents the MPTP-induced loss of dopamine neurons from the substantia nigra pars compacta and preserves striatal dopamine levels in mice [72]. Similarly, oral administration of EGCG to Swedish mutant APP (APPsw) overexpressing transgenic mice decreases amyloid plaque burden and reduces cognitive impairment [73]. All these studies just further emphasize the importance of flavonoid-rich nutraceuticals in improving general health and delaying chronic diseases and the aging process, thus contributing to an increase in life expectancy.

FLAVONOID-RICH NUTRACEUTICALS AND CARDIOVASCULAR DISEASES

CVD remains the number 1 killer disease in the United States of America despite the significant rise in modern conventional medicine to therapeutically manage and improve survival. According to World Health Organization (WHO) statistics, ischemic heart disease is the leading cause of death worldwide. CVDs encompass many heart dysfunctions, including heart failure, hypertension, inflammation, hypertrophy, atherosclerosis ischemia, and disturbance in the electrical activity of the heart, expressed primarily by arrhythmia. As always present marker of CVDs is OS due to over production of ROS relative to antioxidants, and troponins are regulatory proteins and part of the contractile mechanism of the cardiac muscle [74,75]. Numerous reports of research done by studying the effects of consuming flavonoid-rich grade products on CVDs show a lot of beneficial results on the cardiovascular system, including enhancement of endothelial function, decreasing LDL oxidation, altering blood lipids, and modulating inflammatory processes [9,76,77]. Albers et al. reported a study that provided evidence that consumption of flavonoid-rich purple grape juice could attenuate CVDs and inhibit thrombosis. Findings from clinical studies suggest that flavonoid-rich purple grape juice attenuates CVDs and thrombosis by suppressing platelet-dependent inflammation as it significantly decreases the levels of platelet-dependent superoxide and the inflammatory mediator sCD40L after the consumption of the purple grape juice [78]. More research on the consumption of flavonoid-rich grape nutraceutical products shows that it has antioxidative effects and increased levels of anti-inflammatory factors in the absence of dyslipidemias in men with metabolic syndrome [79,80].

Although several identified flavonoid-rich nutraceuticals have been screened and shown to have a beneficial effect in managing CVD, a considerable amount of work still needs to be done to elucidate the safety and actual mechanism of how the active ingredient does alleviate heart disease. Mass production of these phytochemicals in the lab to be added to the diets as supplements would be encouraged as this would balance demand and supply.

FLAVONOID-RICH NUTRACEUTICALS AND METABOLIC SYNDROME-RELATED DISEASES

The cause of obesity and diabetes are numerous and vary by race, age, and genetics. In the United States, they are the most prevalent nutrition-related diseases [81]. Polyphenols and many grape nutraceutical products have proven to reduce metabolic syndrome and prevent the development of obesity and type-2 diabetes by acting as multi-target modulators with antioxidant and anti-inflammatory effects [81,82]. The flavonol, quercetin-3-O-glucoside abundant in grape powder extracts, significantly reduced several inflammatory markers in human adipocytes [83]. Grape skin extract that harbors a considerable number of flavonoids has been shown to possess significant anticancer effects by mitigating various biological activities that maintain the viability of cancer cells [84]. Several other studies on breast cancer and colon cancer cells showed that flavonoid compounds effectively stopped metastasis and exhibited chemopreventive activity via their antioxidant and anti-inflammatory activities [85,86]. An in-depth mechanistic study evaluating the biological activity of grape seed proanthocyanidins extracts on human pancreatic cancer cells showed that the flavonoid significantly reduced cell viability and induced apoptosis in a dose-dependent manner by inactivating the inflammatory transcription factor NF-κB [87]. All these findings continue to add more support and interest in the development of different types of consumable flavonoid-rich nutraceuticals as demands continue to soar.

BIOTECHNOLOGY APPLICATION TO SCALE UP FLAVONOID-RICH NUTRACEUTICALS

The use and application of nutraceuticals continue to be on the rise worldwide, and currently, the nutraceutical industry ears more than $200 billion per year. As the global demand increases, the industry cannot continue to depend solely on the nature to produce phytochemicals needed for nutraceuticals. Several research interests and knowledge in plant biochemistry, plant genomics, molecular biology, and investment in biotechnology are on the rise to scale up the production of nutritional and medical bioactive components from plants, including flavonoids. As results of research findings continue to reveal the potential benefits of flavonoid bioactive components, there is increasing research interest in different methodologies and bioengineering technology to enhance the production of plant flavonoid synthesis in the laboratory. The increasing belief in natural products compared with conventional medicine coupled with the pleiotropic effects of flavonoids on many age-related and metabolic diseases, some discussed above, have activated an exponential growth in the demand for flavonoid-rich nutraceuticals which cannot depend solely on natural plant production. To meet this need for these phytochemicals, numerous research efforts and biotechnological approaches are being applied to step up yields from commercial production of a large quantity of the flavonoid bioactive component from plants [88]. Diverse in vitro and in vivo genomic efforts have been exploited with different plant species to scale up yields of flavonoid biosynthesis in plants. Although very promising results have been reported, it is still a work in progress [89].

Another biotechnological approach is the application of microbes' model systems technic. This technology has great potential for the heterologous production of bioactive flavonoid compounds. *Escherichia coli* and *Saccharomyces cerevisiae* are microbial models that have been widely used to express genes that can convert fed precursors or endogenously produced substrates into valuable end products [90]. Plant-derived flavonoids are examples of such end products' bioconversions in microbes since the interactions between plants and animals' proteins are easy to study and manipulate, and as such, large quantity production of endogenous and heterologous proteins can be done to satisfy the present high demands [90] (Table 2.2).

Another perspective alternative model to maintain continuous production of large quantity flavonods is by application of plant cell cultures under controlled conditions. In recent years, the application of grape cell suspension cultures in mass productions of flavonoids has gained popularity among plants scientists and the industry since reviewed publications demonstrate how grape cell suspensions have been used to study the mechanism of secondary metabolite biosynthesis and in vitro production of valuable polyphenols [29,91]. There are several advantages of culturing plant cells in bioreactors with strictly controlled environmental conditions to produce a biologically active component for flavonoid-rich nutraceuticals. The process minimizes variation in yield and unpredictable metabolite composition compared with conventional breeding. This in vitro production of flavonoid nutraceutical-rich biomass components can be done all year round with no concern about the season, temperature variation, soil types, and

TABLE 2.2   Biotechnology applications engineering to improve yields of flavonoids [90]

FLAVONOID TARGET	TARGET GENES (PLANT DONOR)	ENGINEERED ORGANISMS	METABOLIC EFFECTS
Kaempferol naringenin	C1, LC transcription factors (Zea mays)	L. esculentum	High-flavonol tomatoes (mainly kaempferol, lesser effect for naringerin) resulting to from the heterogenious expression of the maize transcription factor genes LC and C1
Anthocyanins	Del (Delila) transcription factor (Antirrhinum)	L. esculentum	Enhanced anthocyanin pigmentation
Anthocyanins, flavones	P1 transcription factor (Z. mays)	Z. mays	Increased anthocyanins and flavone levels
Anthocyanins	Lc transcription activator (Z. mays)	L. esculentum	Enhanced pigmentation under high light condition
Quercetin	FLS (P. hybrida)	S. cerevisiae	Production of quercetin by conversion of dihydroquercetin
Anthocyanins	ANS (O. sativa)	O. sativa	Overexpression of anthocyanidin synthase accumulate a mixture of flavonoids

climate changes. To sum it all up, in vitro cultivation of plant cells in an eco-friendly bio-safe environment is of great importance [29].

It is important to note that the quantity and quality of in vitro flavonoid biosynthesis in cell suspensions is highly dependent on the composition of the nutrient medium in the bioreactor. Decendit and Merillon's study concluded that to obtain the highest quantity and quality of flavonoid production from plant cell suspensions of *Vitis vinifera*, two media (maintenance and production) were necessary to support or obtain the best growth rate. They also reported that cultures done using only maintenance medium (low sucrose and high nitrate contents) in the cells had maximum growth rate but extremely low levels of flavonoid accumulation. However, when cultures were done using sucrose, ammonium, phosphate, and magnesium concentrations in the nutrient medium were increased (three-, two-, two-, and twofold, respectively), the maximum yields of anthocyanins (1,100 mg/L), proanthocyanidins (300 mg/L) and catechins (25 mg/L) were achieved [92].

The results of the in vitro plant cell suspension cultures by media manipulation technology show a significant contribution to the production of bioactive components such as flavonoids as the quantity is scaled up to meet demand. Also, it can be expected that developing a well-established technology for plant cell cultivation could lead to the development of sustainable technology to produce high-quality flavonoids with increased added value.

Another potential application of in vitro plant cell suspension is in the production of marker compounds that can be used to continue in vivo studies to understand the bioavailability and metabolism of phytonutrients in the human body [29]. Yousef et al. used plant cell suspension culture of *Vitis* hybrid "Bailey Alicant A" to produce radiolabeled anthocyanins, (+)-catechin, and (−)-epicatechin by feeding with ^{14}C-labeled sucrose during cultivation [93]. The radiolabeled flavonoids have great potential as a reliable source of labeled phytochemicals that can be used for in vivo study of bioavailability, catabolism, and the accumulation of these chemicals in animals and humans due to consumption of flavonoid-rich nutraceuticals [29].

Flavonoids derived from grape-rich polyphenols make this plant species a very promising source for the development of flavonoid-rich nutraceutical products. This would be why there has recently been a spike worldwide in the demand and production of food additives and nutritional products from grapes. It should be noted that most commercialized products are obtained during processing pomace, including grape skin or seed extracts, grape skin powder, dry seed powder (capsulated or bulk), pomace powder, and anthocyanin colorants from grape wine and juice production.

CONCLUSION

Flavonoids, without any doubt, exert many beneficial effects on human health. Flavonoids possess solid antioxidant activity that underscores their capability to mitigate OS and promote neuronal cell survival. The ability of flavonoids to reduce OS and promote neuronal cell survival signals through multiple modes of action compared with standard pharmaceutical drugs with one mechanism of action and several side effects are driving the demand for flavonoid-rich nutraceuticals. Natural antioxidants, including flavonoids, are not only active scavengers of free radicals but also function as modulators of pro-survival or pro-apoptotic signaling pathways. Hence, meticulously well-formulated flavonoid-rich nutraceuticals have great potential as novel therapeutics in managing metabolic diseases, CVDs, and neurodegenerative diseases since it is natural.

Several studies show increasing evidence of the benefit of flavonoid-rich nutraceuticals in preventing and alleviating CVDs, and many different age-related diseases. This further underlines the anti-atherogenic and antithrombotic effects due to the strong antioxidation properties of flavonoids. Additionally, several studies also suggest that flavonoids inhibit LDL oxidation and platelet aggregation; hence regular and moderate consumption of flavonoid-rich food and red wine might protect against atherosclerosis and thrombosis.

Effective treatment of neurodegenerative diseases remains a dilemma in the healthcare system with very limited approved drugs available. A lot of funding dollars continue to be directed to AD and PD research in efforts to find potent and safe therapeutics to abate these ailments. Although few palliative therapies have been developed and available, none can boast to significantly slow or halt the underlying pathology of the disease, and they continue to thrive in the communities. Flavonoid-rich nutraceutical antioxidants may be the better option for these categories of patients in the short term since nutraceuticals are subject to fewer regulations than traditional pharmaceuticals. Nutraceuticals could be made available to patients much more rapidly than new prescription drugs.

The future of flavonoid-rich nutraceuticals with their strong antioxidation appears to hold much promise as CVD, AD, and PD continue to dominate the elderly population around the world. It cannot be stressed enough that nutraceuticals provide significant therapeutic benefits to patients suffering from numerous cardiovascular and neurodegenerative diseases compared with pure synthetic pharmaceuticals. It must be noted that the United States does not allow any health claims for nutraceuticals because there is no formal review and approval process for the marketing authorization of nutraceuticals. The only major US regulation related to nutraceuticals is the 1994 passage of the Dietary Supplement Health and Education Act by the US Congress. Based on this act, dietary supplements are classified as foods, not drugs, allowing them to be sold without proof of safety and effectiveness (FDA 1994). Because there is no meticulous and strict regulation of nutraceuticals product, the pharmacology and toxicological information provided on labels cannot be totally trusted. Skeptics of natural products would be given some credit for their doubts about the exact quantity of active components (such as flavonoids) as well as the standardized extraction procedure of the phytochemical constituents. The pharmacological and toxicological evaluation of nutraceuticals, in general, is still overly complex since multiple phytochemicals can be found in a single plant, the variability in plants and their phytochemical constituents due to geography, soil characteristics, and climate, not neglecting human influence by using fertilizers and pesticides and diurnal variation during harvesting. It is highly likely that some or all the above variables would influence the identity, purity, quality, quantity, composition, potency/strength, and safety of the components of flavonoid-rich nutraceuticals, thereby causing a wide variability in product effectiveness from batch to batch and from different companies.

We cannot conclude this chapter without mentioning some of the setbacks facing flavonoid-rich nutraceuticals. The nutraceutical industry as a whole is growing faster than expected, but the following challenges remain a conundrum that must be addressed. They include (a) inadequate knowledge of molecular interaction between bioactive phytochemicals within the same and different plants, (b) lack of authenticity of active ingredients due to limited or no available reference marker compounds, and (c) significant variability in the origin of raw material due to difference in a climate where the plants thrive (e.g., American versus Chinese ginseng), (d) no standardize the process for extracting bioactive phytochemicals, (e) inadequacy and inconsistency in standard quality control in different countries, (f) lack of well-established and evidence-based clinical trials procedures, and (g) inadequate or reliable safety and toxicity data. In addition to these, many challenges are severe adverse effects that could arise from the consumption of nutraceuticals due to adulteration of the nutraceuticals with other pharmaceutical drugs, phytochemicals, and drugs of abuse to maximize profit. Standard, well-established, strict, and comprehensive regulations worldwide would surely improve the safety of nutraceutical, especially flavonoid-rich nutraceuticals, which has proven to be beneficial in alleviating many human diseases.

REFERENCES

1. Potapovich AI, Kostyuk VA. Comparative study of antioxidant properties and cytoprotective activity of flavonoids. *Biochemistry (Mosc).* 2003;68(5):514–9.
2. Rice-Evans CA, Miller NJ, Bolwell PG, Bramley PM, Pridham JB. The relative antioxidant activities of plant-derived polyphenolic flavonoids. *Free Radic Res.* 1995;22(4):375–83.
3. Middleton E, Jr. Effect of plant flavonoids on immune and inflammatory cell function. *Adv Exp Med Biol.* 1998;439:175–82.
4. Kumar S, Pandey AK. Chemistry and biological activities of flavonoids: An overview. *Sci World J.* 2013;2013:162750.
5. de Groot H, Rauen U. Tissue injury by reactive oxygen species and the protective effects of flavonoids. *Fundam Clin Pharmacol.* 1998;12(3):249–55.
6. Havsteen B. Flavonoids, a class of natural products of high pharmacological potency. *Biochem Pharmacol.* 1983;32(7):1141–8.
7. Havsteen BH. The biochemistry and medical significance of flavonoids. *Pharmacol Ther.* 2002;96(2–3):67–202.
8. Kandaswami C, Middleton E, Jr. Free radical scavenging and antioxidant activity of plant flavonoids. *Adv Exp Med Biol.* 1994;366:351–76.
9. Hertog MG, Kromhout D, Aravanis C, Blackburn H, Buzina R, Fidanza F, et al. Flavonoid intake and long-term risk of coronary heart disease and cancer in the seven countries study. *Arch Intern Med.* 1995;155(4):381–6.
10. Hertog MG, Feskens EJ, Hollman PC, Katan MB, Kromhout D. Dietary antioxidant flavonoids and risk of coronary heart disease: The Zutphen elderly study. *Lancet.* 1993;342(8878):1007–11.
11. Keli SO, Hertog MG, Feskens EJ, Kromhout D. Dietary flavonoids, antioxidant vitamins, and incidence of stroke: The Zutphen study. *Arch Intern Med.* 1996;156(6):637–42.
12. Mutagenic food flavonoids. Symposium report. *Fed Proc.* 1984;43(9):2454–8.
13. Hassig A, Liang WX, Schwabl H, Stampfli K. Flavonoids and tannins: Plant-based antioxidants with vitamin character. *Med Hypotheses.* 1999;52(5):479–81.
14. de Vries JH, Janssen PL, Hollman PC, van Staveren WA, Katan MB. Consumption of quercetin and kaempferol in free-living subjects eating a variety of diets. *Cancer Lett.* 1997;114(1–2):141–4.
15. Norbaek R, Brandt K, Kondo T. Identification of flavone C-glycosides including a new flavonoid chromophore from barley leaves (Hordeum vulgare L.) by improved NMR techniques. *J Agric Food Chem.* 2000;48(5):1703–7.
16. Panche AN, Diwan AD, Chandra SR. Flavonoids: An overview. *J Nutr Sci.* 2016;5:e47.
17. Gupta DPaKR. The antioxidant phytochemicals of nutraceutical importance. *Open Nutraceu J.* 2009;2:20–35.
18. Brower V. Nutraceuticals: Poised for a healthy slice of the healthcare market? *Nat Biotechnol.* 1998;16(8):728–31.
19. Jack DB. Keep taking the tomatoes—The exciting world of nutraceuticals. *Mol Med Today.* 1995;1(3):118–21.
20. Das L, Bhaumik E, Raychaudhuri U, Chakraborty R. Role of nutraceuticals in human health. *J Food Sci Technol.* 2012;49(2):173–83.
21. Alfei S, Schito AM, Zuccari G. Nanotechnological manipulation of nutraceuticals and phytochemicals for healthy purposes: Established advantages vs. still undefined risks. *Polymers (Basel).* 2021;13(14).
22. Williamson EM, Liu X, Izzo AA. Trends in use, pharmacology, and clinical applications of emerging herbal nutraceuticals. *Br J Pharmacol.* 2020;177(6):1227–40.

23. Alfei S, Marengo B, Zuccari G. Nanotechnology application in food packaging: A plethora of opportunities versus pending risks assessment and public concerns. *Food Res Int.* 2020;137:109664.
24. Scalbert A, Johnson IT, Saltmarsh M. Polyphenols: Antioxidants and beyond. *Am J Clin Nutr.* 2005;81(1 Suppl):215S–7S.
25. Duthie GGGP, Kyle JAM. Plant polyphenols: Are they the new magic bullet? *Proc Nutr Soc.* 2003;62(3):599–603.
26. Moskaug J, Carlsen H, Myhrstad MC, Blomhoff R. Polyphenols and glutathione synthesis regulation. *Am J Clin Nutr.* 2005;81(1 Suppl):277S–83S.
27. Yang CS, Landau JM, Huang MT, Newmark HL. Inhibition of carcinogenesis by dietary polyphenolic compounds. *Annu Rev Nutr.* 2001;21:381–406.
28. Scalbert A, Manach C, Morand C, Remesy C, Jimenez L. Dietary polyphenols and the prevention of diseases. *Crit Rev Food Sci Nutr.* 2005;45(4):287–306.
29. Georgiev V, Ananga A, Tsolova V. Recent advances and uses of grape flavonoids as nutraceuticals. *Nutrients.* 2014;6(1):391–415.
30. Rice-Evans CA, Miller NJ, Paganga G. Structure-antioxidant activity relationships of flavonoids and phenolic acids. *Free Radic Biol Med.* 1996;20(7):933–56.
31. Rietjens IMCM, Boersma MGHLD, et al. The pro-oxidant chemistry of the natural antioxidants vitamin C, vitamin E, carotenoids, and flavonoids. *Environ Toxicol Pharmacol.* 2002;11:321–33.
32. Kumar G, Dange P, Kailaje V, Vaidya MM, Ramchandani AG, Maru GB. Polymeric black tea polyphenols modulate the localization and activity of 12-O-tetradecanoylphorbol-13-acetate-mediated kinases in mouse skin: Mechanisms of their anti-tumor-promoting action. *Free Radic Biol Med.* 2012;53(6):1358–70.
33. Kumar G, Pillare SP, Maru GB. Black tea polyphenols-mediated in vivo cellular responses during carcinogenesis. *Mini Rev Med Chem.* 2010;10(6):492–505.
34. Maru GB, Hudlikar RR, Kumar G, Gandhi K, Mahimkar MB. Understanding the molecular mechanisms of cancer prevention by dietary phytochemicals: From experimental models to clinical trials. *World J Biol Chem.* 2016;7(1):88–99.
35. Choe E, Min DB. Chemistry and reactions of reactive oxygen species in foods. *Crit Rev Food Sci Nutr.* 2006;46(1):1–22.
36. Marnett LJ. Oxyradicals and DNA damage. *Carcinogenesis.* 2000;21(3):361–70.
37. Xu A, Wu LJ, Santella RM, Hei TK. Role of oxyradicals in mutagenicity and DNA damage induced by crocidolite asbestos in mammalian cells. *Cancer Res.* 1999;59(23):5922–6.
38. Olinski R, Gackowski D, Foksinski M, Rozalski R, Roszkowski K, Jaruga P. Oxidative DNA damage: Assessment of the role in carcinogenesis, atherosclerosis, and acquired immunodeficiency syndrome. *Free Radic Biol Med.* 2002;33(2):192–200.
39. Tiwari AK, Srinivas PV, Kumar SP, Rao JM. Free radical scavenging active components from Cedrus deodara. *J Agric Food Chem.* 2001;49(10):4642–5.
40. Arts IC, Hollman PC. Polyphenols and disease risk in epidemiologic studies. *Am J Clin Nutr.* 2005;81(1 Suppl):317S–25S.
41. Kris-Etherton PM, Hecker KD, Bonanome A, Coval SM, Binkoski AE, Hilpert KF, et al. Bioactive compounds in foods: Their role in the prevention of cardiovascular disease and cancer. *Am J Med.* 2002;113(Suppl 9B):71S–88S.
42. Halliwell B, Whiteman M. Measuring reactive species and oxidative damage in vivo and in cell culture: How should you do it and what do the results mean? *Br J Pharmacol.* 2004;142(2):231–55.
43. Anton D, Matt D, Pedastsaar P, Bender I, Kazimierczak R, Roasto M, et al. Three-year comparative study of polyphenol contents and antioxidant capacities in fruits of tomato (Lycopersicon esculentum Mill.) cultivars grown under organic and conventional conditions. *J Agric Food Chem.* 2014;62(22):5173–80.

44. Arranz S, Saura-Calixto F, Shaha S, Kroon PA. High contents of nonextractable polyphenols in fruits suggest that polyphenol contents of plant foods have been underestimated. *J Agric Food Chem.* 2009;57(16):7298–303.
45. Scalbert A, Williamson G. Dietary intake and bioavailability of polyphenols. *J Nutr.* 2000;130(8S Suppl):2073S–85S.
46. Tapas DS, Kakde RB. Flavonoids as nutraceuticals: A review. *Trop J Pharmac Res.* 2008;7(3):1089–99.
47. Grace PA. Ischemia-reperfusion injury. *Br J Surg.* 1994;81(5):637–47.
48. Gunaratne A, Wu K, Li D, Bentota A, Corke H, Cai YZ. Antioxidant activity and nutritional quality of traditional red-grained rice varieties containing proanthocyanidins. *Food Chem.* 2013;138(2–3):1153–61.
49. Cai Y, Sun M, Xing J, Corke H. Antioxidant phenolic constituents in roots of Rheum officinale and Rubia cordifolia: Structure-radical scavenging activity relationships. *J Agric Food Chem.* 2004;52(26):7884–90.
50. Ferguson LR, Philpott M, Karunasinghe N. Dietary cancer and prevention using antimutagens. *Toxicology.* 2004;198(1–3):147–59.
51. Santos AC, Uyemura SA, Lopes JL, Bazon JN, Mingatto FE, Curti C. Effect of naturally occurring flavonoids on lipid peroxidation and membrane permeability transition in mitochondria. *Free Radic Biol Med.* 1998;24(9):1455–61.
52. Kohlmeier L. Epidemiology of anticarcinogens in food. *Adv Exp Med Biol.* 1995;369:125–39.
53. Aggarwal BB, Shishodia S, Sandur SK, Pandey MK, Sethi G. Inflammation and cancer: How hot is the link? *Biochem Pharmacol.* 2006;72(11):1605–21.
54. Dantzer R, O'Connor JC, Freund GG, Johnson RW, Kelley KW. From inflammation to sickness and depression: When the immune system subjugates the brain. *Nat Rev Neurosci.* 2008;9(1):46–56.
55. Tabas I, Glass CK. Anti-inflammatory therapy in chronic disease: Challenges and opportunities. *Science.* 2013;339(6116):166–72.
56. Rubio-Perez JM, Morillas-Ruiz JM. A review: Inflammatory process in Alzheimer's disease, the role of cytokines. *Sci World J.* 2012;2012:756357.
57. Panico AM, Cardile V, Avondo S, Garufi F, Gentile B, Puglia C, et al. The in vitro effect of a lyophilized extract of wine obtained from Jacquez grapes on human chondrocytes. *Phytomedicine.* 2006;13(7):522–6.
58. Krikorian R, Eliassen JC, Boespflug EL, Nash TA, Shidler MD. Improved cognitive-cerebral function in older adults with chromium supplementation. *Nutr Neurosci.* 2010;13(3):116–22.
59. Krikorian R, Boespflug EL, Fleck DE, Stein AL, Wightman JD, Shidler MD, et al. Concord grape juice supplementation and neurocognitive function in human aging. *J Agric Food Chem.* 2012;60(23):5736–42.
60. Krikorian R, Nash TA, Shidler MD, Shukitt-Hale B, Joseph JA. Concord grape juice supplementation improves memory function in older adults with mild cognitive impairment. *Br J Nutr.* 2010;103(5):730–4.
61. Krikorian R, Shidler MD, Nash TA, Kalt W, Vinqvist-Tymchuk MR, Shukitt-Hale B, et al. Blueberry supplementation improves memory in older adults. *J Agric Food Chem.* 2010;58(7):3996–4000.
62. Ksiezak-Reding H, Ho L, Santa-Maria I, Diaz-Ruiz C, Wang J, Pasinetti GM. Ultrastructural alterations of Alzheimer's disease paired helical filaments by grape seed-derived polyphenols. *Neurobiol Aging.* 2012;33(7):1427–39.
63. Chen TJ, Jeng JY, Lin CW, Wu CY, Chen YC. Quercetin inhibition of ROS-dependent and independent apoptosis in rat glioma C6 cells. *Toxicology.* 2006;223(1–2):113–26.
64. Sharma V, Mishra M, Ghosh S, Tewari R, Basu A, Seth P, et al. Modulation of interleukin-1beta mediated inflammatory response in human astrocytes by flavonoids: Implications in neuroprotection. *Brain Res Bull.* 2007;73(1–3):55–63.

65. Hu P, Wang M, Chen WH, Liu J, Chen L, Yin ST, et al. Quercetin relieves chronic lead exposure-induced impairment of synaptic plasticity in rat dentate gyrus in vivo. *Naunyn Schmiedebergs Arch Pharmacol.* 2008;378(1):43–51.
66. Kumar A, Sehgal N, Kumar P, Padi SS, Naidu PS. Protective effect of quercetin against ICV colchicine-induced cognitive dysfunctions and oxidative damage in rats. *Phytother Res.* 2008;22(12):1563–9.
67. Dajas F, Rivera-Megret F, Blasina F, Arredondo F, Abin-Carriquiry JA, Costa G, et al. Neuroprotection by flavonoids. *Braz J Med Biol Res.* 2003;36(12):1613–20.
68. Schultke E, Kendall E, Kamencic H, Ghong Z, Griebel RW, Juurlink BH. Quercetin promotes functional recovery following acute spinal cord injury. *J Neurotrauma.* 2003;20(6):583–91.
69. Weinreb O, Mandel S, Amit T, Youdim MB. Neurological mechanisms of green tea polyphenols in Alzheimer's and Parkinson's diseases. *J Nutr Biochem.* 2004;15(9):506–16.
70. Paquay JB, Haenen GR, Stender G, Wiseman SA, Tijburg LB, Bast A. Protection against nitric oxide toxicity by tea. *J Agric Food Chem.* 2000;48(11):5768–72.
71. Zimmermann AK, Loucks FA, Schroeder EK, Bouchard RJ, Tyler KL, Linseman DA. Glutathione binding to the Bcl-2 homology-3 domain groove: A molecular basis for Bcl-2 antioxidant function at mitochondria. *J Biol Chem.* 2007;282(40):29296–304.
72. Levites Y, Weinreb O, Maor G, Youdim MB, Mandel S. Green tea polyphenol (–)-epigallocatechin-3-gallate prevents N-methyl-4-phenyl-1,2,3,6-tetrahydropyridine-induced dopaminergic neurodegeneration. *J Neurochem.* 2001;78(5):1073–82.
73. Rezai-Zadeh K, Arendash GW, Hou H, Fernandez F, Jensen M, Runfeldt M, et al. Green tea epigallocatechin-3-gallate (EGCG) reduces beta-amyloid mediated cognitive impairment and modulates tau pathology in Alzheimer transgenic mice. *Brain Res.* 2008;1214:177–87.
74. Selvaraju V, Joshi M, Suresh S, Sanchez JA, Maulik N, Maulik G. Diabetes, oxidative stress, molecular mechanism, and cardiovascular disease—An overview. *Toxicol Mech Methods.* 2012;22(5):330–5.
75. Sorodoc V, Sorodoc L, Ungureanu D, Sava A, Jaba IM. Cardiac troponin T and NT-proBNP as biomarkers of early myocardial damage in amitriptyline-induced cardiovascular toxicity in rats. *Int J Toxicol.* 2013;32(5):351–7.
76. Li H, Forstermann U. Red wine and cardiovascular health. *Circ Res.* 2012;111(8):959–61.
77. Xia EQ, Deng GF, Guo YJ, Li HB. Biological activities of polyphenols from grapes. *Int J Mol Sci.* 2010;11(2):622–46.
78. Albers AR, Varghese S, Vitseva O, Vita JA, Freedman JE. The anti-inflammatory effects of purple grape juice consumption in subjects with stable coronary artery disease. *Arterioscler Thromb Vasc Biol.* 2004;24(11):e179–80.
79. Barona J, Aristizabal JC, Blesso CN, Volek JS, Fernandez ML. Grape polyphenols reduce blood pressure and increase flow-mediated vasodilation in men with metabolic syndrome. *J Nutr.* 2012;142(9):1626–32.
80. Barona J, Blesso CN, Andersen CJ, Park Y, Lee J, Fernandez ML. Grape consumption increases anti-inflammatory markers and upregulates peripheral nitric oxide synthase in the absence of dyslipidemias in men with metabolic syndrome. *Nutrients.* 2012;4(12):1945–57.
81. Chuang CC, McIntosh MK. Potential mechanisms by which polyphenol-rich grapes prevent obesity-mediated inflammation and metabolic diseases. *Annu Rev Nutr.* 2011;31:155–76.
82. Tsuda T. Dietary anthocyanin-rich plants: Biochemical basis and recent progress in health benefits studies. *Mol Nutr Food Res.* 2012;56(1):159–70.
83. Chuang CC, Shen W, Chen H, Xie G, Jia W, Chung S, et al. Differential effects of grape powder and its extract on glucose tolerance and chronic inflammation in high-fat-fed obese mice. *J Agric Food Chem.* 2012;60(51):12458–68.

84. Zhou K, Raffoul JJ. Potential anticancer properties of grape antioxidants. *J Oncol.* 2012;2012:803294.

85. Sun T, Chen QY, Wu LJ, Yao XM, Sun XJ. Antitumor and antimetastatic activities of grape skin polyphenols in a murine model of breast cancer. *Food Chem Toxicol.* 2012;50(10):3462–7.

86. Kountouri AM, Gioxari A, Karvela E, Kaliora AC, Karvelas M, Karathanos VT. Chemopreventive properties of raisins originating from Greece in colon cancer cells. *Food Funct.* 2013;4(3):366–72.

87. Prasad R, Katiyar SK. Grape seed proanthocyanidins inhibit the migration potential of pancreatic cancer cells by promoting mesenchymal-to-epithelial transition and targeting NF-kappaB. *Cancer Lett.* 2013;334(1):118–26.

88. Grotewold E, Chamberlin M, Snook M, Siame B, Butler L, Swenson J, et al. Engineering secondary metabolism in maize cells by ectopic expression of transcription factors. *Plant Cell.* 1998;10(5):721–40.

89. Harmer SL, Hogenesch JB, Straume M, Chang HS, Han B, Zhu T, et al. Orchestrated transcription of key pathways in Arabidopsis by the circadian clock. *Science.* 2000;290(5499):2110–3.

90. Ververidis F, Trantas E, Douglas C, Vollmer G, Kretzschmar G, Panopoulos N. Biotechnology of flavonoids and other phenylpropanoid-derived natural products. Part II: Reconstruction of multienzyme pathways in plants and microbes. *Biotechnol J.* 2007;2(10):1235–49.

91. Davis G, Ananga A, Krastanova S, Sutton S, Ochieng JW, Leong S, et al. Elevated gene expression in chalcone synthase enzyme suggests an increased production of flavonoids in the skin and synchronized red cell cultures of North American native grape berries. *DNA Cell Biol.* 2012;31(6):939–45.

92. Decendit A, Merillon JM. Condensed tannin and anthocyanin production in Vitis vinifera cell suspension cultures. *Plant Cell Rep.* 1996;15(10):762–5.

93. Yousef GG, Seigler DS, Grusak MA, Rogers RB, Knight CT, Kraft TF, et al. Biosynthesis and characterization of 14C-enriched flavonoid fractions from plant cell suspension cultures. *J Agric Food Chem.* 2004;52(5):1138–45.

The Role of Nrf2 in Flavonoids' Anticancer Activity

3

Patricia Mendonca
Florida A&M University

Contents

DOI: 10.1201/9781003225225-3

INTRODUCTION

Cancer is a heterogeneous disease differentiated by multiple stages of pathogenesis. Besides all the progress in developing various anticancer drugs and new strategies, we still do not have the key to selectively destroy malignant cells without affecting the normal ones [1]. With the rising costs of cancer treatment, there is an increasing need to understand the molecular mechanisms that can inhibit cancer, leading to new strategies to prevent cancer progression [2]. Given that neoplastic transformation usually is a relatively extensive process that may take more than decades, there are many strategies to mediate cancer pathogenesis, particularly in the early stages of oncogenesis [1]. One of them is the chemoprevention with naturally occurring or synthetic substances, or their combination, to halt, slow, or reverse the carcinogenesis process. Many of these substances are found in our diets, such as fruits, vegetables, grains, spices, and seeds, which have proven effective in cancer prevention [1]. In vitro and in vivo experiments have evidenced that dietary phytochemicals, such as flavonoids, have anticancer effects interfering with cancer development processes, including inflammation, proliferation, invasion, angiogenesis, and metastasis. The molecular mechanism of flavonoids includes targets such as the mitogen-activated protein kinase (MAPK), protein kinase C (PKC), phosphatidylinositol 3-kinase (PI3K)/Akt, and b-catenin pathways, which are associated with the transformation of normal cells into malignant ones and tumor progress. Besides, flavonoids may modulate the activation of the nuclear factor-kappa B (NF-κB) involved with the expression of proinflammatory mediators [3]. Flavonoids with chemopreventive potential may target redox-sensitive transcription factors and have been described as having chemopreventive effects on inflammation and oxidative stress–associated carcinogenesis, mediating signal transduction associated with diverse redox-regulated transcription factors [4]. Reports have shown that these compounds can activate Nrf2/Keap1 signaling, which is responsible for the transcription of a range of cytoprotective genes against oxidative stress, which may help halt the carcinogenesis process [5,6].

TUMOR MICROENVIRONMENT AND CHEMOPREVENTIVE COMPOUNDS

The tumor microenvironment consists of a multifaceted system crucial to initiating and maintaining tumorigenesis [7], including multipotent stromal cells/mesenchymal stem cells, fibroblasts, blood vessels, endothelial cell precursors, immune cells, and cytokines [7,8]. These changes occur at the molecular and cellular level and entail interactions between developing cancer cells, host structural cells, and adaptive and innate immune cells [9]. The capacity to stimulate proliferation and reduce apoptosis, cause angiogenesis and evade hypoxia, inhibit the immune system, avoid immune detection, and activate immune cells to support invasion and metastasis are some of the "hallmarks of cancer" that alters the tumor microenvironment [10]. Therefore, managing changes in the tumor microenvironment is a useful approach to prevent and treat cancer, with the investigation of specific molecular and cellular mechanisms and then observation of whether or not the inhibition or activation led to the expected results for tumorigenesis [11]. Chemopreventive agents that alter carcinogen metabolism through phase I enzymes and/or increase conjugation and detoxification of activated metabolites through phase II enzymes decrease the chances of cancer initiation [12].

OXIDATIVE STRESS AND INFLAMMATION AS MOLECULAR MECHANISMS OF CANCER

Although the progress in anticancer therapies had significant development, cancer is still considered a global health burden. Current control strategies entail a change from chemotherapy to chemoprevention to prevent cancer progression by inducing carcinogen detoxification and or by causing the blockage, delay, or reversion of proliferation and the consequent transformation of damaged cells into malignant ones [3,4]. Recent studies have demonstrated that intracellular pathway components play a major role in the process of carcinogenesis, mainly when it refers to redox-sensitive transcription factors. These transcription factors control various genes that regulate cell proliferation and growth and protect the cells from oxidative insults. Mechanisms such as increased cellular detoxification and antioxidant activity, induction of carcinogen detoxification, suppression of proinflammatory signaling activated abnormally, reduction of proliferation by decreasing the expression of specific proteins, stimulation of apoptosis in malignant cells, and inhibition of neovascularization may work together to achieve chemoprevention [4].

The overproduction of reactive oxygen species (ROS) as byproducts of aerobic metabolism with an associated decrease in the intrinsic antioxidant capacity of cells creates an oxidative stress state, leading to carcinogenesis. External stimuli such as chemical carcinogens, ultraviolet radiation, and bacterial or viral infection increase ROS levels and can be harmful to human health [13]. The accumulation of ROS in vivo leads to chronic inflammation that plays a role in carcinogenesis development through diverse mechanisms, which include genomic DNA damage and modifications on intracellular signal transduction, causing abnormal cellular growth. Therefore, inflammation and oxidative stress have a role not only in cancer initiation but also in promoting cell proliferation of damaged cells, which produce a tumor microenvironment that induces pre-malignant cells' neoplastic transformation [13,14].

THE ROLE OF NUCLEAR FACTOR E2–RELATED FACTOR-2 IN MODULATING OXIDATIVE STRESS

Many reports have demonstrated that many factors contribute to cancer development, including chronic inflammation, ROS, and/or reactive nitrogen species produced by cells of the immune system as a response to oxidative and xenobiotic stress [15].

Naturally, our body presents cells that own a range of antioxidant and detoxifying enzymes. This is an intrinsic ability to fight against oxidative stress that leads to cellular damage. Enzymes including NAD(P)H: quinone oxidoreductase-1 (NQO1), superoxide dismutase (SOD), glutathione S-transferase (GST), glutathione peroxidase (GPx), heme oxygenase-1 (HO-1), glutamate-cysteine ligase (GCL), and uridine diphosphate glucuronosyltransferase (UGT) can eliminate ROS, protect cellular macromolecules from damage, and consequently protect from carcinogens metabolically activated [13]. The proximal promoter regions of these antioxidant genes present a consensus sequence called antioxidant response element (ARE) or electrophile response element (EpRE), which is known for being the target of nuclear factor E2–related factor-2 (Nrf2) [1]. Nrf2 has a key role in tumorigenesis and cancer progression by mediating various antioxidant genes under oxidative state [16,17].

Nrf2, which represents a crucial cellular defense against oxidative stress and electrophilic insults, stimulates the expression of antioxidant genes or phase-2 detoxifying genes. In the cytoplasm, Keap1 contains many cysteine residues that are sensors of redox modifications and can be modified by oxidation and covalent changes, diminishing the affinity of Nrf2 for Keap1. In normal physiological conditions, the transcription factor Nrf2, which belongs to the Cap-N-Collar (CNC) family, is located in the cytoplasm associated with Kelch-like ECH-associated protein 1 (Keap1), which causes enhanced proteasomal degradation of Nrf2 [5,6]. During oxidative stress, Nrf2 dissociates from Keap1 and translocates into the nucleus of the cell to combine with Maf protein and forms a heterodimer, which interacts with AREs, or EpREs located in the promoter/enhancer regions of genes that code to enzymes with antioxidant and detoxifying activities [1]. This process leads to the transcription of cytoprotective genes, including phase II metabolic enzymes, antioxidant enzymes, proteasome/molecular chaperones, anti-inflammatory factors, and phase III metabolic enzymes [18] (Figure 3.1). Many upstream kinases, including MAPKs, PKC, and PI3K, may also help in the Nrf2-Keap1 complex dissociation by promoting Nrf2 phosphorylation and facilitating the interface of this redox-sensitive transcription factor with CBP/p300 [1].

The regulation of the Keap1/Nrf2 signaling is of crucial importance to control the expression of detoxifying and antioxidant genes and the protection against carcinogenesis and xenobiotic toxicity [2]. Thus, researchers have been interested in Nrf2 activators, mainly phytochemical compounds, which have the ability to reduce cancer risk and could be used as antioxidants or chemopreventive agents [2].

Nrf2/ARE signaling activation has been shown to have chemopreventive cancer effects on normal cells under normal physiological conditions [19–21] through the control of redox homeostasis [22]. This control leads to genomic stability and cell survival, which is assisted by antioxidant defense enzymes and phase 2 and 3 detoxifying enzymes [19,23–26]. These proteins have the ability to reduce DNA damage by diminishing pro-carcinogens activation, inducing higher levels of detoxification of carcinogens, or simply by reducing the exposure of DNA to carcinogens. Hence, Nrf2/ARE pathway inactivation would lead to increased levels of oxidative stress through the generation of ROS, production of mutagenesis, beginning of carcinogenesis, and formation of tumors in non-malignant cells [27–29].

Many researchers have been investigating the potential of Nrf2/ARE pathway activation in cancer prevention [30]. It was reported that, among smokers, a reduced expression of the Nrf2 gene increases the risk of lung cancer [31]. In Nrf2-knockout animals, reduced

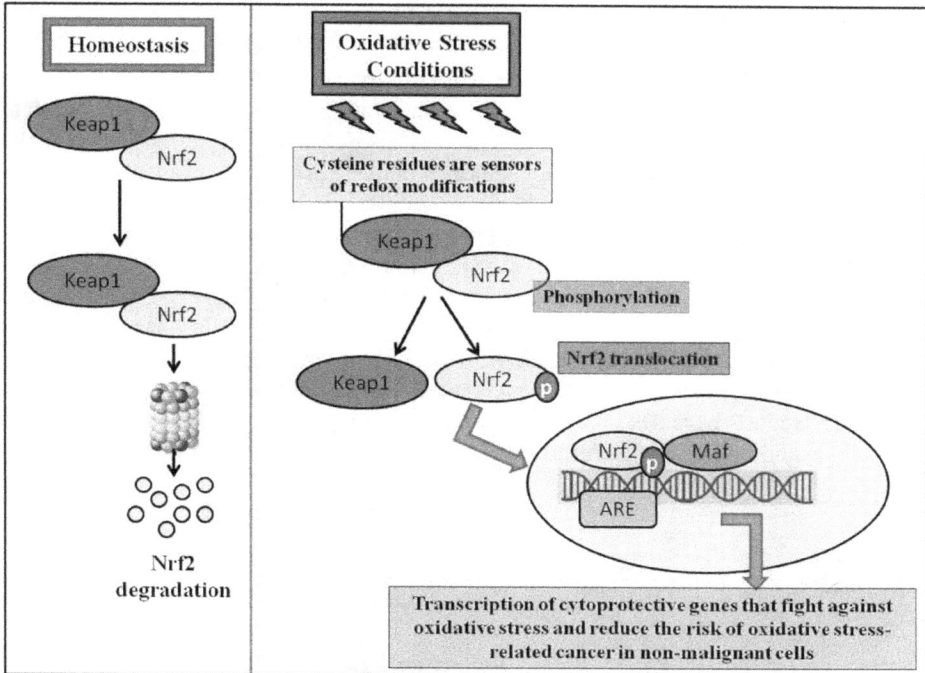

FIGURE 3.1 Nrf2 activation during oxidative stress. The figure shows the Nrf2/Keap1 complex during normal physiological conditions and the activation of Nrf2/ARE signaling in non-malignant cells during oxidative stress conditions.

levels of phase 2 enzymes, including HO-1 and Nrf2 proteins, lead to an increased susceptibility to skin tumorigenesis induced by 7,12-dimethylbenz(a)anthracene [32].

Nrf2 AS THE TARGET FOR CHEMOPREVENTIVE PHYTOCHEMICALS

A vast diversity of dietary phytochemicals are described as Nrf2 activators, exerting chemopreventive effects through the enhancement of cellular antioxidative or detoxification activity [1,13], and/or suppression of inflammation, tumor cell proliferation, and growth signaling mediated by NF-κB, AP-1, or CREB [13,33]. Some of them can induce Nrf2 activation and provide protection against DNA damage originating from oxidative stress and electrophilic carcinogens, thus causing inhibition of tumor initiation. Moreover, phytochemicals that function as negative regulators of signaling modulated by NF-κB, AP-1, CREB, or HIF-1a may prevent tumor promotion and progression [13]. The stimulation of detoxification enzyme expression that is controlled by Nrf2 helps to inactivate and eliminate metabolically activated carcinogenic species. Nrf2 regulates many antioxidant enzymes that help to combat oxidative DNA damage [13].

Several medicinal and dietary plants with antioxidant activities were described to modulate Nrf2/Keap1 signaling, potentiate cellular antioxidant capability, or facilitate the detoxification of carcinogens [34]. There is also a good correlation between the anti-inflammatory activity of some chemopreventive/cytoprotective agents and their capacity to stimulate the expression of antioxidant genes [5]. Nrf2 protects cells from oxidative stress and inflammatory insult [35–40], indicating possible crosstalk between NF-κB signaling and that modulated by Nrf2 action [1].

Polyphenols (Figure 3.2) are examples of compounds that have a great potential to activate Nrf2. They are found in many plants and are composed of the presence of more than one phenol unit per molecule with one or more hydroxyl groups [41]. They are generally combined with sugars and organic acids and classified into flavonoids and non-flavonoids. Reports have described polyphenols as having many pharmacological activities such as antioxidative and antiproliferative effects, induction of cell cycle arrest and

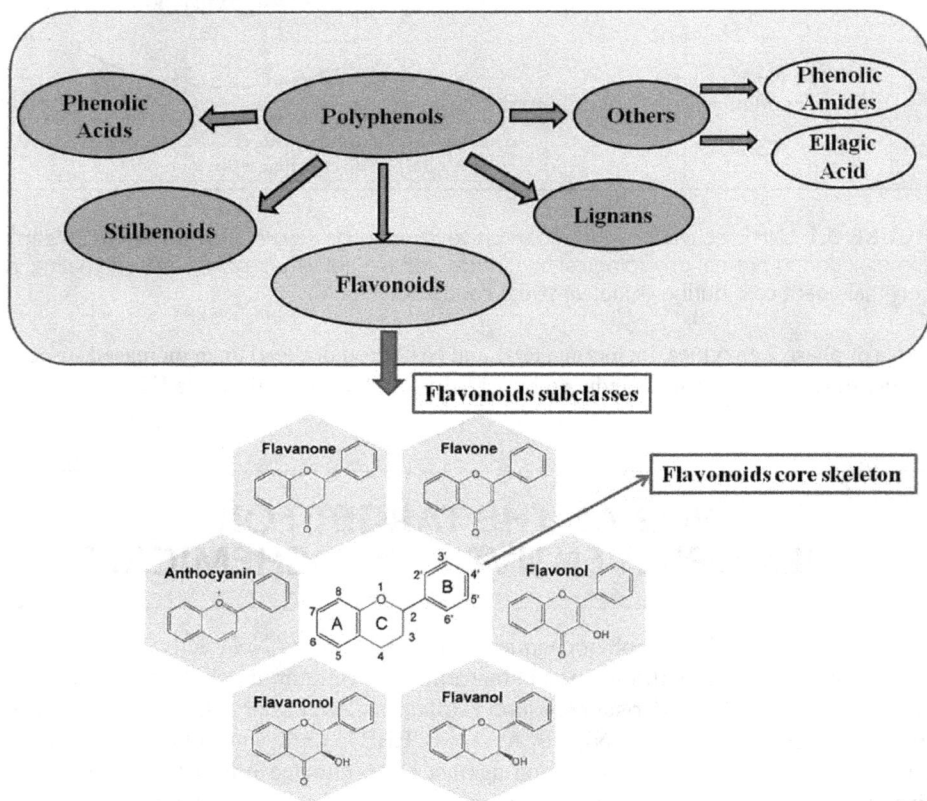

FIGURE 3.2 Polyphenol's classification. The figure shows polyphenol's classification and flavonoids core skeleton containing six subgroups, including flavanone, flavone, flavonol, flavanol, flavanonol, and anthocyanin.

apoptosis, cell differentiation, stimulation of detoxification enzymes, inhibitory effects over bioactivated enzymes, and others. All these together contribute to the chemopreventive activity of these naturally occurring compounds that can interfere with cancer initiation, promotion, and progression [42–44]. The majority of the polyphenols have antioxidant activity, activating nuclear factor-erythroid-2-related factor 2, which regulates the activities of antioxidant enzymes such as glutathione peroxidase (GPx), glutathione S-transferase, catalase, NAD(P)H:quinone oxidoreductase-1 (NQO1), and/or phase II enzymes effectively chelating redox-active metals able of catalyzing lipid peroxidation, which often contributes to their anticancer effects [45–47]. Some polyphenols have shown anticancer effects through mechanisms that change the profile of phase I and II drug-metabolizing enzymes, alter DNA repair rates, and scavenge reactive oxygen [44].

Among dietary phytochemicals that induce the activation of Nrf2/ARE signaling, flavonoids have gained a lot of attention. Flavonoids are a subgroup of polyphenols and present scavenging activity, preventing DNA damage and tumor induction [48,49]. They can regulate oxidative stress by mediating enzyme activity and signaling pathways associated with cancer progression [50,51]. In addition to this antioxidant activity, several phenolic compounds attenuate ROS production by inhibiting redox-sensitive transcription factors, including NF-κB and AP-1, which regulate the expression of the inflammatory enzyme cascade induced by ROS [52–54]. Several subclasses of flavonoids, such as flavones, flavonols, flavanones, flavanols, flavananols, isoflavones, anthocyanidins, and chalcones, induce nuclear translocation of Nrf2, which is required to proceed with ARE-driven gene transcription [55,56] (Figure 3.2).

POLYPHENOLS THAT INDUCE Nrf2 ACTIVATION

Many reports have described the ability of flavonoids in activating and inducing the nuclear translocation of Nrf2, with subsequent transcription of cytoprotective genes (Table 3.1).

RESVERATROL

Resveratrol is a flavonoid that belongs to the subclass of flavonols. It is found in many plants and fruits, including grapes, eucalyptus, spruce, blueberries, mulberries, and peanuts, and it is produced by the plant as a defense against diseases. Reports showed that resveratrol induced expression of GST, GPx, UGT-1A, NQO1, HO-1, and GCL [1,13]. It stimulated Nrf2-driven upregulation of GCL expression in human primary small airway epithelial cells and human alveolar epithelial cells, protecting these cells from oxidative damage [57]. Resveratrol also increased Nrf2 phosphorylation and subsequent translocation and stimulated the NQO1 protein and gene expression in human leukemia K562 cells [58].

TABLE 3.1   Effect of polyphenols over Nrf2 expression

PHYTOCHEMICALS	FLAVONOID SUBCLASS	EFFECTS OVER NRF2 EXPRESSION	EXPERIMENTAL MODELS
Resveratrol	Flavonol	Induced expression of cytoprotective enzymes. Increased Nrf2 phosphorylation.	Human primary small airway epithelial cells and human alveolar epithelial cells. Human leukemia K562 cells.
Curcumin	Flavonoid polyphenol	Increased protein expression, nuclear translocation, and DNA binding of Nrf2. Induced HO-1 expression.	Liver and lung of Swiss albino mice. Liver of mice.
Epigallocatechin gallate (EGCG)	Flavanols	Increased levels of cytoprotective enzymes and decreased lipid peroxidation. Increased Nrf2 translocation and binding to ARE site.	Mouse liver, and mouse skin carcinogenesis. Human mammary epithelial cells.
Quercetin	Flavonols	Induced expression of Nrf2 protein.	Human skin keratinocytes HaCaT, BJ foreskin fibroblast, and human umbilical vein endothelial cells. Intestinal oxidative stress in broiler chicken induced by lipopolysaccharide.
Hesperidin	Flavanones	Showed scavenging properties.	Male Sprague-Dawley rats.
Luteolin	Flavones	Upregulated Nrf2 protein expression in vitro and in pre-clinical investigations.	Rat myoblast H9C2 cells.
Baicalin	Flavones	Upregulated Nrf2 protein expression in vitro and in pre-clinical investigations.	Rat myoblast H9C2 cells and male Sprague-Dawley rats.
Apigenin	Flavones	Upregulated Nrf2 protein expression in vitro and pre-clinical investigations.	Human retinal pigment epithelial ARPE-19 cells and human renal tubular epithelial HK-2 cells.
Naringenin	Flavanones	Upregulated Nrf2 protein expression in vitro and in pre-clinical investigations.	Neuron cells derived from neonatal Sprague-Dawley rats.

Note: The table shows flavonoids and their effects on Nrf2 expression.

CURCUMIN

Curcumin is a flavonoid polyphenol that has been demonstrated to target multiple signaling molecules and has activity at the cellular level, helping to support its multiple health benefits [59]. The antioxidant effect of curcumin is also through the Nrf2-ARE signaling. Reports show that curcumin added to the diet of Swiss albino mice caused an increase in protein expression, nuclear translocation, and DNA binding of Nrf2 in the liver and lung, compared with controls [60]. When administered orally, curcumin also induced Nrf2 nuclear translocation and binding to ARE, inducing HO-1 expression in the liver of mice, leading to effective protection against dimethyl nitrosamine-induced hepatotoxicity [61].

EPIGALLOCATECHIN GALLATE

The catechin epigallocatechin gallate (EGCG) is the main flavonoid compound of green tea and has great pharmacological importance due to its recognized beneficial health effects [62]. EGCG was reported to increase GST, GPx, SOD, and catalase levels in mouse liver and decreased lipid peroxidation and cell proliferation during mouse skin carcinogenesis induced by lipid peroxidation and cell proliferation 12-O-tetradecanoylphorbol13-acetate (TPA) [63]. When given through gavage, EGCG reduced atypical hyperplasia, aberrant crypt foci number, and formation of adenocarcinoma through Nrf2 activation in mouse colon [64]. EGCG also increased GCL and GSTp mRNA expression and Nrf2 nuclear translocation and binding to ARE site in human mammary epithelial cells [65].

QUERCETIN

The flavonol quercetin increased the expression of Nrf2 protein in a range of human cell lines, including human skin keratinocytes HaCaT, BJ foreskin fibroblast, and human umbilical vein endothelial cells [66–69]. Its oral administration upregulated Nrf2 protein levels against intestinal oxidative stress in broiler chicken induced by lipopolysaccharide [70].

HESPERIDIN

Hesperidin, an active bioflavonoid compound, is found in citrus fruits and was described to have a free radical scavenging property and anti-lipid peroxidation effects in biological membranes [71]. Oral administration of hesperidin and intraperitoneal injection of

EGCG demonstrated that comparable upregulations could be obtained at concentrations that are not toxic to male Sprague-Dawley rats with methotrexate (MTX)-induced hepatotoxicity and testicular ischemia-induced oxidative stress, respectively [72–75].

LUTEOLIN, BAICALIN, APIGENIN, AND NARINGENIN

Luteolin, baicalin, and apigenin (subclass flavones) are known to upregulate Nrf2 protein expression in vitro and in pre-clinical investigations [74,76,77]. Luteolin upregulates Nrf2 protein expression in alleviating cell injury in rat myoblast H9C2 cells at rat-physiological concentrations induced by high glucose [74,76–78]. Baicalin increased Nrf2 protein expression against apoptosis induced by hypoxia in rat myoblast H9C2 cells [79,80]. Its intraperitoneal administration showed a similar effect in Sprague-Dawley rats' subsequent induction of subarachnoid hemorrhage through endovascular perforation [76]. Moreover, apigenin upregulated Nrf2 protein level in response to oxidative cell injury in human retinal pigment epithelial ARPE-19 cells in higher concentration than other flavones [77] and upregulated Nrf2 expression at protein and gene levels, against oxidative stress and cell injury induced by hydrogen peroxide in human renal tubular epithelial HK-2 cells [81]. Besides, naringenin, a flavanone found in citrus fruits, increased levels of Nrf2 protein in neuron cells derived from neonatal Sprague-Dawley rats induced by hypoxia [82].

The flavonoids baicalin and baicalein compete with the Nrf2 binding site (Shi et al. [84]). Because of their hydroxyl groups at C5 and C6 of the A-ring, these compounds may be helpful to bind them to the Nrf2 binding site in the Keap1-kelch domain by forming a hydrogen bond [83]. Baicalin and baicalein phosphorylate Nrf2 by phosphorylating ERK1/2 and protein kinase C (PKC) and promote Nrf2 stabilization through the prevention of Nrf2 ubiquitination [84].

Luteolin upregulates Nrf2 nuclear translocation in male Sprague-Dawley rats with intracerebral hemorrhage-induced secondary brain damage (intraperitoneal administration) and male ICR mice (oral administration) in non-toxic concentrations [85–88]. Likewise, baicalein (oral administration) assists Nrf2 nuclear translocation in male type 2 diabetes mellitus Kunming mice with high glucose-induced oxidative stress, in concentrations much lower than tolerable levels for mice [89,90]. Moreover, luteolin, baicalein, myricetin, quercetin, and genistein have been described to possess the ability to upregulate nuclear translocation of Nrf2 [70,85,86,89,91].

The effect of flavonoids was also observed to induce downstream activation of the Nrf2/ARE signaling after Nrf2 nuclear translocation [92]. Flavones such as luteolin, apigenin, baicalin, baicalein, chrysin, flavanones such as naringenin and hesperidin, flavonols such as quercetin, rutin, anthocyanins (C3G), and isoflavones such as genistein promoted the overexpression of antioxidant defense genes (GSH, SOD, GPx, and CAT) and phase 2 detoxifying genes (HO-1 and NQO-1) [92].

CONCLUSION

Carcinogenesis associated with excessive oxidative stress conditions in normal cells leads to the formation of non-malignant cells and induction of cancer progression. Activation of Nrf2/ARE signaling in normal cells has been described as a possible way to prevent oncogenesis; hence, the use of flavonoids to activate Nrf2 signaling may be a potential approach for cancer prevention. In this regard, the crucial role of flavonoids in mediating Nrf2 upregulation in the transcriptional and translational levels has been widely reported. Although it is known that Nrf2 activation is necessary for the progression of the signaling pathway, the molecular mechanism is still unclear. Therefore, more investigations are required to discover novel flavonoids that may activate Nrf2, and more clinical studies are necessary to confirm their beneficial therapeutic effects against oxidative stress–related carcinogenesis (Figure 3.3).

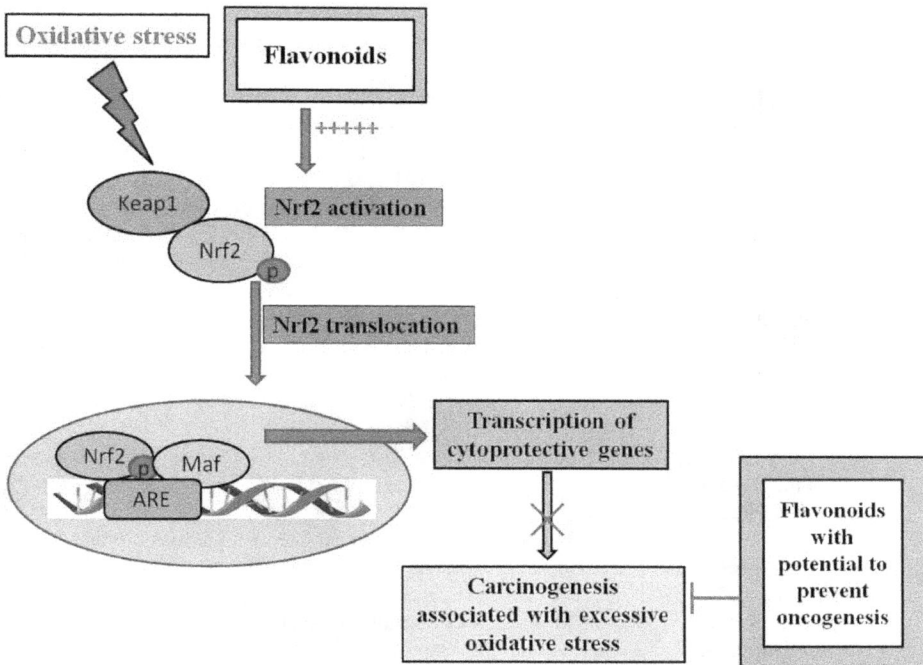

FIGURE 3.3 The role of flavonoids in Nrf2 activation. The diagram shows the effect of flavonoids in Nrf2 activation and consequent transcription of cytoprotective genes and their potential to prevent carcinogenesis associated with excessive oxidative stress.

REFERENCES

1. Surh YJ, Na HK. NF-kappaB and Nrf2 as prime molecular targets for chemoprevention and cytoprotection with anti-inflammatory and antioxidant phytochemicals. *Genes Nutr.* 2008 Feb;2(4):313–17. doi: 10.1007/s12263-007-0063-0. PMID: 18850223; PMCID: PMC2478481.

2. Zhu Y, Yang Q, Liu H, Song Z, Chen W. Phytochemical compounds targeting on Nrf2 for chemoprevention in colorectal cancer. *Eur J Pharmacol.* 2020 Nov 15;887:173588. doi: 10.1016/j.ejphar.2020.173588. Epub 2020 Sep 19. PMID: 32961170.

3. Surh YJ. Cancer chemoprevention with dietary phytochemicals. *Nat Rev Cancer.* 2003;(10):768–80.

4. Kundu JK, Na H-K, Surh Y-J. Intracellular signaling molecules as targets of selected dietary chemopreventive agents. In: Surh Y-J, Packer L, Cadenas E, Dong Z, editors. *Dietary Modulation of Cell Signaling Pathways.* New York: CRC Press, Taylor & Francis Group, 2008: pp. 1–44.

5. Dinkova-Kostova AT, Holtzclaw WD, Wakabayashi N. Keap1, the sensor for electrophiles and oxidants that regulates the phase 2 response, is a zinc metalloprotein. *Biochemistry.* 2005;44:6889–99.

6. Furukawa M, Xiong Y. BTB protein Keap1 targets antioxidant transcription factor Nrf2 for ubiquitination by the Cullin 3-Roc1 ligase. *Mol Cell Biol.* 2005;25:162–71.

7. Kenny PA, Lee GY, Bissell MJ. Targeting the tumor microenvironment. *Front Biosci.* 2007;12:3468–74.

8. Casey SC, Li Y, Fan AC, Felsher DW. Oncogene withdrawal engages the immune system to induce sustained cancer regression. *J Immunother Cancer.* 2014;2:24.

9. Shiao SL, Ganesan AP, Rugo HS, Coussens LM. Immune microenvironments in solid tumors: New targets for therapy. *Genes Dev.* 2011;25:2559–72.

10. Hanahan D, Weinberg RA. Hallmarks of cancer: The next generation. *Cell.* 2011;144:646–74.

11. Casey SC, Amedei A, Aquilano K, et al. Cancer prevention and therapy through the modulation of the tumor microenvironment. *Semin Cancer Biol.* 2015 Dec;35 (Suppl.): S199–S223. doi: 10.1016/j.semcancer.2015.02.007. Epub 2015 Apr 10. PMID: 25865775; PMCID: PMC4930000.

12. Morley N, Clifford T, Salter L, Campbell S, Gould D, Curnow A. The green tea polyphenol (–)-epigallocatechin gallate and green tea can protect human cellular DNA from ultraviolet and visible radiation-induced damage. *Photodermatol Photoimmunol Photomed.* 2005;21:15–22.

13. Surh YJ, Kundu JK, Na HK, Lee JS. Redox-sensitive transcription factors as prime targets for chemoprevention with anti-inflammatory and antioxidative phytochemicals. *J Nutr.* 2005;135:2993S–3001S.

14. Kundu JK, Surh YJ. Molecular basis of chemoprevention with dietary phytochemicals: Redox-regulated transcription factors as relevant targets. *Phytochem Rev.* 2009 Jun;8(2):333–47.

15. Shibata T, Kokubu A, Gotoh M, et al. Genetic alteration of Keap1 confers constitutive Nrf2 activation and resistance to chemotherapy in gallbladder cancer. *Gastroenterology.* 2008:135:1358–68, e1351–1354.

16. Bockmann S, Hinz B. Cannabidiol promotes endothelial cell survival by heme oxygenase-1-mediated autophagy. *Cell.* 2020;9:1703.

17. Mai HN, Pham DT, Chung YH, et al. Glutathione peroxidase-1 knockout potentiates behavioral sensitization induced by cocaine in mice via σ-1 receptor-mediated ERK signaling: A comparison with the case of glutathione peroxidase-1 overexpressing transgenic mice. *Brain Research Bulletin.* 2020;164:107–20.

18. Kobayashi M, Yamamoto M. Molecular mechanisms activating the Nrf2-Keap1 pathway of antioxidant gene regulation. *Antioxid Redox Signal.* 2005;7:385–94.
19. Wu S, Lu H, Bai Y. Nrf2 in cancers: A double-edged sword. *Cancer Med.* 2019:8:2252–67.
20. Fernando W, Rupasinghe HPV, Hoskin DW. Dietary phytochemicals with antioxidant and prooxidant activities: A double-edged sword in relation to adjuvant chemotherapy and radiotherapy? *Cancer Lett.* 2019:452:168–77.
21. Kwak M-K, Kensler TW. Targeting NRF2 signaling for cancer chemoprevention. *Toxicol Appl Pharmacol.* 2010:244:66–76.
22. Basak P, Sadhukhan P, Sarkar P, Sil PC. Perspectives of the Nrf-2 signaling pathway in cancer progression and therapy. *Toxicol Rep.* 2017;4:306–18 doi: 10.1016/j.toxrep.2017.06.002.
23. George VC, Dellaire G, Rupasinghe HPV. Plant flavonoids in cancer chemoprevention: Role in genome stability. *J Nutr Biochem.* 2017;45:1–14.
24. Furfaro AL, Traverso N, Domenicotti C, et al. The Nrf2/HO-1 axis in cancer cell growth and chemoresistance. *Oxid Med Cell Longev.* 2016:2016:1958174.
25. Abed DA, Goldstein M, Albanyan H, Jin H, Hu L. Discovery of direct inhibitors of Keap1–Nrf2 protein–protein interaction as potential therapeutic and preventive agents. *Acta Pharm Sin B.* 2015:5:285–99.
26. Jung K-A, Kwak M-K. The Nrf2 system as a potential target for the development of indirect antioxidants. *Molecules.* 2010:15:7266–91.
27. Jeeva JS, Sunitha J, Ananthalakshmi R, Rajkumari S, Ramesh M, Krishnan R. Enzymatic antioxidants, and its role in oral diseases. *J Pharm Bioallied Sci.* 2015:7:S331–S333.
28. Vogelstein B, Kinzler KW. Cancer genes and the pathways they control. *Nat Med.* 2004:10:789–99.
29. Kensler TW, Wakabayashi N, Biswal S. Cell survival responses to environmental stresses via the Keap1-Nrf2-ARE pathway. *Annu Rev Pharmacol Toxicol.* 2007:47:89–116.
30. Krajka-Ku ´zniak V, Paluszczak J, Baer-Dubowska W. The Nrf2-ARE signaling pathway: An update on its regulation and possible role in cancer prevention and treatment. *Pharmacol Rep.* 2017:69:393–402.
31. Suzuki T, Shibata T, Takaya K, et al. Regulatory nexus of synthesis and degradation deciphers cellular Nrf2 expression levels. *Mol Cell Biol.* 2013:33:2402–12.
32. Xu C, Huang M-T, Shen G, et al. Inhibition of 7,12-dimethylbenz(a)anthracene-induced skin tumorigenesis in C57BL/6 mice by sulforaphane is mediated by nuclear factor E2–related factor 2. *Cancer Res.* 2006:66:8293–96.
33. Kundu JK, Surh YJ. Epigallocatechin gallate inhibits phorbol ester-induced activation of NF-κB and CREB in mouse skin: Role of p38 MAPK. *Ann New York Acad Sci.* 2007 Jan;1095(1):504–12.
34. Lee JS, Surh YJ. Nrf2 as a novel molecular target for chemoprevention. *Cancer Lett* 2005;224:171–84.
35. Chen XL, Dodd G, Thomas S, et al. Activation of Nrf2/ARE pathway protects endothelial cells from oxidant injury and inhibits inflammatory gene expression. *Am J Physiol Heart Circ Physiol.* 2006;290:H1862–H1870.
36. Chen XL, Kunsch C. Induction of cytoprotective genes through Nrf2/antioxidant response element pathway: A new therapeutic approach for the treatment of inflammatory diseases. *Curr Pharm Des.* 2004;10:879–91.
37. Khor TO, Huang MT, Kwon KH, Chan JY, Reddy BS, Kong AN. Nrf2-deficient mice have an increased susceptibility to dextran sulfate sodium-induced colitis. *Cancer Res.* 2006;66:11580–584.
38. Li N, Nel AE. Role of the Nrf2-mediated signaling pathway as a negative regulator of inflammation: Implications for the impact of particulate pollutants on asthma. *Antioxid Redox Signal.* 2006;8:88–98.
39. Rahman I, Biswas SK, Kirkham PA. Regulation of inflammation and redox signaling by dietary polyphenols. *Biochem Pharmacol.* 2006;72:1439–52.

40. Yates MS, Kensler TW. Chemopreventive promise of targeting the Nrf2 pathway. *Drug News Perspect.* 2007;20:109–17.
41. Stevenson DE, Hurst RD. Polyphenolic phytochemicals—Just antioxidants or much more? *Cell Mol Life Sci.* 2007;64:2900–16.
42. Di Domenico F, Foppoli C, Coccia R, Perluigi M. Antioxidants in cervical cancer: Chemopreventive and chemotherapeutic effects of polyphenols. *Biochim Biophys Acta.* 2011. doi: 10.1016/j.bbadis.2011.10.005.
43. Shukla S, Gupta S. Apigenin and cancer chemoprevention. In Watson RR, Pree VR, editors, *Bioactive Foods in Promoting Health: Fruit and Vegetables.* Netherlands: Elsevier, 2010: pp. 663–89.
44. Khan N, Mukhtar H. Cancer chemoprevention. *Comprehensive Toxicol.* 2010;14:417–31.
45. Tyagi S, Singh G, Sharma A, Aggarwal G. Phytochemicals as candidate therapeutics: An overview. *Int J Pharmac Sci Rev Res.* 2010;3(1):53–5.
46. Perron NR, Brumaghim JL. A review of the antioxidant mechanisms of polyphenol compounds related to iron binding. *Cell Biochem Biophys.* 2009;53:75–100.
47. Hu M-L. Dietary polyphenols as antioxidants and anticancer agents: More questions than answers. *Chang Gung Med J.* 2011;34:449–60.
48. Johnson MK, Loo G. Effects of epigallocatechin gallate and quercetin on oxidative damage to cellular DNA. *Mutat Res.* 2000;459:211–18.
49. Heijnen CG, Haenen GR, van Acker FA, van der Vijgh WJ, Bast A. Flavonoids as peroxynitrite scavengers: The role of the hydroxyl groups. *Toxicol In Vitro.* 2001;15:3–6.
50. Rajendran P, Ekambaram G, Sakthisekaran D. Cytoprotective effect of mangiferin on benzo(a)pyrene-induced lung carcinogenesis in Swiss albino mice. *Basic Clin Pharmacol Toxicol.* 2008;103:137–42.
51. Lee DE, Shin BJ, Hur HJ, et al. Quercetin, the active phenolic component in kiwifruit, prevents hydrogen peroxide-induced inhibition of gapjunction intercellular communication. *Br J Nutr.* 2010;104:164–70.
52. Aggarwal BB, Shishodia S. Molecular targets of dietary agents for prevention and therapy of cancer. *Biochem Pharmacol.* 2006;71:1397–1421.
53. Fresco P, Borges F, Diniz C, Marques MP. New insights into the anticancer properties of polyphenols. *Med Res Rev.* 2006;26:747–66.
54. Le Corre L, Chalabi N, Delort L, Bignon Y-J, Bernard-Gallon DJ. Resveratrol and breast cancer chemoprevention: Molecular mechanisms. *Mol Nutr Food Res.* 2005;49:462–71.
55. Joo MS, Kim WD, Lee KY, Kim JH, Koo JH, Kim SG. AMPK facilitates nuclear accumulation of Nrf2 by phosphorylating at Serine 550. *Mol Cell Biol.* 2016:36:1931–42.
56. Zimmermann K, Baldinger J, Mayerhofer B, Atanasov AG, Dirsch VM, Heiss EH. Activated AMPK boosts the Nrf2/HO-1 signaling axis–A role for the unfolded protein response. *Free Rad Biol Med.* 2015:88:417–26.
57. Kode A, Rajendrasozhan S, Caito S, Yang SR, Megson IL, Rahman I. Resveratrol induces glutathione synthesis by activation of Nrf2 and protects against cigarette smoke-mediated oxidative stress in human lung epithelial cells. *Am J Physiol Lung Cell Mol Physiol.* 2008 Mar;294(3): L478–88. doi: 10.1152/ajplung.00361.2007. Epub 2007 Dec 27. PMID: 18162601.
58. Hsieh TC, Lu X, Wang Z, Wu JM. Induction of quinone reductase NQO1 by resveratrol in human K562 cells involves the antioxidant response element ARE and is accompanied by nuclear translocation of transcription factor Nrf2. *Med Chem.* 2006 May;2(3):275–85. doi: 10.2174/157340606776930709. PMID: 16948474.
59. Gupta SC, Patchva S, Aggarwal BB. Therapeutic roles of curcumin: Lessons learned from clinical trials. *AAPS J.* 2013 Jan;15(1):195–218. doi: 10.1208/s12248-012-9432-8. Epub 2012 Nov 10. PMID: 23143785; PMCID: PMC3535097.

60. Garg R, Ramchandani AG, Maru GB. Curcumin decreases 12-O-tetradecanoylphorbol-13-acetate-induced protein kinase C translocation to modulate downstream targets in mouse skin. *Carcinogenesis.* 2008 Jun;29(6):1249–57. doi: 10.1093/carcin/bgn114. Epub 2008 May 13. PMID: 18477648.

61. Farombi EO, Shrotriya S, Na HK, Kim SH, Surh YJ. Curcumin attenuates dimethylnitrosamine-induced liver injury in rats through Nrf2-mediated induction of heme oxygenase-1. *Food Chem Toxicol.* 2008 Apr;46(4):1279–87. doi: 10.1016/j.fct.2007.09.095. Epub 2007 Sep 26. PMID: 18006204.

62. Kelemen K, Kiesecker C, Zitron E, et al. Green tea flavonoid epigallocatechin-3-gallate (EGCG) inhibits cardiac hERG potassium channels. *Biochem Biophys Res Commun.* 2007 Dec 21;364(3):429–35. doi: 10.1016/j.bbrc.2007.10.001. Epub 2007 Oct 9. PMID: 17961513.

63. Saha P, Das S. Elimination of deleterious effects of free radicals in murine skin carcinogenesis by black tea infusion theaflavins epigallocatechin gallate. *Asian Pac J Cancer Prev.* 2002;3:225–30.

64. Yuan JH, Li YQ, Yang XY. Protective effects of epigallocatechin gallate on colon preneoplastic lesions induced by 2-amino-3-methylimidazo [4,5-f] quinoline in mice. *Mol Med.* 2008 Sep–Oct;14(9–10):590–98. doi: 10.2119/2007-00050. PMID: 18596869; PMCID: PMC2442020.

65. Na HK, Kim EH, Jung JH, Lee HH, Hyun JW, Surh YJ. (–)-Epigallocatechin gallate induces Nrf2-mediated antioxidant enzyme expression via activation of PI3K and ERK in human mammary epithelial cells. *Arch Biochem Biophys.* 2008 Aug 15:476(2):171–77.

66. Schadich E, Hlaváč J, Volná T, Varanasi L, Hajdúch M, Džubák P. Effects of ginger phenylpropanoids and quercetin on Nrf2-ARE pathway in human BJ fibroblasts and HaCaT keratinocytes. *BioMed Res Int.* 2016:2016:2173275.

67. Tian R, Yang Z, Lu N, Peng Y-Y. Quercetin, but not rutin, attenuated hydrogen peroxide-induced cell damage via heme oxygenase-1 induction in endothelial cells. *Arch Biochem Biophys.* 2019:676:108157.

68. Egert S. Wolffram S. Bosy-Westphal A. Daily quercetin supplementation dose-dependently increases plasma quercetin concentrations in healthy humans. *J Nutr.* 2008:138:1615–21.

69. Erlund I, Kosonen T, Alfthan G. Pharmacokinetics of quercetin from quercetin aglycone and rutin in healthy volunteers. *Eur J Clin Pharmacol.* 2000:56:545–53.

70. Sun L, Xu G, Dong Y, Li M, Yang L, Lu W. Quercetin protects against lipopolysaccharide-induced intestinal oxidative stress in broiler chickens through activation of Nrf2 pathway. *Molecules.* 2020:25:1053.

71. Hussein M, Othman S. Structure-activity relationship of antioxidative property of hesperidin. *Int J Pharmac Res Devel* 2011;3(8):19–29.

72. Abdelaziz RM, Abdelazem AZ, Hashem KS, Attia YA. Protective effects of hesperidin against MTX-induced hepatotoxicity in male albino rats. *Naunyn Schmiedeberg's Arch Pharmacol.* 2020:393:1405–17.

73. Al-Maghrebi M, Alnajem AS, Esmaeil A. Epigallocatechin-3-gallate modulates germ cell apoptosis through the SAFE/Nrf2 signaling pathway. *Naunyn-Schmiedeberg's Arch Pharmacol.* 2020:393:663–71.

74. Li L, Luo W, Qian Y, et al. Luteolin protects against diabetic cardiomyopathy by inhibiting NF-κB-mediated inflammation and activating the Nrf2-mediated antioxidant responses. *Phytomedicine.* 2019:59:152774.

75. Chen J-H, Tipoe GL, Liong EC, et al. Green tea polyphenols prevent toxin-induced hepatotoxicity in mice by down-regulating inducible nitric oxide-derived prooxidants. *Am J Clin Nutr.* 2004:80:742–51.

76. Zhang H, Tu X, Song S, Liang R, Shi S. Baicalin reduces early brain injury after subarachnoid hemorrhage in rats. *Chin J Integr Med.* 2020:26:510–18.

77. Xu X, Li M, Chen W, Yu H, Yang Y, Hang L. Apigenin attenuates oxidative injury in ARPE-19 cells thorough activation of Nrf2 pathway. *Oxid Med Cell Longev* 2016:2016:4378461.

78. Sarawek S, Derendorf H, Butterweck V. Pharmacokinetics of luteolin and metabolites in rats. *Nat Prod Commun.* 2008:3:2029–36.
79. Yu H, Chen B, Ren Q. Baicalin relieves hypoxia-aroused H9c2 cell apoptosis by activating Nrf2/HO-1-mediated HIF1α/BNIP3 pathway. *Artif Cells Nanomed Biotechnol.* 2019:47:3657–63.
80. Zhao L, Wei Y, Huang Y, He B, Zhou Y, Fu J. Nanoemulsion improves the oral bioavailability of baicalin in rats: In vitro and in vivo evaluation. *Int J Nanomed.* 2013:8:3769–79.
81. Zhang J, Zhao X, Zhu H, Wang J, Ma J, Gu M. Apigenin protects against renal tubular epithelial cell injury and oxidative stress by high glucose via regulation of NF-E2-related factor 2 (Nrf2) pathway. *Med Sci Monit.* 2019:25:5280–88.
82. Wang K, Chen Z, Huang L, et al. Naringenin reduces oxidative stress and improves mitochondrial dysfunction via activation of the Nrf2/ARE signaling pathway in neurons. *Int J Mol Med.* 2017:40:1582–90.
83. Pang C, Zheng Z, Shi L, et al. Caffeic acid prevents acetaminophen-induced liver injury by activating the Keap1-Nrf2 antioxidative defense system. *Free Rad Biol Med.* 2016:91:236–46.
84. Shi L, Hao Z, Zhang S, et al. Baicalein and baicalin alleviate acetaminophen-induced liver injury by activating Nrf2 antioxidant pathway: The involvement of ERK1/2 and PKC. *Biochem Pharmacol.* 2018:150:9–23.
85. Kitakaze T, Makiyama A, Yamashita Y, Ashida H. Low dose of luteolin activates Nrf2 in the liver of mice at start of the active phase but not that of the inactive phase. *PLoS One.* 2020:15:e0231403.
86. Tan X, Yang Y, Xu J, et al. Luteolin exerts neuroprotection via modulation of the p62/Keap1/Nrf2 pathway in intracerebral hemorrhage. *Front Pharmacol.* 2020:10:1551.
87. Yang D, Tan X, Lv Z, et al. Regulation of Sirt1/Nrf2/TNF-α signaling pathway by luteolin is critical to attenuate acute mercuric chloride exposure induced hepatotoxicity. *Sci Rep.* 2016:6:37157.
88. Zhang H, Tan X, Yang D, et al. Dietary luteolin attenuates chronic liver injury induced by mercuric chloride via the Nrf2/NF-κB/P53 signaling pathway in rats. *Oncotarget.* 2017:8:40982–993.
89. Dong Y, Xing Y, Sun J, Sun W, Xu Y, Quan C. Baicalein alleviates liver oxidative stress and apoptosis induced by high-level glucose through the activation of the PERK/Nrf2 signaling pathway. *Molecules.* 2020:25:599.
90. Chen L, Dou J, Su Z, et al. Synergistic activity of baicalein with ribavirin against influenza A (H1N1) virus infections in cell culture and in mice. *Antivir Res.* 2011:91:314–20.
91. Zhang Q, Li Z, Wu S, et al. Myricetin alleviates cuprizone-induced behavioral dysfunction and demyelination in mice by Nrf2 pathway. *Food Funct.* 2016:7:4332–42.
92. Huang C-S, Lii C-K, Lin A-H, et al. Protection by chrysin, apigenin, and luteolin against oxidative stress is mediated by the Nrf2-dependent up-regulation of heme oxygenase 1 and glutamate-cysteine ligase in rat primary hepatocytes. *Arch Toxicol.* 2013;87:167–78.

Role of Flavonoid Activation of Nrf2 in Neurodegenerative Disease and Brain Aging

4

Equar Taka, Getinet M. Adinew, and Karam F.A. Soliman

Florida A&M University

Contents

DOI: 10.1201/9781003225225-4

61

INTRODUCTION

The term "neurodegenerative disease" (ND) refers to a group of neurological conditions that primarily affect neurons in the central nervous system (CNS). These conditions are characterized by the progressive loss of neurons in the CNS, which causes deficits in a number of cognitive, motor, and memory functions [1]. The most common chronic NDs include Alzheimer's disease (AD), Parkinson's disease (PD), Huntington's disease (HD), and amyotrophic lateral sclerosis (ALS) [2]. In the United States, AD affects 5 million people, PD affects 1 million, ALS affects 30,000, and HD affects 30,000. Because NDs most commonly strike people in their middle to late years of life, their prevalence is expected to climb as the population ages. By 2030, one out of every five persons in the United States will be 65 or older, implying that NDs will impact more than 12 million Americans in the next 30 years if they are not addressed [3]. The goal of finding treatments and solutions for ND is becoming more urgent.

To develop therapeutics that can prevent or treat NDs, first, the changes in the aging brain that lead to the development of neurodegenerative disorders should be identified. Several biochemical pathways have been associated with neurodegeneration, including oxidative stress (OS), neuroinflammation, excitotoxicity, mitochondrial dysfunction, aberrant protein misfolding and aggregation, and apoptosis, all of which can lead to cell death [4]. However, age has been identified as the key risk factor for most neurodegenerative disorders, including AD, PD, HD, and frontotemporal lobar dementia; all these conditions are more prevalent in the elderly [5].

This suggests that since multiple changes are associated with the aging brain, it is unlikely that developing drugs that can target a single change will be an effective therapeutic treatment. Therefore, there is a need to develop drugs with multiple biological activities that can affect the various age-related changes in the brain that can contribute to NDs' progression and development. Despite advances in the medical and pharmaceutical fields currently, no ND is curable, and the treatments available only manage the symptoms or halt the progression of the disease. Therefore, a new treatment for this disease is urgently needed [6].

Natural products produced from plants and their bioactive components have been investigated intensively in recent years for their therapeutic potential in various NDs, including AD, HD, and PD [7]. Plant-derived flavonoids are the most widely studied natural products for preventing and treating neurodegenerative disorders. The neuroprotective mechanism of flavonoid action is via suppression of lipid peroxidation, inhibition of inflammatory mediators, modulation of gene expressions, and activation of antioxidant enzymes, making them ideal therapeutic representatives for treating neurodegenerative disorders [8]. However, flavonoids have limited accessibility to the brain; they exert protective effects by modulation of cell signaling pathways and activation of cellular antioxidant defense mechanisms, such as Nrf2 [9].

By stimulating several cytoprotective genes, Nrf2 has emerged as a crucial regulator of flavonoid-mediated protection [10]. Nrf2 is widely expressed in the CNS and is regulated in response to acute cerebral insults and ND. In addition to its crucial regulatory role in the endogenous defense to various cellular stresses, Nrf2 is a well-known regulator of inflammation in the brain [11]. Furthermore, Nrf2 activation mitigates multiple pathogenic processes involved in these neurodegenerative disorders through upregulation of antioxidant defenses, inhibition of inflammation, improvement of mitochondrial function, and maintenance of protein homeostasis [12]. On the other hand, insufficient Nrf2 activation in humans has been linked to chronic diseases such as PD, AD, and ALS [11]. Therefore, targeting Nrf2 signaling could be a promising therapeutic strategy for delaying the development, slowing the progression, and alleviating the symptoms of NDs. Here, in this chapter, we will review the role of flavonoids targeted Nrf2 overexpression in the prevention or slowdown of the aging brain and NDs.

NEURODEGENERATIVE DISEASES AND BRAIN AGING

NDs are associated with several risk factors; however, aging is the primary risk factor for the development of most diseases. Aging is associated with physical deterioration, leading to an increased risk of disease and death [13]. Among the pathophysiological changes in the aging brain that contribute to neurodegeneration include increases in OS, changes in energy metabolism, loss of neurotrophic support, changes in protein processing leading to protein aggregate accumulation, dysfunction of the neurovascular system, and immune system activation [14]. For this and more other reasons, the incidence of NDs is expected to increase as the population ages.

The US population aged greater than 65 is estimated to increase from 53 million in 2018 to 88 million in 2050 [13]. As the elderly population increases, the financial burden of age-related NDs will also increase, devastatingly impacting individuals, families, and society unless effective preventive or therapeutic approaches are introduced to reduce the incidence and progression of these diseases.

BIOLOGICAL PROCESS IMPLICATED IN THE PROGRESSION AND PATHOGENESIS OF NEURODEGENERATIVE DISEASES

OS, neuroinflammation, mitochondrial dysfunction, intracellular calcium excess, protein aggregation, and neuronal degeneration in particular brain regions have been associated to the development and pathophysiology of NDs [4]. Below will be discussed how these biological processes are involved in the pathogenesis of neurodegenerative.

Oxidative Stress

OS plays a role as a regulatory element in aging and various neurological disorders. OS is a condition of imbalance between reactive oxygen species (ROS) formation and cellular antioxidant capacity due to an increase in production of ROS or dysfunction of the antioxidant system [15]. Excess cellular levels of ROS cause damage to proteins, nucleic acids, lipids, membranes, and organelles, which can lead to the activation of cell death processes such as apoptosis [16]. Various NDs, including PD, AD, HD, and ALS, can be caused by biochemical changes in bimolecular components or OS [17].

Neuroinflammation

Neuroinflammation has been linked to several diseases, including PD, ALS, and AD [18]. Inflammation usually results in infection protection, followed by resolution—returning damaged tissues to their normal structural and functional state [19]. In other words, neuroinflammation is a protective system for the brain that removes or inhibits numerous infections [20]. Chronic neuroinflammation and microglia activation, on the other hand, play a key role in ND pathogenesis [21]. The inflammatory and neurotoxic mediators involved in NDs include interleukin-1beta (IL-1β), interleukin-6, IL-8, IL-33, tumor necrosis factor-alpha (TNF-α), chemokine (C-C motif) ligand 2 (CCL2), CCL5, matrix metalloproteinase, granulocyte-macrophage colony-stimulating factor (GM-CSF), glia maturation factor, substance P, ROS, reactive nitrogen species, mast cell–mediated histamine and proteases, protease-activated receptor-2 (PAR-2), CD40, CD40L, CD88, intracellular Ca+ elevation, and activation of mitogen-activated protein kinases (MAPKs) and nuclear factor kappa-B (NF-κB) [22]. These mediators affect neuronal survival and can cause neurodegeneration directly or indirectly via glial and inflammatory cells. As a result, neuroinflammation leads to neurodegeneration, which is exacerbated by neurodegenerative processes.

Mitochondrial Dysfunction

Mitochondrial dysfunction has been associated with many NDs' pathological processes and ethology [23]. Several mitochondrial abnormalities have been found in CNS disorders. Membrane leakage and electrolyte imbalances, activation of the pro-apoptotic pathway, and mycophagy have been linked to NDs such as AD, PD, HD, and ischemic stroke [24]. Mitochondria, a subcellular self-autonomous organelle, perform various activities, the most important of which are energy generation and adenosine triphosphate (ATP) synthesis. Aside from that, mitochondria are involved in amino acid and lipid metabolism and apoptosis regulation [25]. In addition, mitochondria play essential roles in controlling fundamental processes in neuroplasticity, including neural differentiation, neurite outgrowth, neurotransmitter release, and dendritic remodeling [26]. However, mitochondrial dysfunction results in depletion of ATP, halting the activities of enzymes of the electron transport chain, generation of ROS, reduction of mitochondrial DNA (mtDNA), and caspase 3 release [23]. Additionally, aging is the leading risk factor for the onset of NDs. A decline in mitochondrial function has been observed in several age-dependent neurodegenerative disorders and may be a major contributing factor in their progression [27]. In aged subjects, mitochondria are characterized by impaired functions such as lowered oxidative capacity, reduced oxidative phosphorylation, decreased ATP production, a significant increase in ROS generation, and diminished antioxidant [25]. All the factors are associated with the pathological process of many NDs.

Apoptosis

Apoptosis or program cell death (PCD) also plays a role in the pathological process of many NDs. Apoptosis is a type of cell death characterized by cytoplasmic shrinkage, nuclear condensation and fragmentation, and apoptotic bodies in many tissues under physiological or pathological conditions [28]. Apoptosis is essential in various processes, including normal cell turnover, immune system development and function, hormone-dependent atrophy, embryonic development, and chemical-induced cell death. However, either too little or too much apoptosis is a factor in various human diseases, including NDs, ischemia damage, autoimmune disorders, and cancer [29]. Apoptosis or PCD induces neuronal death by causing OS, disrupting calcium homeostasis, mitochondrial malfunction, and activating cysteine proteases known as caspases [30]. For example, aberrant activation of PCD pathways is a common feature in NDs, such as ALS, AD, PD, and HD, resulting in unwanted loss of neuronal cells and function. Conversely, the inactivation of PCDs may contribute to the development of brain cancers and impact their response to therapy [28]. Therefore, agents that may either inhibit or stimulate PCD may provide essential components of future treatment methods, with many disorders of the brain revealing abnormalities in PCD pathways.

Excitotoxicity

Excitotoxicity is a complicated process resulting in dendritic degradation and cell death when glutamate receptors are activated. Excessive glutamate receptor activation by excitatory amino acids has several negative consequences, including calcium buffering impairment, free radical production, stimulation of the mitochondrial permeability transition, and secondary excitotoxicity [31]. The mechanism of excitotoxins is by binding to glutamate receptors and causing a significant amount of Ca^{2+} to be released. Increases in cytoplasmic Ca^{2+} levels in response to glutamate receptor activation can cause Ca^{2+} uptake into mitochondria which, if excessive, can cause the generation of ROS and limit the production of ATP. Ca^{2+} is a critical mediator of excitotoxic cell death because it activates proteases and causes OS [32]. Furthermore, chronic excitotoxicity has been linked to various neuropathological diseases such as PD, HD, AD, and ALS [33]. Therefore, understanding the pathways involved in excitotoxicity is crucial for the future clinical treatment of numerous NDs. We highlight the possible causes of neurodegenerative disorders and brain aging in Figure 4.1.

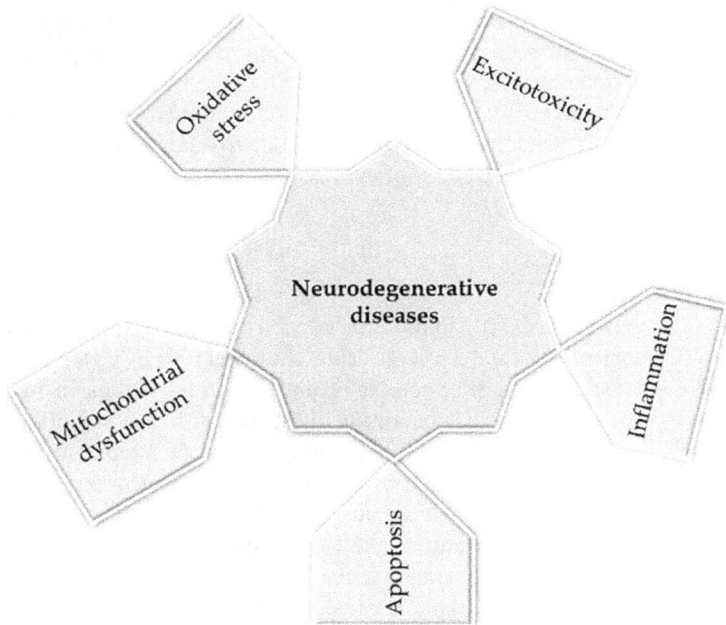

FIGURE 4.1 Possible causes of neurodegenerative diseases and brain aging. As addressed above in this chapter, oxidative stress, neuroinflammation, mitochondrial dysfunction, apoptosis, and excitotoxicity are some of the common pathways implicated in the progression and pathogenesis of neurodegenerative diseases and brain aging.

FLAVONOIDS ALTER MULTIPLE PATHWAYS IMPLICATED IN BRAIN AGING AND NEURODEGENERATIVE

Flavonoids are secondary plant metabolites that are found in some fruits, vegetables, and beverages [34]. Flavonoids have been studied extensively for their antioxidant, neuroprotective, anti-inflammatory, and chemopreventive activities [35]. Flavonoids may help with various ailments, including neurodegenerative disorders [36]. Flavonoids alter multiple pathways implicated in brain aging and NDs. As discussed in this chapter, flavonoids can increase brain cell function and neuronal survival by reducing OS, inhibiting inflammatory responses, and activating Nrf2. Therefore, they have the potential to act as multi-factorial therapeutics for reducing the impact of NDs.

Role of Flavonoids in Oxidative Stress

Flavonoids are phenolic molecules with low molecular weight and a flavan nucleus. So far, approximately 4,000 flavonoids have been found in plant leaves, seeds, bark, and flowers [37]. Humans obtain flavonoids mostly from fruits, vegetables, tea, and wine. Many flavonoids have been proven to have antioxidative, free radical scavenging, coronary heart disease prevention, hepatoprotective, anti-inflammatory, and anticancer activities, while others may have antiviral properties [38,39]. The antioxidant property of flavonoids depends upon the configuration, the total number of hydroxyl groups, and substituting functional groups about their nuclear structure [37]. Flavonoids' antioxidant activity inhibits ROS-producing enzymes, chelates transition metal ions that may stimulate ROS formation, quenches free radical events in lipid peroxidation, and upregulates or protects antioxidant defenses [40]. This evidence suggests that flavonoid antioxidant activity may protect cell constituents against OS and reduce the risk of ND associated with OS.

Role of Flavonoids in Inflammation

Flavonoids have neuroprotective properties connected to their ability to control the inflammatory responses involved in neurodegenerative disorders [41]. To date, evidence suggests that flavonoids inhibit neuroinflammation by playing a role in inhibiting the release of cytokines such as IL-1β and TNF-activated glia; inhibiting iNOS induction and subsequent nitric oxide production in response to glial activation; inhibiting the activation of NADPH oxidase and subsequent ROS generation in activated glia, and downregulate the activity of pro-inflammatory transcription factors such as NF-κB. Furthermore, the influence of several glial and neuronal signaling pathways, such as the MAPK cascade, on these processes appears to be mediated [42]. Citrus flavonoids have neuroprotective properties linked to flavonoids' anti-inflammatory properties in neurodegenerative disorders. Kaempferol, naringin, and nobiletin are citrus flavonoids with inhibitory effects on nuclear factor-B and mitogen-activated protein kinase signaling pathways, altering inflammatory conditions in microglial cells [43]. These findings imply that flavonoids' anti-inflammatory properties may play a role in preventing or slowing neuroinflammation in neurodegenerative disorders.

Role of Flavonoids in Glutathione Increase

Plant compounds can either directly or indirectly scavenge ROS by activating endogenous defense systems to battle insults. Two of these defense systems are phase 2 detoxification and antioxidant enzymes. Glutathione (GSH) is a nonprotein present in all cell types at millimolar concentrations. GSH has two primary functions: maintaining intracellular redox equilibrium and removing xenobiotics and ROS. GSH provides the cell with various defenses, not only against ROS but also against other detrimental toxicants [44].

In several senescent creatures, including humans, GSH levels have been observed to decrease with age. Human GSH concentrations in the cerebral spinal fluid decrease with age, as indicated by induced ectopic GSH production, which extends life duration. Age-related declines in GSH, according to these studies, may be a fundamental factor in the aging process, explaining many changes that occur with normal aging as well as the onset of many diseases [45]. Several neurodegenerative decreases, including PD, AD, and ALS, have been linked to a disruption in GSH homeostasis. GSH can be safely increased through dietary/treatment options such as flavonoids, and an increase in brain GSH results in clinical benefit and/or neuroprotection in animal models and human disorders [46,47].

Many flavonoids' biological effects have been linked to their antioxidant characteristics, either through their reducing capabilities or their impact on the intracellular redox state (GSH: GSSG ratio) [48]. To discover how they affect the antioxidant defense system, flavonoids isolated from *E. pubescens* are being studied in *Drosophila melanogaster*. Because of their antiradical ability and increased expression of GSH-Px, *E. pubescens* has the potential to become a natural antioxidant [49]. Flavonoids such as epigallocatechin-3-gallate (EGCG) and genistein have been shown to increase GSH synthesis via a PI3kinase-dependent antioxidant pathway activated by Nrf2 [50].

Role of Flavonoids in Nrf2 Modulation

Nrf2, encoded by the NFE2L2 gene, controls over 250 genes involved in cellular homeostasis, including antioxidant proteins, detoxifying enzymes, drug transporters, and various cytoprotective proteins [51]. Nrf2 binds to antioxidant response elements (AREs), which include drug-metabolizing enzymes (cytochrome P450s, glutathione S-transferases; GSTs), antioxidant enzymes (glutamate-cysteine ligase), molecular chaperones, proteasome subunits, and DNA repair enzymes [52]. Nrf2 heterodimerization with small Maf proteins is needed for effective binding to the ARE/EpRE (antioxidant response element/electrophilic response element) [53], which is required for transcription of Nrf2-mediated genes. The cell's ability to maintain redox equilibrium

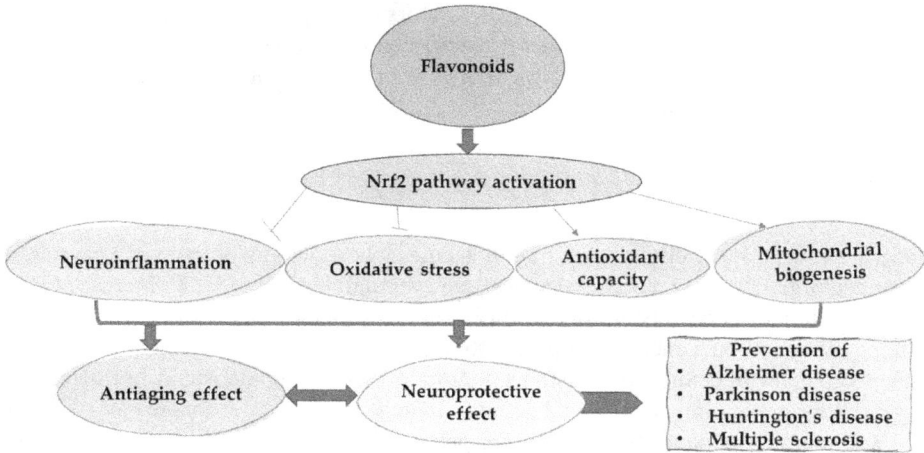

FIGURE 4.2 Flavonoids play a role in preventing numerous degenerative disorders by modulating Nrf2. Flavonoids, through activating Nrf2, counteract various pathogenic processes implicated in neurodegenerative disease and brain aging by upregulating antioxidant defenses, inhibiting neuroinflammation, inhibiting oxidative stress, and improving mitochondrial function, as seen in this diagram.

and remove proteins damaged by xenobiotic and OS is dependent on the transcription of these protective genes [54]. In various studies, flavonoids were found to have Nrf2-stimulating action [55]. Figure 4.2 summarizes the neuroprotective and antiaging effects of flavonoids through Nrf2 activation.

ROLE OF Nrf2 IN NEURODEGENERATIVE DISEASES

Nrf2 is a master regulator of several pathways, including the antioxidant defense system and anti-inflammatory genes that counter stresses in neuronal cells [56]. Nrf2 is a well-known genetic factor involved in the pathophysiology of NDs. Nrf2 is inhibited in several NDs, including AD, PD, HD, and ALS. Conversely, Nrf2 overexpression prevents NDs [57], resulting in that Nrf2 has been shown to improve neuronal function [58,59]. It is commonly accepted that Nrf2 has a protective effect on OS [60]. Evidence has shown that expression of Nrf2 was significantly improved in midbrain regions of marine-treated mice, protecting the animals from oxidative damage [61–63], suggesting Nrf2 modulation afforded significant protection against various neurodegenerative disorders associated with OS.

Targeting Nrf2 signaling could be a promising therapeutic method for delaying the onset of NDs, reducing their course, and alleviating symptoms. Many natural compounds have been identified as Nrf2 regulators in various chronic disorders, including carcinogenic, liver ailments, inflammatory conditions, neurodegenerations, diabetes, and cardiotoxicities [2]. Below, we will go over some of Nrf2's core functions as a means of the mechanism of action to prevent numerous NDs.

Antioxidant Role of Nrf2

ROS are crucial intracellular signaling molecules, but too many of them can cause OS, damaged organelles and macromolecules, and eventually cell death [64]. Increased ROS production and OS have been linked to the pathophysiology of AD, PD, HD, and MS, among other neurodegenerative illnesses [65]. Because the brain is particularly susceptible to changes in cellular redox status, maintaining redox homeostasis in the brain is essential for preventing OS-induced cellular damage [66].

Cellular antioxidants are essential for preventing neuronal death and lowering OS. Cells have multiple defense systems to manage OS-induced damage in response to OS. Nrf2 controls the production of several antioxidant enzymes and proteins that have cytoprotective properties, and there is growing evidence that inducing Nrf2-dependent antioxidant activity improves neurological outcomes in various disease models [67]. The transcription factor Nrf2 regulates the most critical defensive process in cells, called phase II antioxidant response enzymes. Nrf2 regulates both the constitutive and inducible expression of ARE-regulated genes [68].

Anti-Inflammatory Role of Nrf2

Inflammation control is crucial in preventing various diseases, including neurodegenerative disorders. Nrf2, required for OS defense, has reduced inflammation [69]. Nrf2 can control inflammation through multiple mechanisms, including redox homeostasis modulation and inhibition of pro-inflammatory genes, either directly or through interaction with NF-κB. Inflammation raises local and systemic ROS levels, while ROS exacerbates inflammation [70]. This vicious loop can be broken by Nrf2-mediated ROS homeostatic regulation.

Nrf2's anti-inflammatory properties have long been overlooked in favor of its antioxidant properties. For example, OS activates the conventional pro-inflammatory transcription factor NF-κB, which can be inhibited by Nrf2-dependent activation of antioxidant target genes, resulting in lower transcription of pro-inflammatory cytokines [71]. Furthermore, Nrf2 regulates the transcription of Nrf2 itself [72], which inhibits the transcriptional activity of NF-κB, and tunes gene expression in inflammatory macrophages through a bidirectional interaction with the NF-κB transcription factor [73].

Nrf2, on the other hand, has been demonstrated to influence the expression of anti-inflammatory mediators such as interleukin (IL)-17D, CD36, macrophage receptors with collagenous structure, and G protein-coupled receptor kinase [74,75]. Furthermore, Nrf2 has been linked to reducing pro-inflammatory cytokines such as tumor necrosis factor (TNF), IL-1β, IL-6, and IL-8 in microglia, macrophages, monocytes, and astrocytes [76]. Nrf2 also inhibits the recruitment of RNA polymerase II, which is required to initiate gene transcription of the pro-inflammatory cytokines IL-6 and IL-1β [76]. Moreover, Nrf2 has been found to have a key function in controlling inflammatory responses in the peripheral nervous system. Several studies have shown that Nrf2 can modulate chemokine, cytokine, immune cell responsiveness, and prostanoid expression using Nrf2-deficient mice as a model. The administration of lipopolysaccharide or bacterial endotoxin to Nrf2 defective mice increased pro-inflammatory cytokines and NF-κB-binding activities [73].

Role of Nrf2 in Mitochondrial Function

Mitochondrial dysfunction becomes more prominent with age, and several NDs have been associated with mitochondrial dysfunction [77]. Mitochondrial function and antioxidant response have a complicated relationship. Nrf2 protects mitochondria from oxidative damage by triggering free radical scavenging enzymes. Nrf2 can also directly regulate mitochondrial biogenesis and function, reducing intracellular ROS generation by increasing mitochondrial function. Many mitochondrial enzymes required for optimal bioenergetics function are affected by Nrf2 activation, including malic enzyme 1, isocitrate dehydrogenase 1, glucose-6-phosphate dehydrogenase, and 6-phosphogluconate-dehydrogenase [78].

Nrf2 has also been connected to mitochondrial integrity and regulation of mitochondrial biogenesis, improving mitochondrial fatty acid oxidation, and preserving mitochondrial membrane potential and respiration [79]. Activation of Nrf2 has been shown to protect mitochondria by opening the mitochondrial permeability transition pore [80], and decreased Nrf2 signaling has been linked to increased mtDNA damage [81]. Nrf2 activation also affects the expression of ATP synthase subunit and NDUFA4, two-electron transport chain components [82], and Nrf2-deficient animals exhibit lower mtDNA levels [83]. Nrf2 activation also impacts the expression of numerous mitochondrial biogenesis regulators, including Sirt1 (sirtuin 1), PPAR (peroxisome proliferator-activated receptor), and Pgc1 (PPAR coactivator 1), the master regulator of biogenesis [84–86]. Furthermore, most importantly, Nrf2 plays a crucial role in maintaining proper mitochondrial function by mediating the cellular redox balance, fatty acid oxidation, membrane potential, and structural integrity of the mitochondria itself [87].

Mitophagy refers to the process of scavenging mitochondria. Mitophagy is required for mitochondrial homeostasis because defective mitochondria are selectively absorbed by autophagosomes and transferred to lysosomes to be destroyed and recycled by the cell [88]. Nrf2 aids mitochondrial homeostasis by promoting mitophagy. This could be more noticeable in the presence of OS [87]. This evidence suggests that Nrf2 has a significant role in improving mitochondrial function.

Role of Nrf2 in Brain Aging

Nrf2 target genes protect against the development of age-related diseases, both by directly neutralizing free radicals and minimizing the damage produced by ROS. Most NDs are linked to aging, and OS increases with age [89]. A diminished capacity of cellular homeostatic mechanisms that protect the body from a range of oxidative damage is one of the characteristics of aging [90]. Because OS, inflammation, and mitochondrial dysfunction are all hallmarks of aging, Nrf2 has emerged as a promising target for medicinal intervention to extend life expectancy, as Nrf2 expression and activity decline with age [91,92].

Nrf2 pathways are in place to guarantee that ROS are adequately decreased, which reduces the risk of age-related diseases occurring. In addition to its antioxidant function, Nrf2 is crucial for autophagy and the proteasome, which deteriorate with age. Nrf2 controls the production of autophagosomes and proteasomes via regulating multiple autophagy-related proteins. Nrf2 signaling loss could significantly contribute to the proteotoxic phenotype seen in many age-related illnesses. Nrf2 loss would disrupt proteasome assembly, resulting in a buildup of misfolded proteins, autophagy initiation would be reduced, and misfolded or damaged proteins would accumulate, implying that Nrf2 should never be lost [93]. According to systematic review research, the loss of Nrf2 is linked to increased expression of its negative regulators or epigenetic repression, the most common cause of aging. Furthermore, decreased Nrf2 and increased OS contributes to the aging hallmarks: genomic instability, epigenetic changes, telomere attrition, stem cell fatigue, unregulated nutrition sensing, cellular senescence, and altered intercellular communications [94]. Thus, reducing the Nrf2 function is an integral part of aging. As such, it is developing Nrf2-based treatments to combat aging and its associated disorders is a critical area of research.

NEUROPROTECTIVE ACTIVITIES OF FLAVONOID TARGETING Nrf2

Natural products have emerged as a potential strategy for preventing and therapy NDs. Several studies have reported the neuroprotective effects of natural compounds in NDs such as AD, PD, HD, ALS, and brain tumors [4]. Flavonoids are well-studied natural compounds and have a wide range of biological activities that could effectively prevent and treat NDs. Flavonoids are a diversified group of natural compounds with over 6,000 compounds identified. Based on their structural chemistry, they have been classified into six subgroups: flavones, flavanols, flavonols, flavanones, isoflavones, and anthocyanidins [39]. The pharmacological properties of flavonoids include anticancer, anti-inflammatory, immunomodulatory, cardioprotective, and anti-infective, to name a few. They alter various molecular pathways, resulting in attenuated neuronal dysfunction and delaying the onset and progression of neurodegeneration [95]. Thus, because of its potential benefits to human health, flavonoid-enriched extracts should be seriously considered as innovative therapeutics to prevent neurodegenerative disorders. These flavonoids may be able to target various brain regions and prevent against NDs. Activation of Nrf2 is, therefore, increasingly implicated as an attractive target for the prevention of neurodegenerative conditions. Flavonoids that target Nrf2 have shown to be quite effective in treating NDs. Below will be discussed the role of flavonoids in targeting Nrf2 in the most common NDs.

Flavonoid Targeting Nrf2 in Alzheimer's Disease

AD is the most common chronic and progressive ND among the elderly and the primary cause of dementia. The two pathogenic hallmarks of AD are intracellular neurofibrillary tangles and extracellular beta-amyloid (Aβ). These two hallmarks cause neuroinflammation, OS, mitochondrial malfunction, and apoptosis, all of which have a role in the course and pathogenesis of AD [9].

Increased OS is thought to be an early occurrence of AD [96], and decreased antioxidant capacity as well as increased OS indicators can be found in both the blood and the brains of AD patients [97]. Neurons missing Nrf2 are more vulnerable to OS caused by H_2O_2 and non-excitotoxic glutamate [98], which can be alleviated by Nrf2 overexpression [99]. Thus, for protection against AD caused by oxidative death, neurons and astrocytes rely on Nrf2 activation of ARE-containing genes. In AD, Nrf2 nuclear expression is lowered, and a recent meta-analysis of microarray datasets discovered 31 downregulated ARE genes in AD patients [100]. Loss of Nrf2 has been shown to increase levels of Aβ and phosphorylated tau [101], as well as glial activation, OS markers, and neurodegeneration, and accelerate cognitive impairment [102]. In patients with AD, the Nrf2 pathway is disrupted, with lower nuclear levels of Nrf2 in hippocampal neurons [103].

Flavonoid compounds play a significant role in preventing and treating AD by activating Nrf2. Flavonoids have been proven to promote brain-derived neurotrophic factor (BDNF), which improves cognitive functions, stimulates neurogenesis, enhances neuronal formation, and helps to lessen the pathology of AD [104]. Because Nrf2 stimulates synaptogenesis by upregulating BDNF [105], flavonoid products may improve cognitive performance by activating Nrf2. Similarly, studies have revealed that flavonoids lower OS indicators in the brains of AD mice models via activating Nrf2 [106].

Neuroprotective substances include naturally occurring flavonoids such as carnosic acid and sulfuretin, among others. Carnosic acid, found in rosemary and sage, is a naturally occurring pro-electric molecule activated by OS, which triggers the Keap1/Nrf2 transcriptional pathway, producing phase 2 antioxidant enzymes. According to histological investigations, carnosic acid increased dendritic and synaptic markers while lowering astrogliosis, Aβ plaque number, and phospho-tau staining in the hippocampus [107]. Additionally, Sulfuretin, a flavonoid glycoside, increased the expression of the antioxidant Nrf2-target gene heme oxygenase-1 (HO-1) via the PI3K/Akt signaling pathway [108]. Flavonoids that target Nrf2 are becoming more beneficial in preventing and treating AD for these and other reasons.

Flavonoid Targeting Nrf2 in Parkinson's Disease

PD is a chronic, progressive, and the second most common ND. PD is characterized by the loss of dopaminergic neurons in the substantia nigra [109], leading to diminished motor function, including bradykinesia, resting tremor, muscle rigidity, and postural imbalance that develops later [110]. Neuropathological hallmarks of PD include the accumulation of intracellular protein aggregation, Lewy bodies, and Lewy neurites, which are mostly composed of misfolded and aggregated forms of the presynaptic protein alpha (α)-synuclein, and the progressive loss of dopaminergic substantia nigra neurons [111]. In addition, several studies have stated that OS, neuroinflammation, and mitochondrial dysfunction have all been implicated in the development and progression of PD [112,113].

Nrf2 expression and activity are altered in nigra dopaminergic neurons in PD patients [114]. According to postmortem studies, PD patients' Nrf2 translocates into the nucleus, but the expression of phase II antioxidant genes does not increase as expected, suggesting the Nrf2 pathway's dysregulation. Because Nrf2 activity and effectiveness decline with age, and age is one of the key risk factors for PD, it has been shown that Nrf2 can delay the occurrence of the disease [100]. A functional haplotype in the human Nrf2 promoter that increases the transcriptional activity of the gene has been associated with a lower risk of PD and a delayed onset of the disease [115]. pharmacological manipulation of Nrf2 expression levels can mimic this protective haplotype [116]. Nrf2 activation has been associated with neuroprotection in several PD model systems [117].

Flavonoids regulate various essential physiological processes, which may help explain why they have neuroprotective properties in PD. Reduced DA neuronal loss and dopamine depletion, reduced neuroinflammation, better antioxidant status and mitochondrial dysfunction, activated antiapoptotic pathways, activation of neurotrophic factors, and inhibition of a-synuclein aggregation were all results of these reactions [118].

Several studies have recommended naringin, a prominent flavanone glycoside present in citrus fruits, as a potential treatment agent for neurodegenerative illnesses [119]. Through overexpression of Nrf2 and subsequent activation of the ARE pathway, naringenin reduced 6-OHDA-induced neurotoxicity. An in vivo investigation utilizing 6-OHDA–lesioned mice found that naringenin reduced nigrostriatal DA neurodegeneration and oxidative damage via activating the Nrf2/ARE signaling pathway [120]. As a result, the Nrf2/ARE pathway is thought to have a role in ND prevention [121]. Similar studies in MPTP-induced neurotoxicity prevented various classes of flavonoids in the mouse model by reserving dopamine neurons and decreasing inflammation markers [122].

These findings suggested that Nrf2 could be a suitable PD therapeutic target. Flavonoids that target the Nrf2-the pathway to intervene in OS could be effective in treating PD.

Flavonoid Targeting of Nrf2 in Huntington's Disease

HD is a progressive neurological disease that runs in families characterized by a triad of motor, psychiatric and cognitive impairments. The striatum and cortex are the affected brain regions that exhibit dense reciprocal excitatory glutamate and inhibitory gamma-aminobutyric acid (GABA) connections. The excitatory and inhibitory signaling imbalance affects motor and cognitive processes [123]. HD is caused by pathological expansion of trinucleotide repeat of the nucleotides cytosine, adenine, and guanine (a CAG expansion) in the Huntingtin (HTT) gene, located at the short arm of chromosome 4 [124].

Although HD has a complex pathogenic mechanism, compromised OS defense systems have emerged as a contributing factor to the pathogenesis of HD. Studies demonstrated an alteration of the Nrf2 pathway in HD patients [103] and the beneficial effects of pharmacological Nrf2 activators. Thus, activation of Nrf2-suppressed the release of pro-inflammatory cytokines in primary mouse HD microglia and astrocytes and was neuroprotective in HD rat corticostriatal brain slices and an HD Drosophila model [125].

In mouse models of HD, triterpenoids improved the brain pathology and behavior of the animals. Similarly, administration of Nrf2-activating synthetic triterpenoids similarly attenuated motor deficits increased longevity and reduced OS in a transgenic HD mouse model [126]. Indeed, activation of the Nrf2 pathway, which plays a prominent role in mediating antioxidant responses, has been considered as one of the treatment strategies for the management of HD [103].

Mounting studies have shown that several flavonoids have demonstrated beneficial effects on different models of HD through preserving motor function, improving mitochondrial function, reduce markers of inflammation and OS [127–130]; these effects may directly or indirectly relate to the upregulation of Nrf2 or cytoprotective elements or various signaling molecules associated to HD. Altogether, the available evidence suggests that a modest activation of Nrf2 by natural compounds including flavonoids is neuroprotective in the brain.

Flavonoid Targeting Nrf2 in Amyotrophic Lateral Sclerosis

ALS is also a progressive ND caused by motor neuron degeneration in the primary motor cortex, corticospinal tracts, brainstem, and spinal cord, resulting in progressive muscular paralysis, which causes paralysis and death from respiratory failure. One of the disease markers is the loss of upper and lower motor neurons [131,132]. The common clinical symptoms of ALS include muscle weakness, slurred speech, muscle cramps, changes in behavior, and cognitive difficulties [132]. Most people with ALS have a sporadic condition, which means it occurs in people with no history of the disorder in their family. However, about 5%–10% of all ALS cases have an autosomal dominant inheritance or familial form of the disease, termed as fALS [133], and approximately 20% of familial are linked to a toxic gain-of-function mutation in Cu/Zn-superoxide dismutase (SOD1) [134].

According to postmortem investigations, the expression of Nrf2-related genes is reduced in ALS patients. Nrf2 mRNA and protein levels have also been found to be lower in ALS patients' neurons, implying that the Nrf2 pathway is dysfunctional in this condition [135]. Furthermore, postmortem tissue from ALS patients showed higher amounts of oxidative damage to proteins, lipids, and DNA [136]. In models of SOD1-related ALS and in the CNS of ALS patients, Nrf2 signaling is reduced despite the presence of OS [137]. As a result, Nrf2 function appears to be decreased in ALS, suggesting that it may play a role in the disease's pathogenesis. For ALS and other NDs, increasing Nrf2 activity is a primary therapeutic focus [54].

So far, because of the disease's complexity, developing effective treatments has been challenging. The only approved drugs in general use, ri3luzole and edaravone, provide relatively small benefits, and only in a few individuals; therefore, current treatment choices are primarily on symptom management and respiratory support [138,139].

Despite the absence of effective treatments, studies in ALS animal models have revealed that flavonoids reduce age-dependent decrease of motor performance and preserve motor neuron count. They also decrease the rate of disease progression, increase lifespan, increase antioxidant enzymes, and reduce markers of inflammation [140–143]. In various studies, these effects are associated with Nrf2 activation [67,73,137,144,145]. This evidence suggests that using Nrf2 induction agents like flavonoids as a treatment for ALS could be a promising idea.

FLAVONOIDS THAT ACTIVATE THE EXPRESSION OF Nrf2

Nrf2 activation can be induced by exogenous chemicals, which naturally respond to increased OS. Several natural and synthetic substances have also been proven to activate the Nrf2 pathway effectively [146,147]. Several Nrf2 activator compounds have been investigated for their therapeutic potential in ND and brain aging, and a few are listed below.

7, 8-Dihydroxyflavone

7, 8-Dihydroxyflavone [7,8-DHF] is a natural compound flavonoid family that has antioxidant properties [148] and is found in fruits, vegetables, tea, and red wine [149]. The cytoprotective mechanism of 7,8-DHF against OS-induced cell damage is due to its stimulatory effect on the expression of heme oxygenase-1 (HO-1). 7,8-DHF increases HO-1 expression via increased Nrf2 protein expression and causes Nrf2 to translocate from the cytosol to the nucleus. This stimulus activates the ERK/Nrf2/HO-1 signaling pathway, protecting cells from oxidative damage [148]. 7,8-DHF has been identified as a possible pharmacotherapeutic method for PD, AD, high blood pressure, diet-induced obesity, fragile X syndrome, and traumatic brain injury [150].

Luteolin

Luteolin, a dietary flavone obtained from fruits, vegetables, and herbs, has beneficial effects, including anti-inflammatory, antiallergic, anticancer, and antioxidant, to prevent degenerative diseases [151–153]. According to several studies, a high dose of luteolin stimulates the Nrf2/ARE pathway in the liver, then increases the nuclear translocation of Nrf2, resulting in increased production of its target gene, HO-1 [154], which then protects cells from oxidative damage.

Myricetin

Myricetin is a flavonoid found in various foods that have been proven to exhibit biological activity in several studies and may have antibacterial and antioxidant properties. Its antibacterial and antioxidant properties have been extensively researched, and multiple studies have shown neurobiological activity and a potentially positive effect on AD, PD, heart disease, and ALS [155]. Myricetin ameliorates brain injury and neurological deficits via Nrf2 activation after experimental stroke in middle-aged rats [156]. Myricetin also suppresses the generation of pro-inflammatory mediators by inducing Nrf2-mediated HO-1 expression and suppressing NF-κB and STAT1 activation. These findings imply that myricetin could be used to treat a variety of inflammatory diseases as an anti-inflammatory and antioxidant medication [157].

Sulforaphane

Sulforaphane (SFN), an organic isothiocyanate, contains broccoli, Brussels sprouts, cabbage, and cauliflower [146]. SFN stimulates Nrf2 production, as a result, strengthens cellular defenses [74]. SFN plays a vital role in neurodegenerative and aging diseases. SFN treatment enhances Nrf2 transcription, activation, nuclear translocation, DNA-binding, and antioxidant gene expression in epithelial cells isolated from aged rats and humans [158]. In addition, in vivo and in vitro studies have indicated that SFN protects against stroke, traumatic brain injury, AD, PD, HD, and ALS [146]. As a result, SFN, through activation of Nrf2, is an essential inducer of the antioxidant and protective responses in the aging and ND process.

Epigallocatechin Gallate

EGCG, a flavonoid found in green tea, is a powerful antioxidant and an activator of the Nrf2 transcriptional pathway [159]. According to several investigations, this natural compound contains anti-inflammatory and anti-atherogenic activities and protective actions against neuronal injury and brain edema. Furthermore, in vitro and in vivo investigations on AD syndrome revealed that EGCG primarily reduces Aβ buildup by altering multiple biological pathways [160].

Curcumin

Curcumin, derived from *Curcuma longa* rhizomes, is known to be protective in neurons via activation of Nrf2, a master regulator of endogenous defense against OS in cells [161]. In addition, curcumin has a wide range of pharmacological effects such as antioxidant, anti-inflammatory, antimicrobial, antitumor, and hepatoprotective activities [162]. The neuroprotective effect of curcumin involves activation through the Akt/Nrf2 pathway, then activation of Nrf2, which is involved in fighting against oxidative damage [163].

CONCLUSION

Although each ND is described as a separate entity in this chapter, there is often overlap. Neuropathology will remain the gold standard for the foreseeable future because none of the neurodegenerative disorders have complete diagnostic accuracy. Several cellular and molecular processes, such as OS, decreased mitochondrial function, excitotoxicity, neuroinflammation, and activation of apoptotic factors, are the principal drivers of neurodegenerative disorders, in addition to normal brain aging. Flavonoids are plant polyphenols that are found in abundance in all fruits, vegetables, and medicinal plants. They have emerged as a prospective contender in developing therapy techniques for various NDs and brain aging due to their ability to regulate proteins like Nrf2. Given recent evidence of flavonoids' role in brain Nrf2 activation, it is expected that these molecules will one day represent a new generation of bioactive medications for enhancing brain function in various NDs and brain aging.

FUNDING

This research was supported by the National Institute of Minority Health and Health Disparities of the National Institutes of Health through Grant Number U54 MD 007582 and Grant Number P20 MD006738.

INSTITUTIONAL REVIEW BOARD STATEMENT

Not applicable.

INFORMED CONSENT STATEMENT

Not applicable.

AUTHOR CONTRIBUTIONS

Conceptualization, KFAS and ET; methodology, ET and GMA; formal analysis, ET and GMA; writing—original draft preparation, ET and GMA; writing—review and editing, KFAS, GMA, and ET; visualization, KFAS, ET, and GMA. All authors have read and agreed to the published version of the manuscript.

CONFLICT OF INTEREST

The authors declare that there is no conflict of interest.

REFERENCES

1. Gao H-M, Hong J-S. Why neurodegenerative diseases are progressive: Uncontrolled inflammation drives disease progression. *Trends Immunol.* 2008;29(8):357–65.
2. Khan H, Tundis R, Ullah H, Aschner M, Belwal T, Mirzaei H, et al. Flavonoids targeting NRF2 in neurodegenerative disorders. *Food Chem Toxicol.* 2020;146:111817.
3. Harvard NeuroDiscovery Center. *The Challenge of NeurodegenerAeases.* Available online at https://neurodiscoveryharvardedu/challenge (accessed on 12/22/2021).
4. Mohd Sairazi NS, Sirajudeen KNS. Natural products and their bioactive compounds: Neuroprotective potentials against neurodegenerative diseases. *Evidence-Based Complementary Altern Med.* 2020;2020:6565396.
5. Azam S, Haque ME, Balakrishnan R, Kim I-S, Choi D-K. The ageing brain: Molecular and cellular basis of neurodegeneration. *Front Cell Dev Biol.* 2021;9:683459.
6. Durães F, Pinto M, Sousa E. Old drugs as new treatments for neurodegenerative diseases. *Pharmaceuticals (Basel).* 2018;11(2):44.
7. Rahman MH, Bajgai J, Fadriquela A, Sharma S, Trinh TT, Akter R, et al. Therapeutic potential of natural products in treating neurodegenerative disorders and their future prospects and challenges. *Molecules (Basel, Switzerland).* 2021;26(17):5327.
8. Hussain G, Zhang L, Rasul A, Anwar H, Sohail MU, Razzaq A, et al. Role of plant-derived flavonoids and their mechanism in attenuation of Alzheimer's and Parkinson's diseases: An update of recent data. *Molecules (Basel, Switzerland).* 2018;23(4):814.
9. Frandsen JR, Narayanasamy P. Neuroprotection through flavonoid: Enhancement of the glyoxalase pathway. *Redox Biol.* 2018;14:465–73.
10. Leonardo CC, Doré S. Dietary flavonoids are neuroprotective through Nrf2-coordinated induction of endogenous cytoprotective proteins. *Nutr Neurosci.* 2011;14(5):226–36.
11. Sandberg M, Patil J, D'Angelo B, Weber SG, Mallard C. Nrf2-regulation in brain health and disease: Implication of cerebral inflammation. *Neuropharmacology.* 2014;79:298–306.
12. Dinkova-Kostova AT, Kostov RV, Kazantsev AG. The role of Nrf2 signaling in counteracting neurodegenerative diseases. *FEBS J.* 2018;285(19):3576–90.
13. Hou Y, Dan X, Babbar M, Wei Y, Hasselbalch SG, Croteau DL, et al. Ageing as a risk factor for neurodegenerative disease. *Nat Rev Neurol.* 2019;15(10):565–81.
14. Maher P. The potential of flavonoids for the treatment of neurodegenerative diseases. *Int J Mol Sci.* 2019;20(12):3056.
15. Chen X, Guo C, Kong J. Oxidative stress in neurodegenerative diseases. *Neural Regen Res.* 2012;7(5):376–85.
16. Redza-Dutordoir M, Averill-Bates DA. Activation of apoptosis signalling pathways by reactive oxygen species. *Biochimica et Biophysica Acta (BBA) – Mol Cell Res.* 2016;1863(12):2977–92.
17. Singh A, Kukreti R, Saso L, Kukreti S. Oxidative stress: A key modulator in neurodegenerative diseases. *Molecules.* 2019;24(8):1583.
18. Kwon HS, Koh SH. Neuroinflammation in neurodegenerative disorders: The roles of microglia and astrocytes. *Transl Neurodegener.* 2020;9(1):42.

19. Nathan C, Ding A. Nonresolving inflammation. *Cell.* 2010;140(6):871–82.
20. Wyss-Coray T, Mucke L. Inflammation in neurodegenerative disease—A double-edged sword. *Neuron.* 2002;35(3):419–32.
21. Chen W-W, Zhang X, Huang W-J. Role of neuroinflammation in neurodegenerative diseases (review). *Mol Med Rep.* 2016;13(4):3391–6.
22. Kempuraj D, Thangavel R, Natteru PA, Selvakumar GP, Saeed D, Zahoor H, et al. Neuroinflammation induces neurodegeneration. *J Neurol Neurosurg Spine.* 2016;1(1):1003.
23. Wu Y, Chen M, Jiang J. Mitochondrial dysfunction in neurodegenerative diseases and drug targets via apoptotic signaling. *Mitochondrion.* 2019;49:35–45.
24. Norat P, Soldozy S, Sokolowski JD, Gorick CM, Kumar JS, Chae Y, et al. Mitochondrial dysfunction in neurological disorders: Exploring mitochondrial transplantation. *NPJ: Regener Med.* 2020;5(1):22.
25. Chistiakov DA, Sobenin IA, Revin VV, Orekhov AN, Bobryshev YV. Mitochondrial aging and age-related dysfunction of mitochondria. *Biomed Res Int.* 2014;2014:238463.
26. Cheng A, Hou Y, Mattson MP. Mitochondria and neuroplasticity. *ASN Neuro.* 2010;2(5):e00045.
27. Müller M, Ahumada-Castro U, Sanhueza M, Gonzalez-Billault C, Court FA, Cárdenas C. Mitochondria and calcium regulation as basis of neurodegeneration associated with aging. *Front Neurosci.* 2018;12:470.
28. Moujalled D, Strasser A, Liddell JR. Molecular mechanisms of cell death in neurological diseases. *Cell Death Differ.* 2021;28(7):2029–44.
29. Elmore S. Apoptosis: A review of programmed cell death. *Toxicol Pathol.* 2007;35(4):495–516.
30. Mattson MP. Apoptosis in neurodegenerative disorders. *Nat Rev Mol Cell Biol.* 2000;1(2):120–30.
31. Dong X-X, Wang Y, Qin Z-H. Molecular mechanisms of excitotoxicity and their relevance to pathogenesis of neurodegenerative diseases. *Acta Pharmacol Sin.* 2009;30(4):379–87.
32. Mattson MP. Excitotoxic and excitoprotective mechanisms. *Neuro Mol Med.* 2003;3(2):65–94.
33. Salińska E, Danysz W, Łazarewicz JW. The role of excitotoxicity in neurodegeneration. *Folia Neuropathol.* 2005;43(4):322–39.
34. Panche AN, Diwan AD, Chandra SR. Flavonoids: An overview. *J Nutr Sci.* 2016;5:e47.
35. Mansuri ML, Parihar P, Solanki I, Parihar MS. Flavonoids in modulation of cell survival signalling pathways. *Genes Nutr.* 2014;9(3):400.
36. Scalbert A, Manach C, Morand C, Rémésy C, Jiménez L. Dietary polyphenols and the prevention of diseases. *Crit Rev Food Sci Nutr.* 2005;45(4):287–306.
37. Heim KE, Tagliaferro AR, Bobilya DJ. Flavonoid antioxidants: Chemistry, metabolism and structure-activity relationships. *J Nutr Biochem.* 2002;13(10):572–84.
38. Kumar S, Pandey AK. Chemistry and biological activities of flavonoids: An overview. *Sci World J.* 2013;2013:162750.
39. Adinew GM, Taka E, Mendonca P, Messeha SS, Soliman KFA. The Anticancer Effects of Flavonoids through miRNAs Modulations in Triple-Negative Breast Cancer. Nutrients. 2021;13(4):1212.
40. Mierziak J, Kostyn K, Kulma A. Flavonoids as important molecules of plant interactions with the environment. *Molecules.* 2014;19(10):16240-65.
41. Spagnuolo C, Moccia S, Russo GL. Anti-inflammatory effects of flavonoids in neurodegenerative disorders. *Eur J Med Chem.* 2018;153:105–15.
42. Spencer JPE, Vafeiadou K, Williams RJ, Vauzour D. Neuroinflammation: Modulation by flavonoids and mechanisms of action. *Mol Aspects Med.* 2012;33(1):83–97.
43. Heesu L, Baskar S, Ki Yeon Y, Seong-Hee K. Flavonoids as anti-inflammatory and neuroprotective agents. *Int J Oral Biol.* 2020;45(2):33–41.

44. Myhrstad MC, Carlsen H, Nordström O, Blomhoff R, Moskaug J. Flavonoids increase the intracellular glutathione level by transactivation of the gamma-glutamylcysteine synthetase catalytical subunit promoter. *Free Radic Biol Med.* 2002;32(5):386–93.
45. Sohal RS, Weindruch R. Oxidative stress, caloric restriction, and aging. *Science.* 1996;273(5271):59–63.
46. Cudkowicz ME, Sexton PM, Ellis T, Hayden DL, Gwilt PR, Whalen J, et al. The pharmacokinetics and pharmacodynamics of procysteine in amyotrophic lateral sclerosis. *Neurology.* 1999;52(7):1492.
47. Aoyama K, Suh SW, Hamby AM, Liu J, Chan WY, Chen Y, et al. Neuronal glutathione deficiency and age-dependent neurodegeneration in the EAAC1 deficient mouse. *Nature Neurosci.* 2006;9(1):119–26.
48. Rice-Evans CA, Miller NJ, Paganga G. Structure-antioxidant activity relationships of flavonoids and phenolic acids. *Free Radic Biol Med.* 1996;20(7):933–56.
49. Yang X-H, Li L, Xue Y-B, Zhou X-X, Tang J-H. Flavonoids from epimedium pubescens: Extraction and mechanism, antioxidant capacity and effects on CAT and GSH-Px of drosophila melanogaster. *Peer J.* 2020;8:e8361.
50. Hernandez-Montes E, Pollard SE, Vauzour D, Jofre-Montseny L, Rota C, Rimbach G, et al. Activation of glutathione peroxidase via Nrf1 mediates genistein's protection against oxidative endothelial cell injury. *Biochem Biophys Res Commun.* 2006;346(3):851–9.
51. O'Connell MA, Hayes JD. The Keap1/Nrf2 pathway in health and disease: From the bench to the clinic. *Biochem Soc Trans.* 2015;43(4):687–9.
52. Sykiotis GP, Bohmann D. Stress-activated cap 'n' collar transcription factors in aging and human disease. *Sci Signal.* 2010;3(112):re3.
53. Silva-Palacios A, Ostolga-Chavarría M, Zazueta C, Königsberg M. Nrf2: Molecular and epigenetic regulation during aging. *Ageing Res Rev.* 2018;47:31–40.
54. Kerr F, Sofola-Adesakin O, Ivanov DK, Gatliff J, Gomez Perez-Nievas B, Bertrand HC, et al. Direct Keap1-Nrf2 disruption as a potential therapeutic target for Alzheimer's disease. *PLoS Genet.* 2017;13(3):e1006593.
55. Wu X-Y, Chen X-M, Zhou M-X, Hu H-X, Zhang J-Z, Wang X-N, et al. Artocarmitin B enhances intracellular antioxidant capacity via activation of Nrf2 signaling pathway in human lung epithelial cells. *Chem-Biol Interact.* 2019;310:108741.
56. Silva A, Pereira M, Carrascal MA, Brites G, Neves B, Moreira P, et al. Calcium modulation, anti-oxidant and anti-inflammatory effect of skin allergens targeting the Nrf2 signaling pathway in Alzheimer's disease cellular models. *Int J Mol Sci.* 2020;21(20):7791.
57. Kanninen K, Malm TM, Jyrkkänen H-K, Goldsteins G, Keksa-Goldsteine V, Tanila H, et al. Nuclear factor erythroid 2-related factor 2 protects against beta amyloid. *Mol Cell Neurosci.* 2008;39(3):302–13.
58. Sian J, Dexter DT, Lees AJ, Daniel S, Jenner P, Marsden CD. Glutathione-related enzymes in brain in Parkinson's disease. *Ann Neurol.* 1994;36(3):356–61.
59. Rojo AI, Innamorato NG, Martín-Moreno AM, De Ceballos ML, Yamamoto M, Cuadrado A. Nrf2 regulates microglial dynamics and neuroinflammation in experimental Parkinson's disease. *Glia.* 2010;58(5):588–98.
60. Meng F, Wang J, Ding F, Xie Y, Zhang Y, Zhu J. Neuroprotective effect of matrine on MPTP-induced Parkinson's disease and on Nrf2 expression. *Oncol Lett.* 2017;13(1):296–300.
61. Johnson DA, Johnson JA. Nrf2—A therapeutic target for the treatment of neurodegenerative diseases. *Free Radic Biol Med.* 2015;88:253–67.
62. Itoh K, Wakabayashi N, Katoh Y, Ishii T, Igarashi K, Engel JD, et al. Keap1 represses nuclear activation of antioxidant responsive elements by Nrf2 through binding to the amino-terminal Neh2 domain. *Genes Dev.* 1999;13(1):76–86.

63. Calkins MJ, Johnson DA, Townsend JA, Vargas MR, Dowell JA, Williamson TP, et al. The Nrf2/ARE Pathway as a potential therapeutic target in neurodegenerative disease. *Antioxid Redox Signaling.* 2008;11(3):497–508.
64. Zuo L, Zhou T, Pannell BK, Ziegler AC, Best TM. Biological and physiological role of reactive oxygen species—The good, the bad and the ugly. *Acta Physiol.* 2015;214(3):329–48.
65. Holmström KM, Kostov RV, Dinkova-Kostova AT. The multifaceted role of Nrf2 in mitochondrial function. *Curr Opin Toxicol.* 2016;1:80–91.
66. Yamazaki H, Tanji K, Wakabayashi K, Matsuura S, Itoh K. Role of the Keap1/Nrf2 pathway in neurodegenerative diseases. *Pathol Int.* 2015;65(5):210–9.
67. Buendia I, Michalska P, Navarro E, Gameiro I, Egea J, León R. Nrf2-ARE pathway: An emerging target against oxidative stress and neuroinflammation in neurodegenerative diseases. *Pharmacol Ther.* 2016;157:84–104.
68. Danilov CA, Chandrasekaran K, Racz J, Soane L, Zielke C, Fiskum G. Sulforaphane protects astrocytes against oxidative stress and delayed death caused by oxygen and glucose deprivation. *Glia.* 2009;57(6):645–56.
69. Itoh K, Chiba T, Takahashi S, Ishii T, Igarashi K, Katoh Y, et al. An Nrf2/small Maf heterodimer mediates the induction of phase II detoxifying enzyme genes through antioxidant response elements. *Biochem Biophys Res Commun.* 1997;236(2):313–22.
70. Joseph J, Ametepe ES, Haribabu N, Agbayani G, Krishnan L, Blais A, et al. Inhibition of ROS and upregulation of inflammatory cytokines by FoxO3a promotes survival against Salmonella typhimurium. *Nat Commun.* 2016;7:12748.
71. Lee JM, Shih AY, Murphy TH, Johnson JA. NF-E2-related factor-2 mediates neuroprotection against mitochondrial complex I inhibitors and increased concentrations of intracellular calcium in primary cortical neurons. *J Biol Chem.* 2003;278(39):37948–56.
72. Rushworth SA, Zaitseva L, Murray MY, Shah NM, Bowles KM, MacEwan DJ. The high Nrf2 expression in human acute myeloid leukemia is driven by NF-κB and underlies its chemo-resistance. *Blood.* 2012;120(26):5188–98.
73. Thimmulappa RK, Lee H, Rangasamy T, Reddy SP, Yamamoto M, Kensler TW, et al. Nrf2 is a critical regulator of the innate immune response and survival during experimental sepsis. *J Clin Invest.* 2006;116(4):984–95.
74. Thimmulappa RK, Mai KH, Srisuma S, Kensler TW, Yamamoto M, Biswal S. Identification of Nrf2-regulated genes induced by the chemopreventive agent sulforaphane by oligonucleotide microarray. *Cancer Res.* 2002;62(18):5196–203.
75. Saddawi-Konefka R, Seelige R, Gross ET, Levy E, Searles SC, Washington A, Jr., et al. Nrf2 Induces IL-17D to mediate tumor and virus surveillance. *Cell Rep.* 2016;16(9):2348–58.
76. Kobayashi EH, Suzuki T, Funayama R, Nagashima T, Hayashi M, Sekine H, et al. Nrf2 suppresses macrophage inflammatory response by blocking proinflammatory cytokine transcription. *Nat Commun.* 2016;7:11624.
77. Lin MT, Beal MF. Mitochondrial dysfunction and oxidative stress in neurodegenerative diseases. *Nature.* 2006;443(7113):787–95.
78. Morgan B, Ezeriņa D, Amoako TN, Riemer J, Seedorf M, Dick TP. Multiple glutathione disulfide removal pathways mediate cytosolic redox homeostasis. *Nat Chem Biol.* 2013;9(2):119–25.
79. Holmström KM, Baird L, Zhang Y, Hargreaves I, Chalasani A, Land JM, et al. Nrf2 impacts cellular bioenergetics by controlling substrate availability for mitochondrial respiration. *Biol Open.* 2013;2(8):761–70.
80. Greco T, Fiskum G. Brain mitochondria from rats treated with sulforaphane are resistant to redox-regulated permeability transition. *J Bioenerg Biomembr.* 2010;42(6):491–7.
81. Li Y, Zhang H. Soybean isoflavones ameliorate ischemic cardiomyopathy by activating Nrf2-mediated antioxidant responses. *Food Funct.* 2017;8(8):2935–44.

82. Abdullah A, Kitteringham NR, Jenkins RE, Goldring C, Higgins L, Yamamoto M, et al. Analysis of the role of Nrf2 in the expression of liver proteins in mice using two-dimensional gel-based proteomics. *Pharmacol Rep.* 2012;64(3):680–97.
83. Zhang YK, Wu KC, Klaassen CD. Genetic activation of Nrf2 protects against fasting-induced oxidative stress in livers of mice. *PLoS One.* 2013;8(3):e59122.
84. Cho HY, Gladwell W, Wang X, Chorley B, Bell D, Reddy SP, et al. Nrf2-regulated PPAR{gamma} expression is critical to protection against acute lung injury in mice. *Am J Respir Crit Care Med.* 2010;182(2):170–82.
85. Ping Z, Zhang LF, Cui YJ, Chang YM, Jiang CW, Meng ZZ, et al. The protective effects of salidroside from exhaustive exercise-induced heart injury by enhancing the PGC-1 α—NRF1/NRF2 pathway and mitochondrial respiratory function in rats. *Oxid Med Cell Longev.* 2015;2015:876825.
86. Song NY, Lee YH, Na HK, Baek JH, Surh YJ. Leptin induces SIRT1 expression through activation of NF-E2-related factor 2: Implications for obesity-associated colon carcinogenesis. *Biochem Pharmacol.* 2018;153:282–91.
87. Dinkova-Kostova AT, Abramov AY. The emerging role of Nrf2 in mitochondrial function. *Free Radic Biol Med.* 2015;88(Pt B):179–88.
88. Kim I, Rodriguez-Enriquez S, Lemasters JJ. Selective degradation of mitochondria by mitophagy. *Arch Biochem Biophys.* 2007;462(2):245–53.
89. Gandhi S, Abramov AY. Mechanism of oxidative stress in neurodegeneration. *Oxid Med Cell Longev.* 2012;2012:428010.
90. Harman D. Free radical theory of aging. *Mutat Res.* 1992;275(3–6):257–66.
91. Suh JH, Shenvi SV, Dixon BM, Liu H, Jaiswal AK, Liu RM, et al. Decline in transcriptional activity of Nrf2 causes age-related loss of glutathione synthesis, which is reversible with lipoic acid. *Proc Natl Acad Sci USA.* 2004;101(10):3381–6.
92. Collins AR, Lyon CJ, Xia X, Liu JZ, Tangirala RK, Yin F, et al. Age-accelerated atherosclerosis correlates with failure to upregulate antioxidant genes. *Circ Res.* 2009;104(6):e42–54.
93. Pajares M, Jiménez-Moreno N, García-Yagüe ÁJ, Escoll M, de Ceballos ML, Van Leuven F, et al. Transcription factor NFE2L2/NRF2 is a regulator of macroautophagy genes. *Autophagy.* 2016;12(10):1902–16.
94. Schmidlin CJ, Dodson MB, Madhavan L, Zhang DD. Redox regulation by NRF2 in aging and disease. *Free Radic Biol Med.* 2019;134:702–7.
95. Agrawal A. Pharmacological activities of flavonoids: A review. *Int J Pharm Sci Nanotechnol.* 2011;4(2):1394–8.
96. Lovell MA, Markesbery WR. Oxidative damage in mild cognitive impairment and early Alzheimer's disease. *J Neurosci Res.* 2007;85(14):3036–40.
97. Gubandru M, Margina D, Tsitsimpikou C, Goutzourelas N, Tsarouhas K, Ilie M, et al. Alzheimer's disease treated patients showed different patterns for oxidative stress and inflammation markers. *Food Chem Toxicol.* 2013;61:209–14.
98. Kraft AD, Johnson DA, Johnson JA. Nuclear factor E2-related factor 2-dependent antioxidant response element activation by tert-butylhydroquinone and sulforaphane occurring preferentially in astrocytes conditions neurons against oxidative insult. *J Neurosci.* 2004;24(5):1101–12.
99. Lee JM, Johnson JA. An important role of Nrf2-ARE pathway in the cellular defense mechanism. *J Biochem Mol Biol.* 2004;37(2):139–43.
100. Ramsey CP, Glass CA, Montgomery MB, Lindl KA, Ritson GP, Chia LA, et al. Expression of Nrf2 in neurodegenerative diseases. *J Neuropathol Exp Neurol.* 2007;66(1):75–85.
101. Branca C, Ferreira E, Nguyen TV, Doyle K, Caccamo A, Oddo S. Genetic reduction of Nrf2 exacerbates cognitive deficits in a mouse model of Alzheimer's disease. *Hum Mol Genet.* 2017;26(24):4823–35.

102. Rojo AI, Pajares M, García-Yagüe AJ, Buendia I, Van Leuven F, Yamamoto M, et al. Deficiency in the transcription factor NRF2 worsens inflammatory parameters in a mouse model with combined tauopathy and amyloidopathy. *Redox Biol.* 2018;18:173–80.

103. Jin YN, Yu YV, Gundemir S, Jo C, Cui M, Tieu K, et al. Impaired mitochondrial dynamics and Nrf2 signaling contribute to compromised responses to oxidative stress in striatal cells expressing full-length mutant huntingtin. *PLoS One.* 2013;8(3):e57932.

104. Zhang Z, Wu H, Huang H. Epicatechin plus treadmill exercise are neuroprotective against moderate-stage amyloid precursor protein/presenilin 1 mice. *Pharmacogn Mag.* 2016;12(Suppl 2):S139–46.

105. Chen T, Wu Y, Wang Y, Zhu J, Chu H, Kong L, et al. Brain-derived neurotrophic factor increases synaptic protein levels via the MAPK/erk signaling pathway and Nrf2/Trx axis following the transplantation of neural stem cells in a rat model of traumatic brain injury. *Neurochem Res.* 2017;42(11):3073–83.

106. Zhao L, Wang JL, Liu R, Li XX, Li JF, Zhang L. Neuroprotective, anti-amyloidogenic and neurotrophic effects of apigenin in an Alzheimer's disease mouse model. *Molecules.* 2013;18(8):9949–65.

107. Lipton SA, Rezaie T, Nutter A, Lopez KM, Parker J, Kosaka K, et al. Therapeutic advantage of pro-electrophilic drugs to activate the Nrf2/ARE pathway in Alzheimer's disease models. *Cell Death Dis.* 2016;7(12):e2499.

108. Kwon SH, Ma SX, Hwang JY, Lee SY, Jang CG. Involvement of the Nrf2/HO-1 signaling pathway in sulfuretin-induced protection against amyloid beta25–35 neurotoxicity. *Neuroscience.* 2015;304:14–28.

109. Xie A, Gao J, Xu L, Meng D. Shared mechanisms of neurodegeneration in Alzheimer's disease and Parkinson's disease. *Biomed Res Int.* 2014;2014:648740.

110. Kouli A, Torsney KM, Kuan WL. Parkinson's Disease: Etiology, Neuropathology, and Pathogenesis. In: Stoker TB, Greenland JC, editors. *Parkinson's Disease: Pathogenesis and Clinical Aspects*. Brisbane (AU): Codon Publications; Copyright: The Authors; 2018.

111. Xu L, Pu J. Alpha-synuclein in Parkinson's disease: From pathogenetic dysfunction to potential clinical application. *Parkinson's Dis.* 2016;2016:1720621.

112. Navarro A, Boveris A. Brain mitochondrial dysfunction and oxidative damage in Parkinson's disease. *J Bioenerg Biomembr.* 2009;41(6):517–21.

113. Di Filippo M, Chiasserini D, Tozzi A, Picconi B, Calabresi P. Mitochondria and the link between neuroinflammation and neurodegeneration. *J Alzheimers Dis.* 2010;20(Suppl. 2):S369–79.

114. Schipper HM, Liberman A, Stopa EG. Neural heme oxygenase-1 expression in idiopathic Parkinson's disease. *Exp Neurol.* 1998;150(1):60–8.

115. Von Otter M, Landgren S, Nilsson S, Celojevic D, Bergström P, Håkansson A, et al. Association of Nrf2-encoding NFE2L2 haplotypes with Parkinson's disease. *BMC Med Genet.* 2010;11:36.

116. Huang TT, Hao DL, Wu BN, Mao LL, Zhang J. Uric acid demonstrates neuroprotective effect on Parkinson's disease mice through Nrf2-ARE signaling pathway. *Biochem Biophys Res Commun.* 2017;493(4):1443–9.

117. Williamson TP, Johnson DA, Johnson JA. Activation of the Nrf2-ARE pathway by siRNA knockdown of Keap1 reduces oxidative stress and provides partial protection from MPTP-mediated neurotoxicity. *Neurotoxicology.* 2012;33(3):272–9.

118. Jung UJ, Kim SR. Beneficial effects of flavonoids against Parkinson's disease. *J Med Food.* 2018;21(5):421–32.

119. Kim HD, Jeong KH, Jung UJ, Kim SR. Naringin treatment induces neuroprotective effects in a mouse model of Parkinson's disease in vivo, but not enough to restore the lesioned dopaminergic system. *J Nutr Biochem.* 2016;28:140–6.

120. Lou H, Jing X, Wei X, Shi H, Ren D, Zhang X. Naringenin protects against 6-OHDA-induced neurotoxicity via activation of the Nrf2/ARE signaling pathway. *Neuropharmacology*. 2014;79:380–8.

121. Lin S-P, Hou Y-C, Tsai S-Y, Wang M-J, Chao P-DL. Tissue distribution of naringenin conjugated metabolites following repeated dosing of naringin to rats. *BioMedicine*. 2014;4(3):16.

122. Patil SP, Jain PD, Sancheti JS, Ghumatkar PJ, Tambe R, Sathaye S. Neuroprotective and neurotrophic effects of Apigenin and Luteolin in MPTP induced parkinsonism in mice. *Neuropharmacology*. 2014;86:192–202.

123. Hsu YT, Chang YG, Chern Y. Insights into GABA(A)ergic system alteration in Huntington's disease. *Open Biol*. 2018;8(12):180165.

124. Migliore S, Jankovic J, Squitieri F. Genetic counseling in Huntington's disease: Potential new challenges on horizon? *Front Neurol*. 2019;10(453).

125. Cuadrado A, Rojo AI, Wells G, Hayes JD, Cousin SP, Rumsey WL, et al. Therapeutic targeting of the NRF2 and KEAP1 partnership in chronic diseases. *Nat Rev Drug Discovery*. 2019;18(4):295–317.

126. Stack C, Ho D, Wille E, Calingasan NY, Williams C, Liby K, et al. Triterpenoids CDDO-ethyl amide and CDDO-trifluoroethyl amide improve the behavioral phenotype and brain pathology in a transgenic mouse model of Huntington's disease. *Free Radic Biol Med*. 2010;49(2):147–58.

127. Kreilaus F, Spiro AS, Hannan AJ, Garner B, Jenner AM. Therapeutic effects of Anthocyanins and environmental enrichment in R6/1 Huntington's disease mice. *J Huntingtons Dis*. 2016;5(3):285–96.

128. Menze ET, Esmat A, Tadros MG, Khalifa AE, Abdel-Naim AB. Genistein improves sensorimotor gating: Mechanisms related to its neuroprotective effects on the striatum. *Neuropharmacology*. 2016;105:35–46.

129. Lagoa R, Lopez-Sanchez C, Samhan-Arias AK, Gañan CM, Garcia-Martinez V, Gutierrez-Merino C. Kaempferol protects against rat striatal degeneration induced by 3-nitropropionic acid. *J Neurochem*. 2009;111(2):473–87.

130. Menze ET, Tadros MG, Abdel-Tawab AM, Khalifa AE. Potential neuroprotective effects of hesperidin on 3-nitropropionic acid-induced neurotoxicity in rats. *Neurotoxicology*. 2012;33(5):1265–75.

131. Wijesekera LC, Leigh PN. Amyotrophic lateral sclerosis. *Orphanet J Rare Dis*. 2009;4:3.

132. Cho H, Shukla S. Role of edaravone as a treatment option for patients with amyotrophic lateral sclerosis. *Pharmaceuticals (Basel)*. 2020;14(1):29.

133. Dinkova-Kostova AT, Kazantsev AG. Activation of Nrf2 signaling as a common treatment of neurodegenerative diseases. *Neurodegener Dis Manag*. 2017;7(2):97–100.

134. Rosen DR, Siddique T, Patterson D, Figlewicz DA, Sapp P, Hentati A, et al. Mutations in Cu/Zn superoxide dismutase gene are associated with familial amyotrophic lateral sclerosis. *Nature*. 1993;362(6415):59–62.

135. Sarlette A, Krampfl K, Grothe C, Neuhoff NV, Dengler R, Petri S. Nuclear erythroid 2-related factor 2-antioxidative response element signaling pathway in motor cortex and spinal cord in amyotrophic lateral sclerosis. *J Neuropathol Exp Neurol*. 2008;67(11):1055–62.

136. Lyras L, Cairns NJ, Jenner A, Jenner P, Halliwell B. An assessment of oxidative damage to proteins, lipids, and DNA in brain from patients with Alzheimer's disease. *J Neurochem*. 1997;68(5):2061–9.

137. Milani P, Ambrosi G, Gammoh O, Blandini F, Cereda C. SOD1 and DJ-1 converge at Nrf2 pathway: A clue for antioxidant therapeutic potential in neurodegeneration. *Oxid Med Cell Longev*. 2013;2013:836760.

138. Petrov D, Mansfield C, Moussy A, Hermine O. ALS clinical trials review: 20 Years of failure. Are we any closer to registering a new treatment? *Front Aging Neurosci*. 2017;9:68.

139. Sawada H. Clinical efficacy of edaravone for the treatment of amyotrophic lateral sclerosis. *Expert Opin Pharmacother.* 2017;18(7):735–8.
140. Korkmaz OT, Aytan N, Carreras I, Choi JK, Kowall NW, Jenkins BG, et al. 7,8-Dihydroxyflavone improves motor performance and enhances lower motor neuronal survival in a mouse model of amyotrophic lateral sclerosis. *Neurosci Lett.* 2014;566:286–91.
141. Wang TH, Wang SY, Wang XD, Jiang HQ, Yang YQ, Wang Y, et al. Fisetin exerts antioxidant and neuroprotective effects in multiple mutant hSOD1 models of amyotrophic lateral sclerosis by activating ERK. *Neuroscience.* 2018;379:152–66.
142. Xu Z, Chen S, Li X, Luo G, Li L, Le W. Neuroprotective effects of (–)-epigallocatechin-3-gallate in a transgenic mouse model of amyotrophic lateral sclerosis. *Neurochem Res.* 2006;31(10):1263–9.
143. Koh SH, Lee SM, Kim HY, Lee KY, Lee YJ, Kim HT, et al. The effect of epigallocatechin gallate on suppressing disease progression of ALS model mice. *Neurosci Lett.* 2006;395(2):103–7.
144. Vargas MR, Pehar M, Cassina P, Martínez-Palma L, Thompson JA, Beckman JS, et al. Fibroblast growth factor-1 induces heme oxygenase-1 via nuclear factor erythroid 2-related factor 2 (Nrf2) in spinal cord astrocytes: Consequences for motor neuron survival. *J Biol Chem.* 2005;280(27):25571–9.
145. Thimmulappa RK, Lee H, Rangasamy T, Reddy SP, Yamamoto M, Kensler TW, et al. Nrf2 is a critical regulator of the innate immune response and survival during experimental sepsis. *J Clin Invest.* 2006;116(4):984–95.
146. Brandes MS, Gray NE. NRF2 as a therapeutic target in neurodegenerative diseases. *ASN Neuro.* 2020;12:1759091419899782.
147. Adinew G, Messeha SS, Badisa R, Taka E, Soliman KFA. Thymoquinone anticancer effects through the upregulation of NRF2 and the downregulation of PD-L1 in MDA-MB-231 triple-negative breast cancer cells. *FASEB J.* 2022;36(Suppl. 1): 10.1096/fasebj.2022.36. S1.R2586. PMID: 35723877.
148. Ryu MJ, Kang KA, Piao MJ, Kim KC, Zheng J, Yao CW, et al. Effect of 7, 8-dihydroxyflavone on the up-regulation of Nrf2-mediated heme oxygenase-1 expression in hamster lung fibroblasts. *In Vitro Cell Dev Biol Anim.* 2014;50(6):549–54.
149. Spencer JP. Food for thought: The role of dietary flavonoids in enhancing human memory, learning and neuro-cognitive performance. *Proc Nutr Soc.* 2008;67(2):238–52.
150. Nie S, Ma K, Sun M, Lee M, Tan Y, Chen G, et al. 7,8-dihydroxyflavone protects nigrostriatal dopaminergic neurons from rotenone-induced neurotoxicity in rodents. *Parkinson's Dis.* 2019;2019:9193534.
151. Kwon Y. Luteolin as a potential preventive and therapeutic candidate for Alzheimer's disease. *Exp Gerontol.* 2017;95:39–43.
152. Nabavi SF, Braidy N, Gortzi O, Sobarzo-Sanchez E, Daglia M, Skalicka-Woźniak K, et al. Luteolin as an anti-inflammatory and neuroprotective agent: A brief review. *Brain Res Bull.* 2015;119(Pt A):1–11.
153. Pandurangan AK, Esa NM. Luteolin, a bioflavonoid inhibits colorectal cancer through modulation of multiple signaling pathways: A review. *Asian Pac J Cancer Prev.* 2014;15(14):5501–8.
154. Kitakaze T, Makiyama A, Yamashita Y, Ashida H. Low dose of luteolin activates Nrf2 in the liver of mice at start of the active phase but not that of the inactive phase. *PLoS One.* 2020;15(4):e0231403.
155. Taheri Y, Suleria HAR, Martins N, Sytar O, Beyatli A, Yeskaliyeva B, et al. Myricetin bioactive effects: Moving from preclinical evidence to potential clinical applications. *BMC Complementary Med Ther.* 2020;20(1):241.

156. Wu S, Yue Y, Peng A, Zhang L, Xiang J, Cao X, et al. Myricetin ameliorates brain injury and neurological deficits via Nrf2 activation after experimental stroke in middle-aged rats. *Food Funct.* 2016;7(6):2624–34.
157. Cho BO, Yin HH, Park SH, Byun EB, Ha HY, Jang SI. Anti-inflammatory activity of myricetin from diospyros lotus through suppression of NF-κB and STAT1 activation and Nrf2-mediated HO-1 induction in lipopolysaccharide-stimulated RAW264.7 macrophages. *Biosci Biotechnol Biochem.* 2016;80(8):1520–30.
158. Santín-Márquez R, Alarcón-Aguilar A, López-Diazguerrero NE, Chondrogianni N, Königsberg M. Sulforaphane—Role in aging and neurodegeneration. *Geroscience.* 2019;41(5):655–70.
159. Chesser AS, Ganeshan V, Yang J, Johnson GV. Epigallocatechin-3-gallate enhances clearance of phosphorylated tau in primary neurons. *Nutr Neurosci.* 2016;19(1):21–31.
160. Cascella M, Bimonte S, Muzio MR, Schiavone V, Cuomo A. The efficacy of epigallo-catechin-3-gallate (green tea) in the treatment of Alzheimer's disease: An overview of pre-clinical studies and translational perspectives in clinical practice. *Infect Agent Cancer.* 2017;12:36.
161. Park J-Y, Sohn H-Y, Koh YH, Jo C. Curcumin activates Nrf2 through PKCδ-mediated p62 phosphorylation at Ser351. *Sci Rep.* 2021;11(1):8430.
162. Tung BT, Nham DT, Hai NT, Thu DK. Chapter 10: Curcuma longa, the Polyphenolic Curcumin Compound and Pharmacological Effects on Liver. In: Watson RR, Preedy VR, editors. *Dietary Interventions in Liver Disease.* Washington, DC: Academic Press; 2019. pp. 125–34.
163. Wu J, Li Q, Wang X, Yu S, Li L, Wu X, et al. Neuroprotection by curcumin in ischemic brain injury involves the Akt/Nrf2 pathway. *PLoS One.* 2013;8(3):e59843.

Aging-Related Hearing Loss and Nrf2

5

Charles A. Lewis
Florida A&M University

Contents

Aging-related hearing loss (ARHL), also known as presbycusis, is a gradual bilateral hearing loss that commonly accompanies and is accelerated by aging. A quarter of Americans between the ages of 60 and 70 have a hearing loss of greater than 25 dBA. More than one-half of those in their seventies do, and among Americans over the age of 80, more than four out of five have 25 dBA or greater hearing loss. A 25–40 dBA hearing loss is considered a mild hearing loss. As illustrated in Figure 5.1, a greater than 40 dBA hearing loss was present in about 3% of those 50–59 years old, 7% of those in their 60s, and 19% of those in their 70s. Forty-five percent of those older than 80 years had moderate to severe hearing loss [1]. It is estimated that half a billion people worldwide suffer from hearing loss. World Health Organization data shows that the prevalence of adult-onset hearing loss is higher among people living in a band of Morocco, across North Africa and South Asia, to Micronesia. The prevalence of ARHL in India, Afghanistan, and Bangladesh is about twice that in Northern Europe and North and South Americas, suggesting a heritable impact [2]. For example, in a study performed in Turkey, individuals with the NAT2*6A allele were 15 times more likely to have ARHL [3].

DOI: 10.1201/9781003225225-5

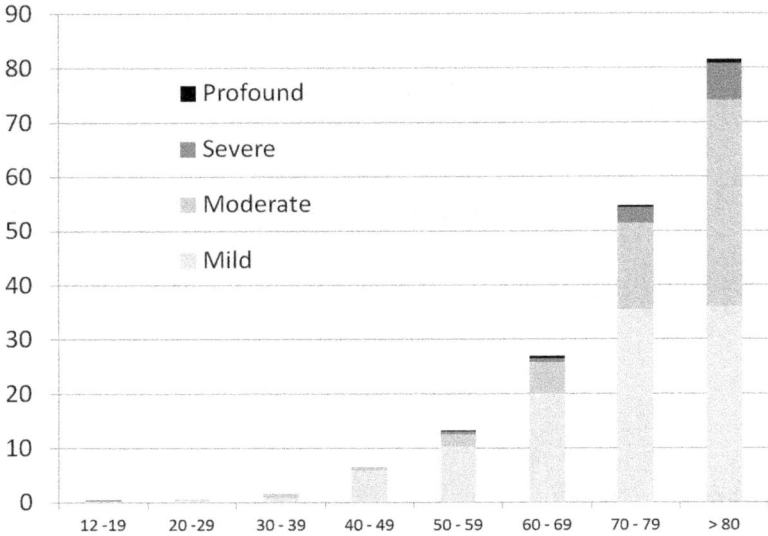

FIGURE 5.1 Hearing loss by age. Data from the 2001 to 2010 NHANES studies [1]. Mild hearing loss: 20–40 dBA loss, moderate hearing loss: >40 dB–60 dBA, severe hearing loss: >60 dBA–80 dB, profound hearing loss: >80 dBA.

N-acetyltransferase2 (NAT2) inactivates certain toxic xenobiotic compounds and aids in eliminating endogenous toxins. Other single-nucleotide polymorphisms (SNPs) are also known to affect the risk of sensorineural hearing loss (SNHL).

Figure 5.1. A graph illustrating an exponential rise in hearing loss with age. Redrawn by the author.

ARHL is dominated by hearing sound loss in the higher-pitched end of the audible sound frequency.

The frequency loss starts at the top, with high-pitch acuity lost earlier, mid-range losses later, and lower frequencies later occurring in older age. Kids can hear a 17,400 Hz sine wave tone, but this sensitivity is lost by age 18. By the age of 40, most adults cannot hear sound frequencies above 15 kHz, and by age 50, most people cannot hear a 12 kHz tone. Between the ages of 50 and 70, hearing sensitivity declines in the 3–8 kHz range, while those over 80 have their greatest loss of hearing in the lower frequencies (500–2,000 Hz). Men have a greater loss in the upper frequencies and at an earlier age than women, likely due to increased occupational and recreational noise exposure [4]. In non-industrialized societies, women and men have similar levels of ARHL [5]. In some animal models, females have milder degeneration of the stria vascularis of the cochlea than do males, but no differences in the survival of hair cells were found between male and female animals [6].

Figure 5.2 shows hearing loss by frequency at different ages and by gender. The high-pitched frequency is more severely affected, and there is more loss with increasing age. The graph shows that men have more severe hearing loss than women with age. The source of the graph is given, adapted by the author.

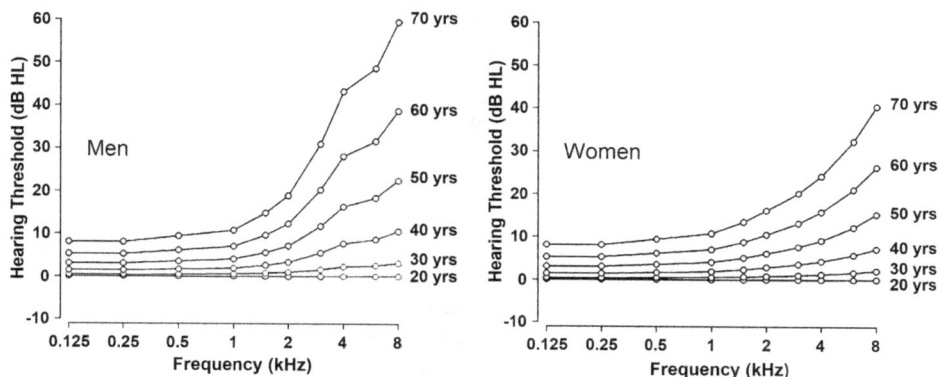

FIGURE 5.2 Average hearing loss by age. Note that age-related hearing loss is greater in the upper frequencies and among men. The hearing threshold increases in the upper frequencies more than in the lower frequencies. Data from ISO 7029 standard [7].

Hearing loss progresses into loss of the upper-middle frequencies, and speech becomes more difficult to decipher. There is a loss in the perception of certain consonants whose dominant sounds are in the upper frequencies; these include those made by the letters s, z, f, and h. This makes speech more difficult to understand. Also, the voices of women and children, being higher pitched, become more difficult to comprehend with ARHL. Thus, while older men with ARHL can hear that their wife is speaking, they have difficulty understanding what is being said, and it creates a higher cognitive load to pay attention to it. With the loss of hearing in the higher frequencies, localizing a source of sounds becomes more difficult. This makes it more difficult to decipher which sounds are salient to the current focus of the listener's attention.

As speech progressively gets more difficult to understand, it can cause isolation, depression, and hearing loss in the elderly and is associated with dementia progression [8]. In animal models, noise exposure has been demonstrated to cause cognitive decline, with tau hyperphosphorylation, the inhibition of neurogenesis, and synaptic loss; pathologic changes present in dementia [9]. There is also human evidence that noise exposure, a major cause of ARHL, promotes Alzheimer's disease.

Noise-induced injury to the middle ear is not limited to hearing. Hearing losses from ARHL, NIHL, and ototoxic agents are common, if not universally, accompanied by damage to vestibular function. Ironworkers that have NIHL have been found to have impaired vestibular function [10], as do soldiers with NIHL from the use of firearms [11]. This vestibular damage usually goes unrecognized, as individuals accommodate by increasing their reliance on visual cues, muscular proprioception, and increasing body sway, which amplifies signaling to the remaining vestibular function. Younger individuals accommodate this loss of vestibular function more easily than older adults. The loss of vestibular function, however, is not without consequence. In a study of audiology patients over the age of 60, half of those seeking treatment for hearing loss reported that they had fallen during the previous 12 months [12].

Hearing loss can be caused by conductive changes in the ear, cerumen impactions (easily reversible), thickening or injury to the tympanic membrane, or changes to the ossicles that transmit sound pressure to the inner ear. Although these are often age-related, ARHL is a different condition. Extremely loud noise can cause mechanical damage to the hair cells; it can cause a breach of the barrier between the endolymph and perilymph, exposing the hair cell population to elevated levels of potassium that can kill the cells and cause deafness. These, however, are not the typical cause of NIHL. ARHL refers to SNHL that progressively develops during aging.

ARHL appears to be intrinsic to aging laboratory animals even when aged in a quiet environment. Nevertheless, the principal ARHL injury in quiet-aged gerbils is to the stria vascularis [13]. The stria vascularis contains capillaries with pericytes (as does the blood–brain barrier, and melanocytes. The stria vascularis produces the endolymph in the scala media, which is high in potassium, in contrast to the perilymph fluid in the scala vestibuli (SV) and scala tympani (ST). The perilymph contains about 5 mM of K while the endolymph has a concentration of 150 mM of K, creating a +80 mV potential between the apex of the hair cells bathed in the endolymph, compared with their bases that are exposed to perilymph. The endolymph thus serves to generate a high resting potential (potassium/sodium gradient) used to create action potentials in the organ of Corti. The function of the stria vascularis can be inhibited with loop diuretics such as furosemide, which can cause reversible hearing loss in patients using this medication. Nevertheless, this medication can increase the risk of permanent hearing loss if the patient is also exposed to noise or ototoxic compounds.

Figure 5.3 shows a cross-sectional diagram of the cochlea, showing the placement of the organ of Corti between the ST and scala vestibule.

However, degeneration of the stria vascularis is not a principal cause of ARHL in humans. The major cause of ARHL in the general population is repetitive injury to the hair cells in the organ of Corti. This is not to say that striatal atrophy does not occur,

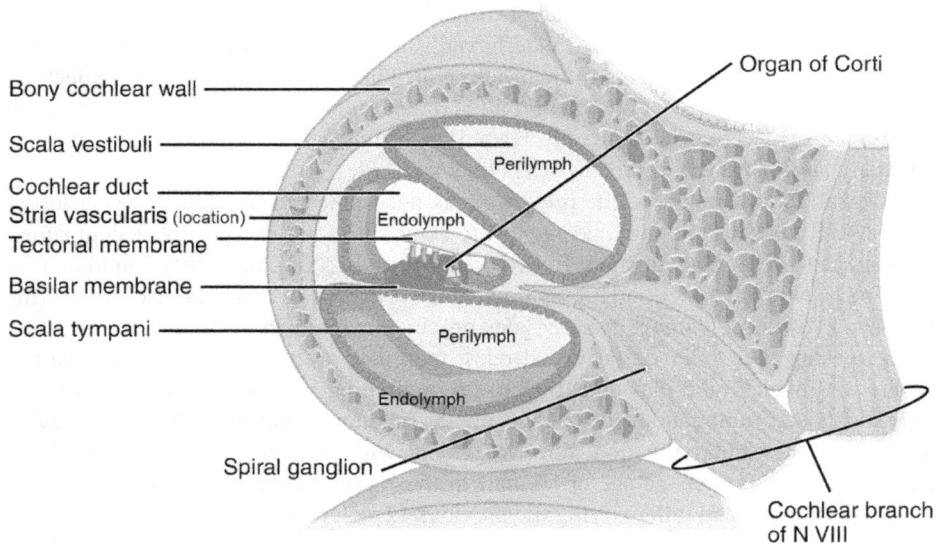

FIGURE 5.3   Diagram showing a section of the cochlea with the organ of Corti [14].

but instead that it is not typically the limiting factor causing ARHL in humans. A recent study, including postmortem histologic analysis of 120 human ears, for which most had audiographic and noise history data, found that the pattern of injury in ARHL was most consistent with noise-induced hearing loss (NIHL). The most severe injury was present in the basal half of the cochlea, with severe loss of outer hair cells (OHCs), with OHCs showing more severe loss than the inner hair cells (IHCs). In animal models of ARHL, there is minimal injury to the IHCs, and OHC loss is principally in the apex and extreme base of the cochlea. In ARHL in humans, there is considerable loss of IHCs, especially at the base of the cochlea, and massive loss of OHCs in the basal half of the cochlea with some loss at the apex in more severe cases. This human pattern is not seen in any of the rodent models of ARHL [15].

This should serve as a reminder that a search for agents to prevent ARHL in humans needs to use a model of ARHL with the same pathological pathways that occur in man. There are several different animal models of ARHL commonly used, and an immortalized mouse outer hair cell (HEI-OC1 cells) is available as an in vitro model.

Hair cells in the basal area of the cochlea are stimulated by higher-pitched frequencies, while lower-pitched frequencies activate sound perception in the apex. Sound waves from the outer ear are mechanically transferred from the tympanic membrane via the ossicles to the cochlea's oval window at the base of the SV. The SV canal spirals around 2¾ times, for a length of about 3.5 cm, to the apex where it is in open communication with the ST, rewinding down to the base to the round window. The scala media, containing the organ of Corti, is positioned between these fluid-filled chambers. The transmission of the sound pressure waves up the SV and back down the ST causes cancellation of the pressure wave except at the areas in which the frequency resonates the basal membrane and the adjacent areas of the organ of Corti. The pressure wave transmitted by the ossicle is allowed to equalize by the free movement of the membrane at the round window at the base of the ST.

Figure 5.4 shows a cross-sectional diagram of the cochlea, showing further details of the organ of the Corti.

Each human cochlea has about 3,500 IHC and 12,000 OHC in youth [16]. This is a vastly smaller number than the million photoreceptors in each eye. Hair cells in the ear are unusual because they use K influx for polarization rather than Naas do most neurons and muscle cells.

Each hair bears 30–300 stereocilia. The multiple stereocilia are fused at their apices and work in concert with each other, providing stability. Pressure waves transmitted through the organ of Corti stimulate OHC activation with elongation of the stereocilia, which vibrates the tectorial membrane. This amplifies the movement of the IHC stereocilia, causing depolarization of the IHCs activating neuronal transmission.

The OHCs both amplify and dampen the mechanical energy present in the frequencies that are transmitted to them by pressure waves carried in the perilymph, which cause resonant vibrations at different areas along the basilar membrane of the cochlea according to their pitch, with lower frequencies vibrating the basilar membrane in the apex and higher-pitched frequencies resonating the base of the cochlea. The gain is about 20 dB at low frequencies, and at higher frequencies, it is around 50–60 dB [17].

The stereocilia of the OHC extend through a rigid cuticle plate. These unusual cells are pressurized so that the stereocilia elongate when they are hyperpolarized and relax

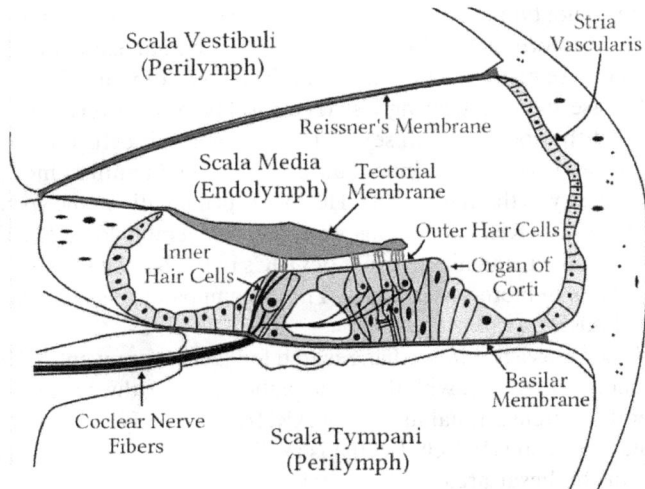

FIGURE 5.4 Cross section of the cochlea. The stria vascularis has capillaries with pericytes and melanocytes; it is not a single layer of cells as illustrated [14].

and contract when they are depolarized, pushing and pulling the tectorial membrane as they pressurize and relax. The OHC stereocilia movement of the tectorial membrane increases the motion of the stereocilia of the IHCs.

The variation in turgor within OHCs relies on intracellular pressure created by conformational changes in the transmembrane protein, prestin, which encircles the walls of these cylindrical cells. Prestin has two voltage-dependent steps, and thus three different contraction levels depend on hyperpolarization or depolarization and binding of chloride ions to prestin. The OHC can contract and relax 70,000 times per second, and by doing so, they amplify the sound wave. Salicylate, the active metabolite of aspirin, can cause reversible hearing loss by competitively inhibiting the chloride binding area of prestin, immobilizing it in its elongated state [18]. The OHCs are innervated and release the neurotransmitter acetylcholine from synapses increase amplifies these cells' motility. This allows us to actively focus our hearing so that we can actively listen to certain sound sources [19].

These OHC cells are most susceptible to NIHL and other types of hearing loss.

Depending on the direction of the motion of the IHC stereocilia, it causes or inhibits depolarization of the IHCs, which have afferent synapses with dendrites of the spiral ganglion neuron (SGN). The SGN process the stimuli and connect them with the cochlear nerves that transmit the signal to the brain.

ARHL results from the accumulation of injuries over a lifetime, with hair cell injuries being the primary lesions. OHCs have great energetic activity, which places them at greater risk for ischemic and oxidative injury than the IHCs; hair cells in humans are irreplaceable. When hair cells can be irrevocably injured by noise, toxins, ischemia-reperfusion injury, or as the result of oxidative injury, they are not replaced. Birds, reptiles, and fish, which only have IHCs, can replace damaged hair cells. Once ours are gone, there is no replacement.

Exposure to loud and percussive noise, which occurs more commonly during youth, is an important cause of injury to the cochlea. Men are more commonly exposed to loud noise from occupational exposure to machinery, military training with the live ordinance, and loud music, and thus more likely to develop NIHL. Another cause of SNHL is exposure to ototoxic compounds, including certain medications, solvents, and toxic metals. The third principal cause of ARHL is chronic oxidative injury, the susceptibility of which increases with age. Cigarette smoking and the consumption of a Western diet may contribute to oxidative stress and the progression of ARHL. Prevention of ARHL thus requires prevention of injury to the organ of Corti.

Although any cell type in the cochlea can be damaged and result in hearing loss, there are two primary lesions causing NIHL and thus ARHL. The first is injuries to the OHCs, with loss of the stereocilia, and eventually the death of these cells. Noise causes more damage in the base of the cochlea, which causes more loss to higher-pitched sound, and this loss can be detected with an audiogram. With ARHL in humans, there is typically a much greater loss of OHCs; however, most IHCs survive.

The IHCs, however, also participate in NIHL. At the base of the IHCs are organelles called synaptic ribbons. These synaptic ribbons bind and coordinate the transfer of synaptic vesicles to the synaptic cleft. The ribbons allow for an organized, rapid sequence of synaptic discharge, like a machine gun shooting directly into the synaptic cleft, thus allowing for consistent, sustained transmission of sound without tachyphylaxis or fatigue. Photoreceptor cells in the retina and the cells' vestibular system have similar synaptic ribbons. Spiral ganglion cell dendrites connect with the IHC, abutting the ribbons to form ribbon synapses.

Excessive, prolonged stimulation of the IHCs and ribbon synapse activity, especially with prolonged exposure to loud noise, can cause glutamate-induced excitotoxic injury to the dendritic receptor, causing breakage of the dendritic terminals or other degeneration of the SGN fibers; this can occur without loss of any OHCs or apparent damage to the IHCs. The SGN nerve terminals can recover. Nevertheless, the SGN soma begins to collect products of lipid peroxidation when the excessive stimuli become excitotoxic. With the repeated injury to the SGN, there can be a loss of afferent connections to the spiral ganglion cells and eventual culling of SGN cells. The loss of synaptic connections causes a degradation in hearing, referred to as "hidden" hearing loss, as it cannot be diagnosed with an audiogram. This type of hearing loss affects the entire range of hearing, degrading hearing acuity [20]. The effect of hidden hearing loss might be compared to a lens that allows light to enter the eye but blurs the image. Thus, the hidden hearing loss impairs speech-sound discrimination, making it sound garbled. Hearing aids that amplify sound can increase audition to overcome the loss of OHCs which function as sound amplifiers but do little to improve the sound processing lost with ribbon synapse and SGN loss.

Unfortunately, even though acute NIHL caused by injury to the ribbon synapses is often temporary and often recovers within a few days, this reversible hearing loss from acoustic overexposure has been found to be associated with delayed loss of afferent nerve terminals and degeneration of SGNs when assessed 2 years later [21].

Thus, in this simplified model, there are two principal types of NIHL injury, one to the OHC and the other to the ribbon synapse that leads to loss of auditory nerve fibers of the SGN. Even to 70 dB of white noise, long-term exposure appears sufficient to cause ribbon synapse injury, which causes noise-induced hidden hearing loss (NIHHL), while loud noise above 90 dB seems most responsible for OHC loss. Both of these contribute to ARHL.

The metabolic pathways for injury to the ribbon synapses involve glutamatergic excitotoxicity with an increased flux of calcium ions into the neurons, promoting activation of lytic enzymes (proteases, lipases, and endonucleases) and the production of reactive oxygen species (ROS) by the mitochondria. Failure of an injured synapse to re-uptake glutamate from the synapse may also poison nearby cells.

Unfortunately, very few human or animal studies evaluate NIHHL or other forms of ribbon synapse hearing loss. Mild to moderate ribbon synapse-related hearing loss cannot be detected with the usual tests of auditory brainstem response or distortion product otoacoustic emissions used in animal studies or audiograms used in humans. Most studies of hearing loss have not specifically looked for losses in SGN dendrite numbers, which is the best indicator of early hidden hearing loss. Thus, many human and animal studies have only sufficiently evaluated OHC injury in NIHL and ARHL, thus limiting the information available on the causation of hidden hearing loss and its mitigation.

OTOTOXIC COMPOUNDS

Ototoxic agents are an important contributor to ARHL. More importantly, understanding the mechanism of action of ototoxic agents gives us clues to understanding ARHL. Many medications pose an ototoxic risk. Aspirin notably causes tinnitus, but the effect is reversible with the withdrawal of the medication. Loop diuretics interfere with creating the potassium-sodium gradient in the endolymph of the cochlea, but this too is reversible if other injury does not occur. The most well-known ototoxic medications are aminoglycoside antibiotics and the chemotherapy drug cisplatin.

Long-term treatment with salicylate, a well-known cause of tinnitus, can also cause loss of ribbon synapse without injury to the IHCs and OHCs due to inhibition of GABAergic activity, promoting excitotoxic injury to the SGN. This causes tinnitus with hidden hearing loss [22,23].

Exposure to toxic metals such as cobalt, manganese, lead, mercury, cadmium, arsenic, and barium is associated with hearing loss, especially when combined with exposure to organic solvents and noise [24–27]. Although various metals interfere with specific enzymes or protein functions, the induction of oxidative stress is a common mechanism of injury for toxic metals, including excess iron. In a case-control study of individuals with tinnitus, plasma cadmium, manganese, and chromium levels were higher, and selenium levels were lower in those with tinnitus than controls [28].

Selenium is required for the antioxidant activity of glutathione peroxidase (GPx). In an animal model, selenium has been demonstrated to prevent aminoglycoside-induced damage to cochlear hair cells [29]. Nevertheless, sodium selenite is toxic and can activate endoplasmic reticulum (ER) stress and promote KEAP1 expression that impedes Nrf2 mediated expression of GPx and other antioxidant response element (ARE) proteins, thus inhibiting cellular stress protective mechanisms and promoting cell injury and death [30].

The solvents ethyl benzene toluene, styrene, p-xylene, and methyl ethyl ketone cause hearing loss by causing injury to the OHCs, especially those in the outermost row. The solvent trichloroethylene is ototoxic, but rather than injuring OHCs; it damages spiral ganglion cells. Many solvents also cause injury to the vestibular system [31–33]. Many ototoxic compounds have been found to have a synergistic effect with noise in causing hair cell loss. Thus, for example, workers exposed to both ototoxic compounds and high noise levels are at greater risk of hearing loss.

Cigarettes, alcohol abuse, and malnutrition increase susceptibility to hearing loss [34]. Cigarette smoking increases the risk of severe NIHL by more than sevenfold [35,36].

CISPLATIN

The cancer chemotherapeutic agent cisplatin has been extensively studied as an ototoxic agent, as it needs to be used in such high doses to be effective against cancer that it causes hearing loss in many patients. Eighty percent of patients completing a course of chemotherapy with cisplatin have a hearing loss of at least 20 dB, and 40% suffer from tinnitus. In one patient series, 78% of children receiving 120 mg/m of cisplatin in 1 day suffered hearing loss, compared with 30% of children that had the dose split over 2 days [37]. Sixty-three percent of children were found to have a hearing threshold over 40 dB after cisplatin chemotherapy [38], and hearing loss continues to progress after the end of treatment [39]. Children younger than five were more than 20 times more susceptible to cisplatin ototoxicity than children over the age of 15 [40]. These children suffer from this loss of hearing for their entire life.

Cisplatin accumulates in and is toxic to the spiral ganglion cells, the stria vascularis, and the organ of Corti; however, the hair cells are particularly susceptible to cisplatin injury [41]. Cisplatin induces oxidative stress and the production of hydrogen peroxide (H_2O_2) and causes the depletion of glutathione and SOD [42]. An In vitro study of cisplatin used in HEI-OC1 auditory hair cells found that cisplatin induces the expression of NADPH oxidase (NOX). Complete inhibition of this enzyme prevented hair cell death from cisplatin, giving survival levels on par with untreated cells. NADPH oxidases are enzyme complexes that assemble and activate the outward-facing cellular membrane. The NOX complex produces H_2O_2 in the cytosol of the cell. NOX acts in the phagosomes in neutrophils, catalyzing the production of superoxide free radicals used to kill bacteria and fungi the neutrophils have captured. NOX is constitutively inactive but assembles into an active complex in the cell membrane during certain cell stress signaling, creating ROS and reactive nitrogen species (RNS) [43].

The NOX protein complex components p47 and p67 (a.k.a. neutrophil cytosol factors 1 and 2) of NOX1 and NOX4 were specifically more highly expressed and transported from the cytosol to the NOX membrane complex in cisplatin-treated HEI-OC1 hair cells. TNF causes the phosphorylation of these p47 and p67, which activates NOX1 and NOX4. Blocking TNF also attenuated cisplatin-induced NOX activation. DPI[1] and apocynin, compounds that block the assembly or activity of NOX, prevented OHC death in mouse cochlear explants, with DPI demonstrated to be more effective than apocynin in preventing hair cell loss. Etanercept, a biologic agent that blocks TNF, was able to attenuate cisplatin-induced NOX1 and NOX4 in the cochlea of mice, preventing injury to the organ of Corti [44].

Cisplatin thus activates TNF and other proinflammatory cytokines (e.g., IL-6 and IL1β) that promote the activation of NOXs, via MEK1/ERK. NOX creates reactive oxygen species that cause damage resulting in hair cell injury and death. Moreover, the compound sodium thiosulfate has been demonstrated to reduce cisplatin-induced hearing loss by about 50% in some small trials [45].

NOISE-INDUCED HEARING LOSS

Figure 5.5 shows electron micrograph images of the organ of Corti hair cells. On the left, intact, orderly hair cells can be seen with neat rows of stereocilia. On the right is the organ of Corti from an individual that had a severe hearing loss; most of the outer and many of the IHC stereocilia are missing.

In Wistar rats exposed to 8–12 kHz noise at 100 dB or 110 dB, 24 hours per day for 8–10 weeks, there was cochlear injury, hearing loss, and the induction of the NADPH

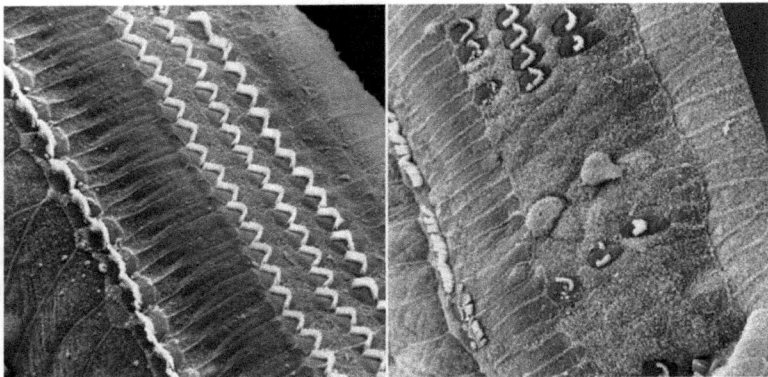

FIGURE 5.5   On the left, healthy hair cells in a section of the organ of Corti; on the right, damaged hair cells. The triple row of hair cells, each with a chevron of stereocilia, are the outer hair cells that mechanically amplify the sound pressure waves. The single row of hair cells in the inner hair cells transform sound vibrations into nerve impulses relayed by the spiral ganglion neurons to the cochlear nerve. Note in the image on the right the greater loss of outer hair cells compared with inner hair cells [46].

---

[1] Diphenyleneiodonium chloride (DPI) inhibits the assembly of the NADPH oxidase complex. The mechanism of action for the inhibition of NOX by apocynin has not been determined.

oxidase enzymes NOX1 and DUOX2, while NOX3 was downregulated, compared with rats exposed to ambient noise (45–55 dB). Pretreatment with DPI mitigated the NIHL [47]. Another investigation found an increase in Nox3 expression in the OHCs of mice exposed to cisplatin > aging > noise exposure [48]. These data suggest that while NOX participates in it, it may not be a principal cause of NIHL.

It should be noted that some studies used octave band noise. This is different from the effect of white noise, which is noise with the power distributed across the audible spectrum, or pink noise, which is like white noise but with a descending power into the higher frequencies. Octave band noise concentrates the power into a single octave. It, thus, can cause more injury to the hearing in that octave than noise evenly distributed across 10 octaves, the human hearing range. Narrowband or even more, a pure sine wave at a signal frequency of similar dB power would easily cause significantly more injury to a smaller area of the cochlea. If white noise is analogous to full-spectrum white light, a single-frequency sine wave is like a laser beam. Narrowband noise concentrates injury to the OHCs that respond to that frequency range.

Sound, even at levels that are not uncomfortable, can cause hearing loss. Rats exposed to 70–85 dB SPL of octave band noise for 6 hours a day for 3 months had spiral ganglion neuronal degeneration to cells in the receptive area for the sound, even though IHCs and OHCs survived. Accumulations of lipofuscin-like aggregates were present in the cytoplasm of the surviving cochlear neurons, suggesting oxidative stress and lipid peroxidation [49]. These results are frightening when one considers that levels below 85 dBA are regarded as safe, and OSHA's permissible exposure limit is 90 dBA for an 8-hour day.

Another study induced cochlear ribbon synapse injury with long-term exposure to 70 dB of white noise 8 hour a day for up to 3 months. There were hearing losses in the animals due to disruption of ribbon synapses caused by glutamate excitotoxicity and activation of the NLRP3 inflammasome. Both the IHCs and OHCs were left intact. However, ribbon synapses were lost in the IHCs, auditory nerve fibers and damage to the SGN cells [50].

Thus, "hidden" NIHL, using the mouse as a model, occurs with long-term exposure to 70 dB of white noise. After short-term exposure to loud noise sufficient to cause injury, there can be temporary threshold shift with tinnitus, hearing loss, ear pain, and other symptoms, which may be recovered in hours to a few days. Short-term exposure to loud noise can cause a temporary hearing loss that may be recovered. As with traumatic brain injury, if another injury occurs before healing can occur, there is less chance for recovery and a higher risk of more severe permanent injury. If loud noise exposure recurs or is chronic, the risk of permanent hearing damage increases [51].

Noise has been found to increase malondialdehyde (MDA) in the cochlea of rats. MDA is a marker of oxidation resulting in lipid peroxidation. Lower superoxide dismutase (SOD) activity was also found in the cochlea of the noise-exposed rats. Noise increases the expression of TGF-β1 (transforming growth factor β1), prestin, and HSP-70 in the rat cochlea. Pre-noise administration of a low dose of the flavonoid myricetin was able to attenuate the noise-induced changes in gene expression and oxidative status induced by noise [52]. The lower dose, 5 mg/kg, was more effective than the 10 mg/kg dose of myricetin, suggesting a hormetic effect. Unfortunately, these doses did not prevent permanent hearing loss in the animals used in this model of NIHL [53].

NIHL is primarily caused by oxidative injury. With oxidative stress, toxic metabolites such as 4-hydroxynonenal (4-HNE) are formed. Glutathione transferase (GST) participates in the detoxification of 4-HNE and other oxidation products. GST binds certain waste products to glutathione, allowing them to be exported from the cell via MPR2 (ABCC2). Thus, GST protects the ear from cochlear aging and ototoxicity [54].

AGING AND HEARING LOSS

Mitochondrial dysfunction is a common cause of oxidative injury. Mitochondria become inefficient and leak ROS with senescence. Mitochondrial DNA (mtDNA) only encodes 13 mitochondrial proteins, with the other proteins in the mitochondria being encoded in the nuclear DNA. This separation helps protect the survival of the mitochondria, as it is the site of high oxidative activity and thus exposes the mtDNA to high oxidative risk. mtDNA is at higher risk of damage, as it is not protected by histones, as is nuclear DNA. As the mitochondria and their DNA get damaged by ROS, they become less efficient and further increase ROS generation, in a vicious cycle in which there is increasing ROS generation and oxidative damage.

In health, mitochondria undergo fusion and fission, where they merge into large, sometimes branched mitochondria, share copies of the mtDNA, and then bud off into small mitochondria. Newly budded mitochondria that get defective copies of mtDNA are weak and leak ROS. This causes a cascade of events under which the effete mitochondria are eliminated in a process called mitophagy. Meanwhile, the new mitochondria with good-quality DNA survive the Darwinian pressure and live on to create clean energy and healthy progeny. This selective pressure on the mitochondria is essential for the survival of post-mitotic cells such as neurons and auditory hair cells that cannot be replaced. As we age, the process of fission, fusion, and culling becomes less efficient.

In a study of archival cochlear tissue samples from elderly persons with and without ARHL, patients with presbycusis had 2.25 times the frequency of mtDNA deletions as did those with typical age-related hearing levels [55]. In another study, patients with ARHL were found to have fewer copies of mtDNA in their peripheral white blood cells, and lower mtDNA copy numbers were associated with more severe hearing loss [56].

The mtDNA is inherited from an animal's mother, and there is a passive drift (one mutation every 8,000 years) in mtDNA, which can be used to assess maternal lineage. There are over 20 common mtDNA haplogroups. An Australian study of ARHL and mtDNA haplogroups found that individuals with haplogroup U mitochondria were 63% more likely to develop moderate to severe ARHL, and those with the haplogroup K were at three times the risk. ARHL severity was further increased in this study with other known risk factors such as noise exposure and diabetes [57]. Another study has found that mutations in the control region of the mtDNA were more common in individuals with ARHL. Mutations in this area can reduce the number of mtDNA copies in the mitochondria and thus put downward pressure on mitophagy and on maintaining the stability of mtDNA [58].

A 30% lifetime caloric restriction in rats prevents mtDNA damage and reduces age-related hearing loss. Supplementation with the antioxidant vitamins C and E also mitigated these changes less efficiently than caloric restriction [59]. In animal models, the antioxidant alpha-lipoic acid is more effective than vitamin E in preventing acoustic trauma-induced hearing loss [60]. Alpha-lipoic acid has also been found to reduce age-related hearing deterioration; acetyl-carnitine improved auditory thresholds and both compounds reduced mtDNA age-related deletions in an animal model [61]. In another study, 50 mg/kg of L-carnitine daily was effective in lowering presbycusis in rats [62], equivalent to about 500 mg of L-carnitine for a 60 kg adult man. L-carnitine protects the ear from NIHL by protecting the mitochondria from oxidative damage, including damage to the mtDNA [63].

The sugar D-galactose is sometimes used to accelerate the process of aging in lab animals. D-galactose can be used to induce oxidative stress and to age in fruit flies [64]. Generally, D-galactose (D-gal) is used as a model of accelerated aging by injecting it subcutaneously into mice or rats daily. For example, injection of 500 mg/kg/day for 8 weeks in rats at the age of 2 months will accelerate aging and thus promote the development of age-related diseases across the animal's life span. It causes oxidative stress, mitochondrial dysfunction, cognitive decline, and ARHL typical of aging. A rat treated with D-gal for 2 months during youth has the mitochondrial function at age 10 months (young adult) similar to that of an untreated rat at 16 months (late adulthood), and by 16 months has the functioning of an elderly rat.

D-gal treatment has been found to promote certain common deletions (CDs) in the mtDNA and significantly reduce mitochondrial base excision repair capacity in the inner ear of D-gal-treated rats compared with those of D-gal-treated rats' controls. Mitochondrial transcription factor A was over-expressed in D-gal-treated animals; this stimulates mtDNA replication and number. Thus, D-gal promotes increased mtDNA replication while reducing its repair capacity [65]. This should be a recipe for disaster; more replications with less repair cause more uncorrected errors. With more mtDNA deletions, there is a decline in mitochondrial efficiency, an increase in oxidative injury, and the development of presbycusis in these animals. A study specifically investigating mtDNA base pair deletions in the middle ear of rats caused by D-gal found that the 4,834 bp deletion comprised two-thirds of all mtDNA deletions in the inner ear of rats and that all four of the most CDs involved cytochrome c oxidase subunit III (COX3) [66]. MtDNA 4,834 bp deletion, abnormal ultrastructure, and cell apoptosis in the auditory cortex were also found in naturally aged geriatric rats and the D-gal age-accelerated rats [67].

The D-gal-treated rats were also found to have a decreased expression of Sirt3. Sirt3 is a mitochondrial NAD-dependent deacetylase. D-gal treatment was associated with an increased association of MnSOD2 (manganese superoxide dismutase) acetylation, which decreases MnSOD activity and reduces ROS clearance.

When cochlear basement membranes, including the organ of Corti, were harvested from juvenile mice, and cultured in growth media with varying concentrations of D-gal, there were dose-dependent increases in mitochondrial superoxide activity, caspase-3 expression, and mtDNA 3,860 bp deletions. The mtDNA 3,860 bp deletions are related to aging in mice and correspond to the 4,977 bp "CD" in human aging and the 4,834 bp deletion in aging rats [68,69]. Furthermore, culturing the cochlear basement membrane cells with D-galactose causes a dose-dependent increase in CD mutations, a decline in ATP production and mitochondrial membrane potential, and a loss of hair cell stereocilia. D-galactose causes dose-dependent breakage and degeneration of the stereocilia and, at higher doses, induces hair cell apoptosis. D-galactose also causes a dose-dependent loss in the number of IHC ribbon synapses, with 82% fewer ribbon synapses present in the high-D-galactose than the control group [70].

D-galactose treatment increased the expression of NOX2 and H_2O_2 levels in the ventral cochlear nucleus (VCN) of rats. NADPH oxidase subunits P22, P47, and P67 were increased. D-gal treatment caused increased cytochrome c (Cyt c) translocation to the cytoplasm and activation of caspase-3. 8-OHdG, a marker of DNA damage due to oxidative stress, was elevated compared with untreated animals [71]. When D-gal-treated rats were treated with apocynin, an NADPH oxidase inhibitor, it reduced H_2O_2 levels, mtDNA CD, 8-OHdG expression; and increased GPx and SOD activity in the VCN of D-gal-treated rats. Apocynin treatment decreased P47, TNF, and uncoupling protein 2 (UCP2); inhibited Cyt c translocation from the mitochondria to the cytosol, and suppressed caspase 3 in the VCN of the D-gal-treated animals [72].

D-gal was found to activate the NLRP3 inflammasome in mice [50]. The NLRP3 inflammasome is also activated by mitochondrial ROS and RNS [73], extracellular ATP, advanced glycation end products (AGEs), PAMPs, and DAMPs [74]. Several of these explain the loss of hearing associated with aging, and the reactivity to PAMPs may explain the hearing loss after certain infections such as influenza. Excitotoxicity may indirectly injure other SGN due to NLRP3 inflammasome activation, the production of caspase 1, and the increase in hyperexcitability within the spiral ganglion [75,76] (Figure 5.6).

ARHL may be accelerated by a high-fat diet (HFD). Two-month-old rats were randomly assigned into 2×2 groupings, with half were placed on a HFD and the other half a normal chow diet (ND); half of the animals in each group were treated with injected D-gal for 8 weeks, and the animals stayed on a diet for 12 months. Hearing loss was greatest in the upper frequencies, and hearing loss was greatest for the HFD-D-gal rats > ND-D-gal > HFD > ND rats. The Unfolded protein UCP2 and UCP3 levels were lowest in the ND < ND-D-gal < HFD < HFD-D-gal-treated rats. The HFD-D-gal-treated rats had about 3.5 times the NOX3 protein expression as did the other three groups, which all had similar levels. The relative amount of the CD in mtDNA was elevated in both the HFD and ND-D-gal rats and even higher in the HFD-D-gal-treated rats. The most striking finding of this study was the profound increase in activated caspase-3 levels associated with the HFD and D-galactose. The cleaved caspase-3 levels in the inner ear were 16.7 times higher in the HFD group, 36.5 times higher in the D-gal group, and 64.8 times higher in the HFD + D-gal-treated groups than in the 14-month-old control rats consuming a normal chow diet [77].

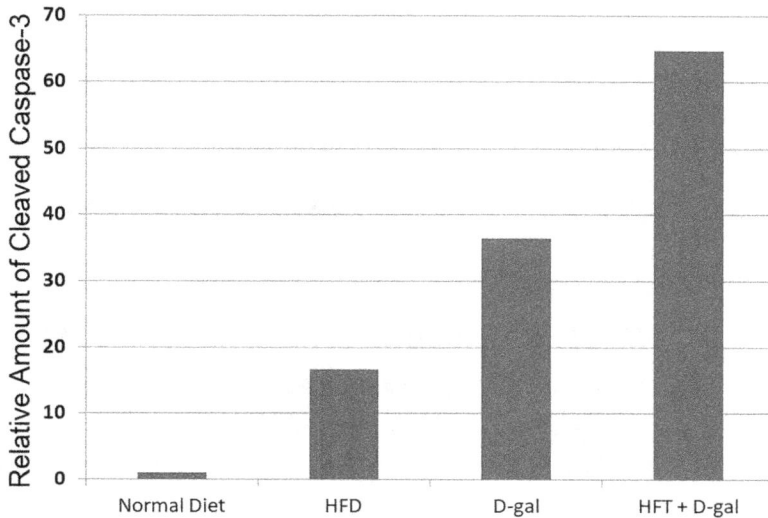

FIGURE 5.6 The relative amounts of cleaved caspase-3 in the inner ear of animals on a normal diet compared with a high-fat diet (HFD) and those treated with D-galactose or both D-gal and HFD.

The gradual rise of cytosolic Keap1 in the auditory cortex of rats with age was greater among the rats treated with D-gal at 4, 10, and 16 months and was accompanied by an accelerated decline in Nrf2 in those treated with D-gal. Along with it, there were reductions in the Nrf2-induced enzymes MnSOD, NQO1, and HO-1, assessed as representative ARE proteins. Using an Nrf2 activating agent inhibited auditory cortex cell apoptosis and delayed senescence [78].

MnSOD protects the mitochondria from ROS, NQO1 catalyzes the reduction of quinones that otherwise create ROS, and HO-1 produces the gasotransmitter CO from heme, which can stimulate neuronal repair and the production of neuroprotective proteins. At low levels, HO-1 promotes tau and α-synuclein degradation, which helps protect the neuron, but in oxidative stress, HO-1 can participate in neurodegeneration [79]. At physiological concentration, CO acts as a gasotransmitter that activates Nrf2, promoting the ARE, and prevents glutamate-induced excitotoxicity. Nevertheless, at higher levels, CO alone or in combination with other agents can activate NF-κB promoting an inflammatory reaction, and at still higher levels, CO can activate AP-1 and apoptosis [80].

Several proteins are differentially expressed in the cochlea with hearing loss during aging in mice. Glutathione peroxidase 6 (Gpx6); thioredoxin reductase 1 (Txnrd1); isocitrate dehydrogenase 1 (Idh1); and heat shock protein 1, Hspb1 [81]. GPX6 and TXNRD1 are important antioxidant system enzymes, with GPX6 recycling oxidized glutathione (GSSH) back into glutathione (2 GSH) and TXNRD1 recycling thioredoxin (Trx). IDH1 converts isocitrate$+$NADP to $\rightleftharpoons$ {\displaystyle\rightleftharpoons} to ttt2-oxoglutarate$+CO_2+$NADPH$+$H. NADPH is required for GPX, TXNRD, and NOX activity. Hspb1 (HSP 27) is expressed under cellular stress and is located at the cuticle plate at the attachment of the roots of the stereocilia; with aging, the expression of Gpx6 increases. The expression of Txnrd1 and Idh1 fell with aging and was more limited among animals with severe hearing loss. Hspb1 fell with aging but was increased in old mice with severe hearing loss.

Hyperuricemia [82,83] and gout are risk factors for ARHL [84]. The enzyme xanthine oxidase (XO) converts hypoxanthine to xanthine plus H_2O_2 and converts xanthine to uric acid plus H_2O_2. Thus, XO promotes the creation of ROS. The medication allopurinol inhibits XO and has been found to attenuate NIHL in animal models.

MOLECULAR INJURY PATHWAYS IN AGING-RELATED HEARING LOSS

Noise-induced OHC injury has a different initiating mechanism for injury from that which occurs in the ribbon synapses, but the molecular pathways converge in how they cause oxidative injury.

Overstimulation of the OHCs depletes energy and antioxidants within the hair cells. The injury may be similar to reperfusion injury wherein NO reacts with superoxide to produce peroxynitrite. Peroxynitrite attacks cell membrane lipids and proteins, damaging the stereocilia and OHCs. During the injury, calcium levels rise in the hair cells. Sufficient calcium influx can cause Cyt C release from the mitochondria and promote apoptosis.

With excessive exposure to noise, the hair cell becomes exhausted. Calcium ions are released from the cell's ER. This may occur from the depletion of glutathione in the ER or energy depletion, and it results in the unfolded protein response (UPR). Animals exposed to noise were found to have lower cochlear levels of GSH and higher GSSG: GSH ratios, documenting the depletion of GSH antioxidant capacity by noise exposure [85].

In the ER, ER oxidoreductin-1α (ERO1α) interacts with protein disulfide isomerase (PDI) to form double sulfide bonds essential to protein folding and post-translational protein modification. As a byproduct of this process, ERO1α generates H_2O_2. This H_2O_2 is then consumed by oxidoreductase enzymes such as GPx, peroxiredoxin, and ascorbate peroxidase. However, in ischemia, energy deficits, or under oxidative stress, these agents can fail to rid the ER of H_2O_2, creating signaling for the UPR. The UPR promotes energy conservation with autophagy and downregulation of protein transcription.

During oxidative stress in the ER, ERO1α is activated by CHOP and causes IP3R-mediated Ca leakage. Hypoxia can also induce ERO1α by way of HIF-1. The ototoxic metal cobalt can also induce ERO1α activity [86]. The calcium release from the ER also activates Ca sensing kinase CaMKII in the cytosol, which induces NOX activation [87]. The ER is the major source of ROS in the cell. Cisplatin induces oxidative stress and apoptosis through ROS production independent of the mitochondria [88], from the ER.

Notably, noise-induced injury of the OHCs appears to follow as a similar cascade of events as does aminoglycoside ototoxicity to the hair cells. Aminoglycoside ototoxicity causes the release of Ca2 from the ER via the inositol-1,4,5-trisphosphate receptor

(IP_3R) channels which provide direct uptake of Ca to mitochondria, which are tethered to the ER. The uptake of Ca by the mitochondria is via voltage-dependent anion channels (VDAC1) in the outer mitochondrial membrane [89]. While low calcium levels enhance mitochondrial production of ATP, high levels can cause a toxic overload that disrupts the electron transport chain, causing loss of mitochondrial transmembrane potential. This initiates a proteolytic sequence causing ROS production and release and the leakage of cytochrome c [90]. Cytochrome c in the cytosol can activate caspase 3 and thus initiate apoptosis.

Noise similarly causes ER stress, the release of Ca with uptake by the mitochondria, loss of mitochondrial membrane potential, loss of mitochondrial glutathione, the leaking of protons, loss of ATP production, and leakage of Cyt c. The influx of Ca into the mitochondria causes an increase in ROS and RNS, with further stimulates the activation of NADPH oxidase and thus promotes the even greater formation of free radicals and the formation of peroxynitrite (ONOO−) lipid peroxides and other toxic compounds in the cell. ROS can activate NF-κB and AP-1, the inflammatory cascade, and promote apoptosis.

The elevation in ROS and RNS induced by noise exposure can persist in the cochlea for 6–10 days after noise exposure. Some lipid peroxidation products, such as isoprostanes, are vasoactive and can potentially lead to reduced cochlear blood flow, further compromising oxygenation and cochlear metabolism, putting it at risk of ischemia-reperfusion injury. Noise has also been found to activate the JNK-MAPK pathway [91].

UPR-mediated Nrf2 activation can also limit or inhibit the inflammatory response caused by excessive ROS. Under ER stress, Nrf2 is phosphorylated by PERK, causing dissociation from KEAP1 and the migration of Nrf2 to the nucleus, promoting the transcription of antioxidant proteins. Nrf2 also represses the transcription of certain pro-oxidant proteins, including TXNIP (thioredoxin interacting protein). A P62/SQSTM1 complex also binds KEAP1 promoting Nrf2-dependent gene expression.

Nrf2 AND THE PREVENTION OF HEARING LOSS

The mechanisms by which Nrf2 is activated and the description of its transcriptional targets have been extensively reviewed in other chapters. Thus, they will not be detailed here, except where Nrf2 is specific to the ear and hearing loss.

Nrf2 is expressed in the human cochlea, at a higher concentration in the organ of Corti, especially in the hair cells and in Hensens' cells which act as support cells for the hair cells. Nrf2 was not detected in the SGN. In the hair cells, Nrf2 was found in the cytoplasm but was present in the nuclei of some specimens. There was a decrease in the presence of Nrf2 in cochlear specimens from autopsies of older individuals. In contrast, Nrf2 was only found in the supporting cells of the organ of Corti in normal rats and only in the cytoplasm and the cytoplasm of the SGN [92].

In a study in mice, noise exposure was found to deplete glutathione in the cochlea and increase the GSSG to GSH ratio; this effect was more pronounced in Nrf2-knockout mice. Nevertheless, noise exposure did not increase the expression of Nrf2 in the cochlea and did not increase the expression of typical Nrf2-target proteins. The use of a chemical compound that activated Nrf2 prior to noise exposure, however, increased the production of Nrf2-target antioxidant proteins and mitigated the production of 4-HNE, a product of lipid peroxidation, in the cochlea, and partially protected the mice from NIHL. Nrf2-knockout mice were highly sensitive to NIHL; they lost more hair cells and had larger shifts in threshold loss than the wild-type animals [85].

NIHL is exacerbated in lab animals with Nrf2-knockout [93,94]. In contrast, mice with an SNP that knockdown of KEAP1 function, and thus have enhanced Nrf2 transcription, were protected from oxidative injury to the cochlea and had reduced loss of OHCs and reduced threshold shifts in hearing with age. Thus, activation of Nrf2 can protect the hearing from ARHL [95].

Nrf2 may be constitutively expressed; however, oddly, noise or the effects of noise may not activate Nrf2. Nevertheless, Nrf2 appears to protect hearing from ARHL and NIHL. Nrf2 needs to be activated *before* the injury to prevent reperfusion, UPR, or oxidative stress injury to the cochlea. Noise does not appear to activate Nrf2. Nrf2 levels in humans also apparently fall with aging.

In a study of members of the Japanese Self-Defense Force, 195 of 602 soldiers were found to have hearing loss typical of NIHL, with an elevation in the hearing threshold at 4 kHz. The men were tested for the common Nrf2 SNP (rs6721961), which is located in the promoter region of the gene. The more common "G" allele is associated with a higher expression of Nrf2 mRNA than is the "T" allele of this SNP. Men with at least one T allele were 33% more likely to have NIHL [96].

In a genome-wide association study including 4,091 European Caucasians, and 1,076 patients with presbycusis, four SNPs were found to be significantly associated with ARHL; two SNPs in each of two genes, PRKCE (protein kinase Cε; PKCε), and TGFB1 (Tissue Growth Factor β1). In both these variants, the less active variant was associated with *decreased* risk of ARHL. Both these genes are members of the Nrf2 pathway [97].

Nrf2-target genes have higher expression in the cochlea of mice treated with aminoglycoside and gentamicin, and as expected, Nrf2 was not induced by this compound in Nfr2-knockout mice. In contrast, cisplatin has been demonstrated to inhibit Nrf2 expression and nuclear translocation of Nrf2 in HEI-OC1 hair cells in vitro [89].

As noted above, nutrient depletion may cause energy deficits that promote the UPR. However, less extreme deficits in glucose should inhibit KEAP1 sequestration of Nrf2 [98].

One of the Nrf2-target enzymes is heme oxidase 1 (HO-1). HO-1 has its salutary action through its release of the gasotransmitter carbon monoxide (CO), which has antioxidant, anti-apoptotic, and anti-inflammatory activity. In a study of aminoglycoside-induced ototoxicity, the aminoglycoside-induced JNK phosphorylation and pro-apoptotic signaling resulted in hair cell loss. An increased expression of HO-1, mediated by celastrol, an Nrf2-inducing agent, mitigated the loss of hair cells in the animals. When HO-1 enzymatic function was inhibited, the protective effect was lost. Incubation of the hair cells with a CO donor was also found to provide significant protection from apoptosis [99].

HO-1 primarily acts on heme from bilirubin from the breakdown of hemoglobin from RBCs that have leaked into the tissue from injury, for example. There should not be bleeding into the cochlea, other than devastating air pressure levels. The cochlea does express neuroglobin, a heme-containing protein that helps protect the CNS from transient oxygen deficits. Neuroglobin is expressed in the SGN and organ of Corti hair cell support cells but not in the hair cells. Thus, neuroglobin may be a source of heme for the production of CO in the middle ear. Neuroglobin is neuroprotective, and higher levels are expressed during oxidative stress. Levels of neuroglobin, however, were significantly lower in autopsies of persons with hearing loss [100]. Heme-containing proteins that may be sources for CO in the hair cells include Cyt c, NOXs, and certain other peroxidases, sulfite oxidase, and catalase. However, CO easily crosses the cell membrane from one cell to another.

Carbon monoxide has profound anti-inflammatory effects and downregulates the NLRP3 inflammasome [101]. CO is now an experimental treatment for sepsis [102].

At higher levels, CO is a well-known toxin. CO, at toxic levels, can injure the SGN, as it amplifies signaling and induces hypoxemia. The toxicity is mediated by glutamate excitotoxicity [103]. CO at toxic levels also amplifies noise-induced shifts in hearing threshold and injury of OHCs at the base of the cochlea. CO alone does appear to not cause permanent hearing loss [104]. The injuries are the result of CO-induced hypoxia and ROS generation, in contrast to CO acting as a local signaling molecule at physiological levels. CO binds to hemoglobin, preventing it from delivering O_2 to the tissues. CO can also bind to Cyt c in the mitochondria inhibiting oxidative phosphorylation and promoting ROS. Interestingly, the combination of noise and environmental CO exposure may increase the risk of Alzheimer's disease [105].

Some of the other enzymes induced by Nrf2 that are important to protect the cochlea include GPx, GCLC, TXNRD1, NQO1, and SOD2. As noted, Nrf2 expression in the cochlea declines with age. In mice with accelerated aging from D-gal, SOD2 expression in the cochlea was also diminished [67]. GPx catalyzes the reaction in which glutathione converts the ROS H_2O_2 into water. The enzyme glutamate-cysteine ligase (GCLC), the rate-limiting enzyme for the production of glutathione, is also upregulated by Nrf2. Thioredoxin reductase 1 (Txnrd1) reduces the redox protein thioredoxin, which acts to reduce oxidative stress.

Typically, in both NIHL and ARHL, there is a more significant injury to the basal cochlea. Limited data indicate that Nrf2 is more active in the apical and middle turns of the cochlea. For example, SOD2 expression was found to be higher in the spiral ganglion cells near the apex and lower for the SGN cells at the base of the cochlea [106]. This may explain the greater injury to the basal cochlea in ARHL. Nevertheless, the mechanical forces and metabolic demand on the OHCs may be greater in the base of the cochlea.

Nrf2 activation needs to be in place before events that induce oxidative injury to the cochlea. Constitutive Nrf2 expression/activation declines with aging, leaving the ear more susceptible to injury. In animal models, Nrf2 activators have been shown to be protective against hearing loss induced by cisplatin [89], gentamicin [100], and noise.

Only Nrf2-inducing agents that have substantial penetrance into the perilymph are likely to be effective in protecting the ear. The entry of compounds into the peri-lymph is limited, similar to the passage of compounds across the blood–brain bar-rier. The entry of molecules into the endolymph fluid is even more tightly controlled [107]. Thus, hair cell culture can help screen agents that induce Nrf2. However, only those that are bioavailable to the organ of Corti would have the potential for clinical efficacy.

Since we are aging on a daily basis, and they MUST be pre-activated before noise-induced, ototoxic, or another cochlear injury occurs, an effective Nrf2-inducing agent for preventing ARHL needs to have minimal toxicity, be highly effective, and have near-automatic compliance. For example, an ideal Nrf2 inducer for the prevention of ARHL might be one that is present in a food item that could easily be consumed on a regular basis, such as tea, coffee, or the author's favored source of anti-aging phenolic compounds, chocolate. Unfortunately, it is highly unlikely that any of these are espe-cially effective at preventing NIHL or ARHL; as if they were, NIHL and ARHL would not be so prevalent.

Several natural compounds that induce Nrf2 and which have been demonstrated in hair cell culture or in animal models to protect the cochlea from injury include sulfora-phane, curcumin, ferulic acid, ginkgolide B, rosmarinic acid, celastrol, piperine, lipoic acid, peanut sprout extract, kaempferol, and phloretin [108–112]. S-allyl mercaptocys-teine and diallyl disulfide from aged garlic and vitamin B12 were found to protect the ear from NIHL in rats. However, induction of Nrf2 was not explored in this study [113]. Medications that have been demonstrated to induce Nrf2 and offer protection from hair cell injury in animal or cell culture models of hearing loss include bucillamine, ebselen, flunarizine, and rapamycin [114–117].

While there have been several studies on the efficacy of antioxidant compounds for the prevention of hearing loss in animals, only a few studies on the use of antioxi-dants for the prevention or treatment of hearing loss or tinnitus are available in humans. Antioxidants have been found to help reduce the subjective loudness and discomfort from existing tinnitus [118]. A systematic review, including 446 published papers, found three placebo control trials on the use of antioxidants for the treatment of sudden SNHL; the use of the antioxidant vitamins and selenium increased the success of treatment [119]. ARHL is slowed with the use of oral antioxidant administration in animal models. Still, there is insufficient data from human studies to conclude that it is helpful or makes treatment recommendations [120].

Prevention of hearing loss needs to include avoidance of loud noise. Metabolic interventions need to prevent oxidative injury and damage to the mitochondria and their DNA. Loud noise causes excitotoxicity, and the UPR appears to be an intermediate pathway in most causes of SNHL. Thus, protecting the SNG nerves from excitotoxicity and the OHCs from the UPR may prevent ARHL. Compounds that induce Nrf2 can help mitigate injury by upregulating the enzymes that protect the cell from oxidative stress and glutathione depletion.

Additionally, nutrients that support the formation of glutathione, such as cysteine, perhaps best when used as a supplement in the form of acetyl-n-cysteine, may help ensure glutathione sufficiency. Selenium adequacy is essential for the function of GPx and thioredoxin reductase. R-Lipoic acid and L-carnitine (best supplemented as acetyl-l-carnitine) protect the mtDNA from oxidative damage [121,122].

Taurine as a supplement may also help protect the cochlea. Taurine reduces calcium influx into the SGN, protecting them from aminoglycoside-induced toxicity [123]. Taurine stimulates the proliferation of cochlear neural stem cells in mice [124], enhances the survival of glial cells and neurons, and enhances neurite outgrowth [125]. Taurine concentrates in the OHCs in the organ of Corti [126] and acts as a partial agonist at inhibitory glycine and GABA receptors, and thus may protect the OHCs and SGN from excitotoxicity. Taurine was found to decrease the evidence of tinnitus in noise-exposed rats and improve auditory discrimination in both taurine-treated noise-exposed and taurine-treated noise-unexposed rats [127].

Magnesium helps prevent excitotoxicity. Mg also protects the ear from NIHL [128] and helps recover after acoustic trauma [129] and idiopathic sudden SNHL hearing loss [130]. In an open-label study, Mg gave significant relief of tinnitus [131].

Finally, folate and the methionine cycle are needed for DNA repair. Several studies have found that persons with SNP alleles that reduce the function of the enzyme 5,10-methylenetetrahydrofolate reductase (MTHFR) are at increased risk of SNHL [132] and ARHL [133]. In a study of otherwise healthy women, those with lower levels of vitamin B_{12} and folate had greater ARHL [134] and tinnitus [135], and folate supplementation appeared to slow the rate of hearing loss [136]. However, vitamin B12 administration after the injury is not effective in treating tinnitus [137]. Since those with genetic alleles for reduced MTHFR are at increased risk of SNHL, the use of the natural, active form of folate, L-5-MTHF (levomefolic acid), should be more effective, at least for those with allelic variants that impair the conversion of folic acid to MTHF.

REFERENCES

1. Goman AM, Lin FR. Prevalence of hearing loss by severity in the United States. *Am J Public Health.* 2016 Oct;106(10):1820–2. doi: 10.2105/AJPH.2016.303299. Epub 2016 Aug 23. PMID: 27552261; PMCID: PMC5024365.
2. *Data from Death and DALY Estimates for 2004 by Cause for WHO Member States (Persons, All Ages)* (2009-11-12), WHO. http://www.who.int/entity/healthinfo/global_burden_disease/gbddeathdalycountryestimates2004.xls.
3. Unal M, Tamer L, Doğruer ZN, Yildirim H, Vayisoğlu Y, Camdeviren H. N-acetyltransferase 2 gene polymorphism and presbycusis. *Laryngoscope.* 2005 Dec;115(12):2238–41. doi: 10.1097/01.mlg.0000183694.10583.12. PMID: 16369173.
4. Wiley TL, Chappell R, Carmichael L, Nondahl DM, Cruickshanks KJ. Changes in hearing thresholds over 10 years in older adults. *J Am Acad Audiol.* 2008 Apr;19(4):281–92; quiz 371. doi: 10.3766/jaaa.19.4.2. PMID: 18795468; PMCID: PMC2802451.

5. Goycoolea MV, Goycoolea HG, Farfan CR, Rodriguez LG, Martinez GC, Vidal R. Effect of life in industrialized societies on hearing in natives of Easter Island. *Laryngoscope.* 1986 Dec;96(12):1391–6. doi: 10.1288/00005537-198612000-00015. PMID: 3784745.
6. Balogová Z, Popelář J, Chiumenti F, Chumak T, Burianová JS, Rybalko N, Syka J. Age-related differences in hearing function and cochlear morphology between male and female fischer 344 rats. *Front Aging Neurosci.* 2018 Jan 4;9:428. doi: 10.3389/fnagi.2017.00428. PMID: 29354051; PMCID: PMC5758597.
7. Wang J, Puel JL. Presbycusis: An update on cochlear mechanisms and therapies. *J Clin Med.* 2020 Jan 14;9(1):218. doi: 10.3390/jcm9010218. PMID: 31947524; PMCID: PMC7019248.
8. Peracino A, Pecorelli S. The epidemiology of cognitive impairment in the aging population: Implications for hearing loss. *Audiol Neurootol.* 2016;21(Suppl. 1):3–9. doi: 10.1159/000448346. Epub 2016 Nov 3. PMID: 27806351.
9. Nadhimi Y, Llano DA. Does hearing loss lead to dementia? A review of the literature. *Hear Res.* 2021 Mar 15;402:108038. doi: 10.1016/j.heares.2020.108038. Epub 2020 Jul 30. PMID: 32814645.
10. Kilburn KH, Warshaw RH, Hanscom B. Are hearing loss and balance dysfunction linked in construction iron workers? *Br J Ind Med.* 1992 Feb;49(2):138–41. doi: 10.1136/oem.49.2.138. PMID: 1536822; PMCID: PMC1012079.
11. Juntunen J, Matikainen E, Ylikoski J, Ylikoski M, Ojala M, Vaheri E. Postural body sway and exposure to high-energy impulse noise. *Lancet.* 1987 Aug 1;2(8553):261–4. PMID: 2886727.
12. Criter RE, Honaker JA. Falls in the audiology clinic: A pilot study. *J Am Acad Audiol.* 2013 Nov–Dec;24(10):1001–5. PMID: 24384085.
13. Gratton MA, Schulte BA. Alterations in microvasculature are associated with atrophy of the stria vascularis in quiet-aged gerbils. *Hear Res.* 1995 Jan;82(1):44–52. doi: 10.1016/0378-5955(94)00161-i. PMID: 7744712.
14. *Image Modified from Wikimedia Creative Commons*, OpenStax. https://cnx.org/contents/FPtK1zmh@8.25:fEI3C8Ot@10/Preface.
15. Wu PZ, O'Malley JT, de Gruttola V, Liberman MC. Age-related hearing loss is dominated by damage to inner ear sensory cells, not the cellular battery that powers them. *J Neurosci.* 2020 Aug 12;40(33):6357–66. doi: 10.1523/JNEUROSCI.0937-20.2020. Epub 2020 Jul 20. PMID: 32690619; PMCID: PMC7424870.
16. Sendowski I. Magnesium therapy in acoustic trauma. *Magnes Res.* 2006 Dec;19(4):244–54. PMID: 17402292.
17. Schmiedt RA. Chapter 2: The physiology of cochlear presbycusis. In Sandra Grodon S et al. (eds.), *The Aging Auditory System.* New York: Springer, 2010. ISBN: 978-1-4419-0993-0.
18. Homma K, Dallos P. Evidence that prestin has at least two voltage-dependent steps. *J Biol Chem.* 2011 Jan 21;286(3):2297–307. doi: 10.1074/jbc.M110.185694. Epub 2010 Nov 11. PMID: 21071769; PMCID: PMC3023524.
19. Frolenkov GI. Regulation of electromotility in the cochlear outer hair cell. *J Physiol.* 2006 Oct 1;576(Pt 1):43–8. doi: 10.1113/jphysiol.2006.114975. Epub 2006 Aug 3. PMID: 16887876; PMCID: PMC1995623.
20. Shi L, Chang Y, Li X, Aiken S, Liu L, Wang J. Cochlear synaptopathy and noise-induced hidden hearing loss. *Neural Plast.* 2016;2016:6143164. doi: 10.1155/2016/6143164. Epub 2016 Sep 21. PMID: 27738526; PMCID: PMC5050381.
21. Kujawa SG, Liberman MC. Adding insult to injury: Cochlear nerve degeneration after "temporary" noise-induced hearing loss. *J Neurosci.* 2009 Nov 11;29(45):14077–85. doi: 10.1523/JNEUROSCI.2845-09.2009. PMID: 19906956; PMCID: PMC2812055.
22. Zhang W, Peng Z, Yu S, Song QL, Qu TF, He L, Liu K, Gong SS. Loss of cochlear ribbon synapse is a critical contributor to chronic salicylate sodium treatment-induced tinnitus without change hearing threshold. *Neural Plast.* 2020 Jul 25;2020:3949161. doi: 10.1155/2020/3949161. PMID: 32774354; PMCID: PMC7397434.

23. Sheppard A, Hayes SH, Chen GD, Ralli M, Salvi R. Review of salicylate-induced hearing loss, neurotoxicity, tinnitus and neuropathophysiology. *Acta Otorhinolaryngol Ital.* 2014 Apr;34(2):79–93. PMID: 24843217; PMCID: PMC4025186.
24. Roth JA, Salvi R. Ototoxicity of divalent metals. *Neurotox Res.* 2016 Aug;30(2):268–82. doi: 10.1007/s12640-016-9627-3. Epub 2016 May 3. PMID: 27142062.
25. Castellanos MJ, Fuente A. The adverse effects of heavy metals with and without noise exposure on the human peripheral and central auditory system: A literature review. *Int J Environ Res Public Health.* 2016 Dec 9;13(12):1223. doi: 10.3390/ijerph13121223. PMID: 27941700; PMCID: PMC5201364.
26. Li X, Ohgami N, Yajima I, Xu H, Iida M, Oshino R, Ninomiya H, Shen D, Ahsan N, Akhand AA, Kato M. Arsenic level in toenails is associated with hearing loss in humans. *PLoS One.* 2018 Jul 5;13(7):e0198743. doi: 10.1371/journal.pone.0198743. PMID: 29975704; PMCID: PMC6033376.
27. Ohgami N, Mitsumatsu Y, Ahsan N, Akhand AA, Li X, Iida M, Yajima I, Naito M, Wakai K, Ohnuma S, Kato M. Epidemiological analysis of the association between hearing and barium in humans. *J Expo Sci Environ Epidemiol.* 2016 Sep;26(5):488–93. doi: 10.1038/jes.2015.62. Epub 2015 Oct 14. PMID: 26464097.
28. Atila NE, Atila A, Kaya Z, Bulut YE, Oner F, Topal K, Bayraktutan Z, Bakan E. The role of manganese, cadmium, chromium and selenium on subjective tinnitus. *Biol Trace Elem Res.* 2021 Aug;199(8):2844–50. doi: 10.1007/s12011-020-02420-4. Epub 2020 Oct 9. PMID: 33037493.
29. Chang J, Choi J, Rah YC, Yoo MH, Oh KH, Im GJ, Lee SH, Kwon SY, Park HC, Chae SW, Jung HH. Sodium selenite acts as an otoprotectant against neomycin-induced hair cell damage in a zebrafish model. *PLoS One.* 2016 Mar 14;11(3):e0151557. doi: 10.1371/journal.pone.0151557. PMID: 26974429; PMCID: PMC4790947.
30. Palsamy P, Bidasee KR, Shinohara T. Selenite cataracts: Activation of endoplasmic reticulum stress and loss of Nrf2/Keap1-dependent stress protection. *Biochim Biophys Acta.* 2014 Sep;1842(9):1794–805. doi: 10.1016/j.bbadis.2014.06.028. Epub 2014 Jul 2. PMID: 24997453; PMCID: PMC4293018.
31. Rabinowitz PM, Galusha D, Slade MD, Dixon-Ernst C, O'Neill A, Fiellin M, Cullen MR. Organic solvent exposure and hearing loss in a cohort of aluminium workers. *Occup Environ Med.* 2008 Apr;65(4):230–5. doi: 10.1136/oem.2006.031047. Epub 2007 Jun 13. PMID: 17567727.
32. Hodgkinson L, Prasher D. Effects of industrial solvents on hearing and balance: A review. *Noise Health.* 2006 Jul–Sep;8(32):114–33. doi: 10.4103/1463-1741.33952. PMID: 17704602.
33. Mohammadi S, Labbafinejad Y, Attarchi M. Combined effects of ototoxic solvents and noise on hearing in automobile plant workers in Iran. *Arh Hig Rada Toksikol.* 2010 Sep;61(3):267–74. doi: 10.2478/10004-1254-61-2010-2013. PMID: 20860967.
34. Van Eyken E, Van Camp G, Fransen E, Topsakal V, Hendrickx JJ, Demeester K, Van de Heyning P, Mäki-Torkko E, Hannula S, Sorri M, Jensen M, Parving A, Bille M, Baur M, Pfister M, Bonaconsa A, Mazzoli M, Orzan E, Espeso A, Stephens D, Verbruggen K, Huyghe J, Dhooge I, Huygen P, Kremer H, Cremers CW, Kunst S, Manninen M, Pyykkö I, Lacava A, Steffens M, Wienker TF, Van Laer L. Contribution of the N-acetyltransferase 2 polymorphism NAT2*6A to age-related hearing impairment. *J Med Genet.* 2007 Sep;44(9):570–8. doi: 10.1136/jmg.2007.049205. Epub 2007 May 18. PMID: 17513527; PMCID: PMC2597944.
35. Pouryaghoub G, Mehrdad R, Mohammadi S. Interaction of smoking and occupational noise exposure on hearing loss: A cross-sectional study. *BMC Public Health.* 2007 Jul 3;7:137. doi: 10.1186/1471-2458-7-137. PMID: 17605828; PMCID: PMC1925081.
36. Mohammadi S, Mazhari MM, Mehrparvar AH, Attarchi MS. Cigarette smoking and occupational noise-induced hearing loss. *Eur J Public Health.* 2010 Aug;20(4):452–5. doi: 10.1093/eurpub/ckp167. Epub 2009 Nov 3. PMID: 19887518.

37. Lewis MJ, DuBois SG, Fligor B, Li X, Goorin A, Grier HE. Ototoxicity in children treated for osteosarcoma. *Pediatr Blood Cancer.* 2009 Mar;52(3):387–91. doi: 10.1002/pbc.21875. PMID: 19061216.
38. Brock PR, Maibach R, Childs M, Rajput K, Roebuck D, Sullivan MJ, Laithier V, Ronghe M, Dall'Igna P, Hiyama E, Brichard B, Skeen J, Mateos ME, Capra M, Rangaswami AA, Ansari M, Rechnitzer C, Veal GJ, Covezzoli A, Brugières L, Perilongo G, Czauderna P, Morland B, Neuwelt EA. Sodium thiosulfate for protection from cisplatin-induced hearing loss. *N Engl J Med.* 2018 Jun 21;378(25):2376–85. doi: 10.1056/NEJMoa1801109. PMID: 29924955; PMCID: PMC6117111.
39. Bertolini P, Lassalle M, Mercier G, Raquin MA, Izzi G, Corradini N, Hartmann O. Platinum compound-related ototoxicity in children: Long-term follow-up reveals continuous worsening of hearing loss. *J Pediatr Hematol Oncol.* 2004 Oct;26(10):649–55. PMID: 15454836.
40. Li Y, Womer RB, Silber JH. Predicting cisplatin ototoxicity in children: The influence of age and the cumulative dose. *Eur J Cancer.* 2004 Nov;40(16):2445–51. doi: 10.1016/j.ejca.2003.08.009. PMID: 15519518.
41. Pang J, Xiong H, Zhan T, Cheng G, Jia H, Ye Y, Su Z, Chen H, Lin H, Lai L, Ou Y, Xu Y, Chen S, Huang Q, Liang M, Cai Y, Zhang X, Xu X, Zheng Y, Yang H. Sirtuin 1 and autophagy attenuate cisplatin-induced hair cell death in the mouse cochlea and zebrafish lateral line. *Front Cell Neurosci.* 2019 Jan 14;12:515. doi: 10.3389/fncel.2018.00515. PMID: 30692914; PMCID: PMC6339946.
42. Sheth S, Mukherjea D, Rybak LP, Ramkumar V. Mechanisms of cisplatin-induced ototoxicity and otoprotection. *Front Cell Neurosci.* 2017 Oct 27;11:338. doi: 10.3389/fncel.2017.00338. PMID: 29163050; PMCID: PMC5663723.
43. Herb M, Gluschko A, Wiegmann K, Farid A, Wolf A, Utermöhlen O, Krut O, Krönke M, Schramm M. Mitochondrial reactive oxygen species enable proinflammatory signaling through disulfide linkage of NEMO. *Sci Signal.* 2019 Feb 12;12(568):eaar5926. doi: 10.1126/scisignal.aar5926. PMID: 30755476.
44. Kim HJ, Lee JH, Kim SJ, Oh GS, Moon HD, Kwon KB, Park C, Park BH, Lee HK, Chung SY, Park R, So HS. Roles of NADPH oxidases in cisplatin-induced reactive oxygen species generation and ototoxicity. *J Neurosci.* 2010 Mar 17;30(11):3933–46. doi: 10.1523/JNEUROSCI.6054-09.2010. PMID: 20237264; PMCID: PMC6632278.
45. Yu D, Gu J, Chen Y, Kang W, Wang X, Wu H. Current strategies to combat cisplatin-induced ototoxicity. *Front Pharmacol.* 2020 Jul 3;11:999. doi: 10.3389/fphar.2020.00999. PMID: 32719605; PMCID: PMC7350523.
46. *Electron Micrograph Courtesy of the House Ear Institute*, Los Angeles, California.
47. Vlajkovic SM, Lin SC, Wong AC, Wackrow B, Thorne PR. Noise-induced changes in expression levels of NADPH oxidases in the cochlea. *Hear Res.* 2013 Oct;304:145–52. doi: 10.1016/j.heares.2013.07.012. Epub 2013 Jul 27. PMID: 23899412.
48. Mohri H, Ninoyu Y, Sakaguchi H, Hirano S, Saito N, Ueyama T. Nox3-derived superoxide in cochleae induces sensorineural hearing loss. *J Neurosci.* 2021 May 26;41(21):4716–31. doi: 10.1523/JNEUROSCI.2672-20.2021. Epub 2021 Apr 13. PMID: 33849947; PMCID: PMC8260246.
49. Gannouni N, Lenoir M, Ben Rhouma K, El May M, Tebourbi O, Puel JL, Mhamdi A. Cochlear neuropathy in the rat exposed for an extended period to moderate-intensity noises. *J Neurosci Res.* 2015 Jun;93(6):848–58. doi: 10.1002/jnr.23567. Epub 2015 Feb 3. PMID: 25648717.
50. Feng S, Yang L, Hui L, Luo Y, Du Z, Xiong W, Liu K, Jiang X. Long-term exposure to low-intensity environmental noise aggravates age-related hearing loss via disruption of cochlear ribbon synapses. *Am J Transl Res.* 2020 Jul 15;12(7):3674–87. PMID: 32774726; PMCID: PMC7407738.

51. Parham K, Sohal M, Petremann M, Romanet C, Broussy A, Tran Van Ba C, Dyhrfjeld-Johnsen J. Noise-induced trauma produces a temporal pattern of change in blood levels of the outer hair cell biomarker prestin. *Hear Res.* 2019 Jan;371:98–104. doi: 10.1016/j.heares.2018.11.013. Epub 2018 Nov 30. PMID: 30529910.

52. Bahaloo M, Rezvani ME, Farashahi Yazd E, Zare Mehrjerdi F, Davari MH, Roohbakhsh A, Mollasadeghi A, Nikkhah H, Vafaei M, Mehrparvar AH. Effect of myricetin on the gene expressions of NOX3, TGF-β1, prestin, and HSP-70 and antioxidant activity in the cochlea of noise-exposed rats. *Iran J Basic Med Sci.* 2020 May;23(5):594–99. doi: 10.22038/IJBMS.2020.41007.9693. PMID: 32742596; PMCID: PMC7374988.

53. Bahaloo M, Rezvani ME, Farashahi Yazd E, Davari MH, Mehrparvar AH. Effect of myricetin on the prevention of noise-induced hearing loss-an animal model. *Iran J Otorhinolaryngol.* 2019 Sep;31(106):273–79. PMID: 31598494; PMCID: PMC6764812.

54. Someya S, Kim MJ. Cochlear detoxification: Role of alpha class glutathione transferases in protection against oxidative lipid damage, ototoxicity, and cochlear aging. *Hear Res.* 2021 Mar 15;402:108002. doi: 10.1016/j.heares.2020.108002. Epub 2020 May 28. PMID: 32600853; PMCID: PMC7704621.

55. Markaryan A, Nelson EG, Hinojosa R. Quantification of the mitochondrial DNA common deletion in presbycusis. *Laryngoscope.* 2009 Jun;119(6):1184–9. doi: 10.1002/lary.20218. PMID: 19358252.

56. Falah M, Houshmand M, Najafi M, Balali M, Mahmoudian S, Asghari A, Emamdjomeh H, Farhadi M. The potential role for use of mitochondrial DNA copy number as predictive biomarker in presbycusis. *Ther Clin Risk Manag.* 2016 Oct 19;12:1573–78. doi: 10.2147/TCRM.S117491. PMID: 27799778; PMCID: PMC5077262.

57. Manwaring N, Jones MM, Wang JJ, Rochtchina E, Howard C, Newall P, Mitchell P, Sue CM. Mitochondrial DNA haplogroups and age-related hearing loss. *Arch Otolaryngol Head Neck Surg.* 2007 Sep;133(9):929–33. doi: 10.1001/archotol.133.9.929. PMID: 17875861.

58. Falah M, Farhadi M, Kamrava SK, Mahmoudian S, Daneshi A, Balali M, Asghari A, Houshmand M. Association of genetic variations in the mitochondrial DNA control region with presbycusis. *Clin Interv Aging.* 2017 Mar 3;12:459–65. doi: 10.2147/CIA.S123278. PMID: 28424544; PMCID: PMC5344408.

59. Seidman MD. Effects of dietary restriction and antioxidants on presbyacusis. *Laryngoscope.* 2000 May;110(5 Pt 1):727–38. PMID: 10807352.

60. Xiong M, Lai H, Yang C, Huang W, Wang J, Fu X, He Q. Comparison of the protective effects of radix astragali, α-lipoic acid, and vitamin E on acute acoustic trauma. *Clin Med Insights Ear Nose Throat.* 2012 Nov 29;5:25–31. doi: 10.4137/CMENT.S10711. PMID: 24179406; PMCID: PMC3791952.

61. Seidman MD, Khan MJ, Bai U, Shirwany N, Quirk WS. Biologic activity of mitochondrial metabolites on aging and age-related hearing loss. *Am J Otol.* 2000 Mar;21(2):161–7. PMID: 10733178.

62. Derin A, Agirdir B, Derin N, et al. The effects of L-carnitine on presbyacusis in the rat model. *Clin Otolaryngol Allied Sci.* 2004 Jun;29(3):238–41. PMID: 15142068.

63. Kopke RD, Coleman JK, Liu J, Campbell KC, Riffenburgh RH. Candidate's thesis: Enhancing intrinsic cochlear stress defenses to reduce noise-induced hearing loss. *Laryngoscope.* 2002 Sep;112(9):1515–32. PMID: 12356659.

64. Cui X, Wang L, Zuo P, Han Z, Fang Z, Li W, Liu J. D-galactose-caused life shortening in Drosophila melanogaster and Musca domestica is associated with oxidative stress. *Biogerontology.* 2004;5(5):317–25. doi: 10.1007/s10522-004-2570-3. PMID: 15547319.

65. Zhong Y, Hu YJ, Chen B, Peng W, Sun Y, Yang Y, Zhao XY, Fan GR, Huang X, Kong WJ. Mitochondrial transcription factor: A overexpression and base excision repair deficiency in the inner ear of rats with D-galactose-induced aging. *FEBS J.* 2011 Jul;278(14):2500–10. doi: 10.1111/j.1742-4658.2011.08176.x. Epub 2011 Jun 5. PMID: 21575134.

66. Zhong Y, Hu YJ, Yang Y, Peng W, Sun Y, Chen B, Huang X, Kong WJ. Contribution of common deletion to total deletion burden in mitochondrial DNA from inner ear of d-galactose-induced aging rats. *Mutat Res.* 2011 Jul 1;712(1–2):11–9. doi: 10.1016/j. mrfmmm.2011.03.013. Epub 2011 Apr 5. PMID: 21473872.

67. Zeng L, Yang Y, Hu Y, Sun Y, Du Z, Xie Z, Zhou T, Kong W. Age-related decrease in the mitochondrial sirtuin deacetylase Sirt3 expression associated with ROS accumulation in the auditory cortex of the mimetic aging rat model. *PLoS One.* 2014 Feb 4;9(2):e88019. doi: 10.1371/journal.pone.0088019. Erratum in: *PLoS One.* 2014;9(5): e98726. PMID: 24505357; PMCID: PMC3913718.

68. Zhang SB, Maguire D, Zhang M, Zhang Z, Zhang A, Yin L, Zhang L, Huang L, Vidyasagar S, Swarts S, Okunieff P. The murine common deletion: Mitochondrial DNA 3,860-bp deletion after irradiation. *Radiat Res.* 2013 Oct;180(4):407–13. doi: 10.1667/RR3373.1. Epub 2013 Sep 23. PMID: 24059680.

69. Meissner C, Bruse P, Mohamed SA, Schulz A, Warnk H, Storm T, Oehmichen M. The 4977 bp deletion of mitochondrial DNA in human skeletal muscle, heart, and different areas of the brain: A useful biomarker or more? *Exp Gerontol.* 2008 Jul;43(7):645–52. doi: 10.1016/j.exger.2008.03.004. Epub 2008 Mar 20. PMID: 18439778.

70. Guo B, Guo Q, Wang Z, Shao JB, Liu K, Du ZD, Gong SS. D-galactose-induced oxidative stress and mitochondrial dysfunction in the cochlear basilar membrane: An in vitro aging model. *Biogerontology.* 2020 Jun;21(3):311–23. doi: 10.1007/s10522-020-09859-x. Epub 2020 Feb 5. PMID: 32026209; PMCID: PMC7196095.

71. Du Z, Yang Q, Liu L, Li S, Zhao J, Hu J, Liu C, Qian D, Gao C. NADPH oxidase 2-dependent oxidative stress, mitochondrial damage, and apoptosis in the ventral cochlear nucleus of D-galactose-induced aging rats. *Neuroscience.* 2015 Feb 12;286:281–92. doi: 10.1016/j.neuroscience.2014.11.061. Epub 2014 Dec 8. PMID: 25499316.

72. Du ZD, Yu S, Qi Y, Qu TF, He L, Wei W, Liu K, Gong SS. NADPH oxidase inhibitor apocynin decreases mitochondrial dysfunction and apoptosis in the ventral cochlear nucleus of D-galactose-induced aging model in rats. *Neurochem Int.* 2019 Mar;124:31–40. doi: 10.1016/j.neuint.2018.12.008. Epub 2018 Dec 20. PMID: 30578839.

73. Hoyt LR, Randall MJ, Ather JL, DePuccio DP, Landry CC, Qian X, Janssen-Heininger YM, van der Vliet A, Dixon AE, Amiel E, Poynter ME. Mitochondrial ROS induced by chronic ethanol exposure promote hyper-activation of the NLRP3 inflammasome. *Redox Biol.* 2017 Aug;12:883–96. doi: 10.1016/j.redox.2017.04.020. Epub 2017 Apr 25. PMID: 28463821; PMCID: PMC5413213.

74. Rathinam VA, Fitzgerald KA. Inflammasome complexes: Emerging mechanisms and effector functions. *Cell.* 2016 May 5;165(4):792–800. doi: 10.1016/j.cell.2016.03.046. PMID: 27153493; PMCID: PMC5503689.

75. Tsoka P, Barbisan PR, Kataoka K, Chen XN, Tian B, Bouzika P, Miller JW, Paschalis EI, Vavvas DG. NLRP3 inflammasome in NMDA-induced retinal excitotoxicity. *Exp Eye Res.* 2019 Apr;181:136–44. doi: 10.1016/j.exer.2019.01.018. Epub 2019 Jan 29. PMID: 30707890; PMCID: PMC6443491.

76. Meng XF, Tan L, Tan MS, Jiang T, Tan CC, Li MM, Wang HF, Yu JT. Inhibition of the NLRP3 inflammasome provides neuroprotection in rats following amygdala kindling-induced status epilepticus. *J Neuroinflammation.* 2014 Dec 17;11:212. doi: 10.1186/s12974-014-0212-5. PMID: 25516224; PMCID: PMC4275944.

77. Du Z, Yang Y, Hu Y, Sun Y, Zhang S, Peng W, Zhong Y, Huang X, Kong W. A long-term high-fat diet increases oxidative stress, mitochondrial damage, and apoptosis in the inner ear of D-galactose-induced aging rats. *Hear Res.* 2012 May;287(1–2):15–24. doi: 10.1016/j. heares.2012.04.012. Epub 2012 Apr 21. PMID: 22543089.

78. Li Y, Zhao X, Hu Y, Sun H, He Z, Yuan J, Cai H, Sun Y, Huang X, Kong W, Kong W. Age-associated decline in Nrf2 signaling and associated mtDNA damage may be involved in the degeneration of the auditory cortex: Implications for central presbycusis. *Int J Mol Med.* 2018 Dec;42(6):3371–85. doi: 10.3892/ijmm.2018.3907. Epub 2018 Oct 1. PMID: 30272261; PMCID: PMC6202109.

79. Schipper HM, Song W. A heme oxygenase-1 transducer model of degenerative and developmental brain disorders. *Int J Mol Sci.* 2015 Mar 9;16(3):5400–19. doi: 10.3390/ijms16035400. PMID: 25761244; PMCID: PMC4394483.

80. Nitti M, Piras S, Brondolo L, Marinari UM, Pronzato MA, Furfaro AL. Heme oxygenase 1 in the nervous system: Does it favor neuronal cell survival or induce neurodegeneration? *Int J Mol Sci.* 2018 Aug 1;19(8):2260. doi: 10.3390/ijms19082260. PMID: 30071692; PMCID: PMC6121636.

81. Tadros SF, D'Souza M, Zhu X, Frisina RD. Gene expression changes for antioxidants pathways in the mouse cochlea: Relations to age-related hearing deficits. *PLoS One.* 2014 Feb 28;9(2):e90279. doi: 10.1371/journal.pone.0090279. PMID: 24587312; PMCID: PMC3938674.

82. Moon IJ, Byun H, Woo SY, Gwak GY, Hong SH, Chung WH, Cho YS. Factors associated with age-related hearing impairment: A retrospective cohort study. *Medicine (Baltimore).* 2015 Oct;94(43):e1846. doi: 10.1097/MD.0000000000001846. PMID: 26512592; PMCID: PMC4985406.

83. Hamed SA, El-Attar AM. Cochlear dysfunction in hyperuricemia: Otoacoustic emission analysis. *Am J Otolaryngol.* 2010 May–Jun;31(3):154–61. doi: 10.1016/j.amjoto.2008.12.002. Epub 2009 Mar 27. PMID: 20015733.

84. Singh JA, Cleveland JD. Gout and hearing impairment in the elderly: A retrospective cohort study using the US Medicare claims data. *BMJ Open.* 2018 Aug 20;8(8):e022854. doi: 10.1136/bmjopen-2018-022854. PMID: 30127053; PMCID: PMC6104764.

85. Honkura Y, Matsuo H, Murakami S, Sakiyama M, Mizutari K, Shiotani A, Yamamoto M, Morita I, Shinomiya N, Kawase T, Katori Y, Motohashi H. NRF2 is a key target for prevention of noise-induced hearing loss by reducing oxidative damage of cochlea. *Sci Rep.* 2016 Jan 18;6:19329. doi: 10.1038/srep19329. PMID: 26776972; PMCID: PMC4726010.

86. Gess B, Hofbauer KH, Wenger RH, Lohaus C, Meyer HE, Kurtz A. The cellular oxygen tension regulates expression of the endoplasmic oxidoreductase ERO1-Lalpha. *Eur J Biochem.* 2003 May;270(10):2228–35. doi: 10.1046/j.1432-1033.2003.03590.x. PMID: 12752442.

87. Zhang Z, Zhang L, Zhou L, Lei Y, Zhang Y, Huang C. Redox signaling and unfolded protein response coordinate cell fate decisions under ER stress. *Redox Biol.* 2019 Jul;25:101047. doi: 10.1016/j.redox.2018.11.005. Epub 2018 Nov 14. PMID: 30470534; PMCID: PMC6859529.

88. Zhang W, Xiong H, Pang J, Su Z, Lai L, Lin H, Jian B, He W, Yang H, Zheng Y. Nrf2 activation protects auditory hair cells from cisplatin-induced ototoxicity independent on mitochondrial ROS production. *Toxicol Lett.* 2020 Oct 1;331:1–10. doi: 10.1016/j.toxlet.2020.04.005. Epub 2020 May 16. PMID: 32428544.

89. Bartok A, Weaver D, Golenár T, Nichtova Z, Katona M, Bánsághi S, Alzayady KJ, Thomas VK, Ando H, Mikoshiba K, Joseph SK, Yule DI, Csordás G, Hajnóczky G. IP3 receptor isoforms differently regulate ER-mitochondrial contacts and local calcium transfer. *Nat Commun.* 2019 Aug 19;10(1):3726. doi: 10.1038/s41467-019-11646-3. PMID: 31427578; PMCID: PMC6700175.

90. Esterberg R, Hailey DW, Rubel EW, Raible DW. ER-mitochondrial calcium flow underlies vulnerability of mechanosensory hair cells to damage. *J Neurosci.* 2014 Jul 16;34(29):9703–19. doi: 10.1523/JNEUROSCI.0281-14.2014. PMID: 25031409; PMCID: PMC4099547.

91. Kurabi A, Keithley EM, Housley GD, Ryan AF, Wong AC. Cellular mechanisms of noise-induced hearing loss. *Hear Res.* 2017 Jun;349:129–37. doi: 10.1016/j.heares.2016.11.013. Epub 2016 Dec 2. PMID: 27916698; PMCID: PMC6750278.

92. Hosokawa K, Hosokawa S, Ishiyama G, Ishiyama A, Lopez IA. Immunohistochemical localization of Nrf2 in the human cochlea. *Brain Res.* 2018 Dec 1;1700:1–8. doi: 10.1016/j.brainres.2018.07.004. Epub 2018 Jul 5. PMID: 29981724; PMCID: PMC6231984.

93. Ibid Reference 97.

94. Hoshino T, Tabuchi K, Nishimura B, Tanaka S, Nakayama M, Ishii T, Warabi E, Yanagawa T, Shimizu R, Yamamoto M, Hara A. Protective role of Nrf2 in age-related hearing loss and gentamicin ototoxicity. *Biochem Biophys Res Commun.* 2011 Nov 11;415(1):94–8. doi: 10.1016/j.bbrc.2011.10.019. Epub 2011 Oct 12. PMID: 22020098.

95. Oishi T, Matsumaru D, Ota N, Kitamura H, Zhang T, Honkura Y, Katori Y, Motohashi H. Activation of the NRF2 pathway in Keap1-knockdown mice attenuates progression of age-related hearing loss. *NPJ Aging Mech Dis.* 2020 Dec 14;6(1):14. doi: 10.1038/s41514-020-00053-4. PMID: 33318486; PMCID: PMC7736866.
96. Ibid Reference 97.
97. Fetoni AR, Zorzi V, Paciello F, Ziraldo G, Peres C, Raspa M, Scavizzi F, Salvatore AM, Crispino G, Tognola G, Gentile G, Spampinato AG, Cuccaro D, Guarnaccia M, Morello G, Van Camp G, Fransen E, Brumat M, Girotto G, Paludetti G, Gasparini P, Cavallaro S, Mammano F. Cx26 partial loss causes accelerated presbycusis by redox imbalance and dysregulation of Nfr2 pathway. *Redox Biol.* 2018 Oct;19:301–17. doi: 10.1016/j.redox.2018.08.002. Epub 2018 Aug 7. PMID: 30199819; PMCID: PMC6129666.
98. Chen PH, Smith TJ, Wu J, Siesser PF, Bisnett BJ, Khan F, Hogue M, Soderblom E, Tang F, Marks JR, Major MB, Swarts BM, Boyce M, Chi JT. Glycosylation of KEAP1 links nutrient sensing to redox stress signaling. *EMBO J.* 2017 Aug 1;36(15):2233–50. doi: 10.15252/embj.201696113. Epub 2017 Jun 29. PMID: 28663241; PMCID: PMC5538768.
99. Francis SP, Kramarenko II, Brandon CS, Lee FS, Baker TG, Cunningham LL. Celastrol inhibits aminoglycoside-induced ototoxicity via heat shock protein 32. *Cell Death Dis.* 2011 Aug 25;2(8):e195. doi: 10.1038/cddis.2011.76. PMID: 21866174; PMCID: PMC3181421.
100. Vorasubin N, Hosokawa S, Hosokawa K, Ishiyama G, Ishiyama A, Lopez IA. Neuroglobin immunoreactivity in the human cochlea. *Brain Res.* 2016 Jan 1;1630:56–63. doi: 10.1016/j.brainres.2015.11.002. Epub 2015 Nov 7. PMID: 26556771; PMCID: PMC4966546.
101. Chen RJ, Lee YH, Chen TH, Chen YY, Yeh YL, Chang CP, Huang CC, Guo HR, Wang YJ. Carbon monoxide-triggered health effects: The key role of the inflammasome and its crosstalk with autophagy and exosomes. *Arch Toxicol.* 2021 Apr;95(4):1141–59. doi: 10.1007/s00204-021-02976-7. Epub 2021 Feb 8. PMID: 33554280.
102. Nakahira K, Choi AM. Carbon monoxide in the treatment of sepsis. *Am J Physiol Lung Cell Mol Physiol.* 2015 Dec 15;309(12):L1387–93. doi: 10.1152/ajplung.00311.2015. Epub 2015 Oct 23. PMID: 26498251; PMCID: PMC4683310.
103. Liu Y, Fechter LD. MK-801 protects against carbon monoxide-induced hearing loss. *Toxicol Appl Pharmacol.* 1995 Jun;132(2):196–202. doi: 10.1006/taap.1995.1099. PMID: 7785048.
104. Fechter LD, Young JS, Carlisle L. Potentiation of noise induced threshold shifts and hair cell loss by carbon monoxide. *Hear Res.* 1988 Jul 1;34(1):39–47. doi: 10.1016/0378-5955(88)90049-4. PMID: 3403384.
105. Bagheri F, Rashedi V. Simultaneous exposure to noise and carbon monoxide increases the risk of Alzheimer's disease: A literature review. *Med Gas Res.* 2020 Apr–Jun;10(2):85–90. doi: 10.4103/2045-9912.285562. PMID: 32541134; PMCID: PMC7885712.
106. Ying YL, Balaban CD. Regional distribution of manganese superoxide dismutase 2 (Mn SOD2) expression in rodent and primate spiral ganglion cells. *Hear Res.* 2009 Jul;253(1–2):116–24. doi: 10.1016/j.heares.2009.04.006. Epub 2009 Apr 17. PMID: 19376215.
107. Sun W, Wang W. Advances in research on labyrinth membranous barriers. *J Otol.* 2015 Sep;10(3):99–104. doi: 10.1016/j.joto.2015.11.003. Epub 2015 Dec 1. PMID: 29937790; PMCID: PMC6002577.
108. Ma W, Hu J, Cheng Y, Wang J, Zhang X, Xu M. Ginkgolide B protects against cisplatin-induced ototoxicity: Enhancement of Akt-Nrf2-HO-1 signaling and reduction of NADPH oxidase. *Cancer Chemother Pharmacol.* 2015 May;75(5):949–59. doi: 10.1007/s00280-015-2716-9. Epub 2015 Mar 7. PMID: 25749575.
109. Fetoni AR, Paciello F, Rolesi R, Eramo SL, Mancuso C, Troiani D, Paludetti G. Rosmarinic acid up-regulates the noise-activated Nrf2/HO-1 pathway and protects against noise-induced injury in rat cochlea. *Free Radic Biol Med.* 2015 Aug;85:269–81. doi: 10.1016/j.freeradbiomed.2015.04.021. Epub 2015 Apr 30. PMID: 25936352.

110. Lee J, Jung SY, Yang KJ, Kim Y, Lee D, Lee MH, Kim DK. α-Lipoic acid prevents against cisplatin cytotoxicity via activation of the NRF2/HO-1 antioxidant pathway. *PLoS One.* 2019 Dec 26;14(12):e0226769. doi: 10.1371/journal.pone.0226769. PMID: 31877176; PMCID: PMC6932784.

111. Youn CK, Jo ER, Sim JH, Cho SI. Peanut sprout extract attenuates cisplatin-induced ototoxicity by induction of the Akt/Nrf2-mediated redox pathway. *Int J Pediatr Otorhinolaryngol.* 2017 Jan;92:61–66. doi: 10.1016/j.ijporl.2016.11.004. Epub 2016 Nov 10. PMID: 28012535.

112. Gao SS, Choi BM, Chen XY, Zhu RZ, Kim Y, So H, Park R, Sung M, Kim BR. Kaempferol suppresses cisplatin-induced apoptosis via inductions of heme oxygenase-1 and glutamate-cysteine ligase catalytic subunit in HEI-OC1 cell. *Pharm Res.* 2010 Feb;27(2):235–45. doi: 10.1007/s11095-009-0003-3. PMID: 19937094.

113. Şahin MM, Uğur MB, Karamert R, Aytekin S, Kabiş B, Düzlü M, Seymen C, Elmas Ç, Gökdoğan Ç, Ünlü S. Evaluation of effect of garlic aged extracts and vitamin B12 on noise-induced hearing loss. *Noise Health.* 2018 Nov–Dec;20(97):232–39. doi: 10.4103/nah. NAH_33_18. PMID: 31823910; PMCID: PMC6924192.

114. Li D, Zhao H, Cui ZK, Tian G. The role of Nrf2 in hearing loss. *Front Pharmacol.* 2021 Apr 12;12:620921. doi: 10.3389/fphar.2021.620921. PMID: 33912042; PMCID: PMC8072655.

115. Kim SJ, Ho Hur J, Park C, Kim HJ, Oh GS, Lee JN, Yoo SJ, Choe SK, So HS, Lim DJ, Moon SK, Park R. Bucillamine prevents cisplatin-induced ototoxicity through induction of glutathione and antioxidant genes. *Exp Mol Med.* 2015 Feb 20;47(2):e142. doi: 10.1038/emm.2014.112. PMID: 25697147; PMCID: PMC4346486.

116. So, H, Kim H, Kim Y, Kim E, Pae HO, Chung HT, Kim HJ, Kwon KB, Lee KM, Lee HY, Moon SK, Park R. Evidence that cisplatin-induced auditory damage is attenuated by down-regulation of pro-inflammatory cytokines via Nrf2/HO-1. *J Assoc Res Otolaryngol.* 2008 Sep;9(3):290–306. doi: 10.1007/s10162-008-0126-y. Epub 2008 Jun 27. PMID: 18584244; PMCID: PMC2538144.

117. Kim SJ, Park C, Han AL, Youn MJ, Lee JH, Kim Y, Kim ES, Kim HJ, Kim JK, Lee HK, Chung SY, So H, Park R. Ebselen attenuates cisplatin-induced ROS generation through Nrf2 activation in auditory cells. *Hear Res.* 2009 May;251(1–2):70–82. doi: 10.1016/j. heares.2009.03.003. Epub 2009 Mar 13. PMID: 19286452.

118. Petridou AI, Zagora ET, Petridis P, Korres GS, Gazouli M, Xenelis I, Kyrodimos E, Kontothanasi G, Kaliora AC. The effect of antioxidant supplementation in patients with tinnitus and normal hearing or hearing loss: A randomized, double-blind, placebo controlled trial. *Nutrients.* 2019 Dec 12;11(12):3037. doi: 10.3390/nu11123037. PMID: 31842394; PMCID: PMC6950042.

119. Ibrahim I, Zeitouni A, da Silva SD. Effect of antioxidant vitamins as adjuvant therapy for sudden sensorineural hearing loss: Systematic review study. *Audiol Neurootol.* 2018;23(1):1–7. doi: 10.1159/000486274. Epub 2018 Jun 22. PMID: 29929192.

120. Tavanai E, Mohammadkhani G. Role of antioxidants in prevention of age-related hearing loss: A review of literature. *Eur Arch Otorhinolaryngol.* 2017 Apr;274(4):1821–34. doi: 10.1007/s00405-016-4378-6. Epub 2016 Nov 17. PMID: 27858145.

121. Tutelyan VA, Makhova AA, Pogozheva AV, Shikh EV, Elizarova EV, Khotimchenko SA. Lipoic acid: Physiological role and prospects for clinical application. *Vopr Pitan.* 2019;88(4):6–11. Russian. doi: 10.24411/0042-8833-2019-10035. Epub 2019 Jul 15. PMID: 31722135.

122. Keshavarz-Bahaghighat H, Sepand MR, Ghahremani MH, Aghsami M, Sanadgol N, Omidi A, Bodaghi-Namileh V, Sabzevari O. Acetyl-L-carnitine attenuates arsenic-induced oxidative stress and hippocampal mitochondrial dysfunction. *Biol Trace Elem Res.* 2018 Aug;184(2):422–35. doi: 10.1007/s12011-017-1210-0. Epub 2017 Nov 30. PMID: 29189995.

123. Liu HY, Chi FL, Gao WY. Taurine modulates calcium influx under normal and oto-toxic conditions in isolated cochlear spiral ganglion neurons. *Pharmacol Rep.* 2008 Jul–Aug;60(4):508–13. PMID: 18799819.

124. Huang X, Wu W, Hu P, Wang Q. Taurine enhances mouse cochlear neural stem cells pro-liferation and differentiation to sprial gangli through activating sonic hedgehog signaling pathway. *Organogenesis.* 2018;14(3):147–57. doi: 10.1080/15476278.2018.1477462. Epub 2018 Aug 13. PMID: 30102120; PMCID: PMC6300102.

125. Rak K, Völker J, Jürgens L, Scherzad A, Schendzielorz P, Radeloff A, Jablonka S, Mlynski R, Hagen R. Neurotrophic effects of taurine on spiral ganglion neurons in vitro. *Neuroreport.* 2014 Nov 12;25(16):1250–4. doi: 10.1097/WNR.0000000000000254. PMID: 25202928.

126. Harding NJ, Davies WE. Cellular localisation of taurine in the organ of Corti. *Hear Res.* 1993 Feb;65(1–2):211–5. doi: 10.1016/0378-5955(93)90214-l. PMID: 8458752.

127. Brozoski TJ, Caspary DM, Bauer CA, Richardson BD. The effect of supplemental dietary taurine on tinnitus and auditory discrimination in an animal model. *Hear Res.* 2010 Dec 1;270(1–2):71–80. doi: 10.1016/j.heares.2010.09.006. Epub 2010 Sep 22. PMID: 20868734; PMCID: PMC2997922.

128. Scheibe F, Haupt H, Ising H. Preventive effect of magnesium supplement on noise-induced hearing loss in the guinea pig. *Eur Arch Otorhinolaryngol.* 2000;257(1):10–6. doi: 10.1007/pl00007505. PMID: 10664038.

129. Sendowski I, Raffin F, Braillon-Cros A. Therapeutic efficacy of magnesium after acoustic trauma caused by gunshot noise in guinea pigs. *Acta Otolaryngol.* 2006 Feb;126(2):122–9. doi: 10.1080/00016480500312547. PMID: 16428187.

130. Gordin A, Goldenberg D, Golz A, Netzer A, Joachims HZ. Magnesium: A new therapy for idiopathic sudden sensorineural hearing loss. *Otol Neurotol.* 2002 Jul;23(4):447–51. doi: 10.1097/00129492-200207000-00009. PMID: 12170143.

131. Cevette MJ, Barrs DM, Patel A, Conroy KP, Sydlowski S, Noble BN, Nelson GA, Stepanek J. Phase 2 study examining magnesium-dependent tinnitus. *Int Tinnitus J.* 2011;16(2):168–73. PMID: 22249877.

132. Pollak A, Mueller-Malesinska M, Lechowicz U, Skorka A, Korniszewski L, Sobczyk-Kopciol A, Waskiewicz A, Broda G, Iwanicka-Pronicka K, Oldak M, Skarzynski H, Płoski R. MTHFR 677T is a strong determinant of the degree of hearing loss among Polish males with postlingual sensorineural hearing impairment. *DNA Cell Biol.* 2012 Jul;31(7):1267–73. doi: 10.1089/dna.2012.1607. Epub 2012 Mar 16. PMID: 22424391; PMCID: PMC3391488.

133. Manche SK, Jangala M, Dudekula D, Koralla M, Akka J. Polymorphisms in folate metabo-lism genes are associated with susceptibility to presbycusis. *Life Sci.* 2018 Mar 1;196:77–83. doi: 10.1016/j.lfs.2018.01.015. Epub 2018 Jan 31. PMID: 29369772.

134. Houston DK, Johnson MA, Nozza RJ, Gunter EW, Shea KJ, Cutler GM, Edmonds JT. Age-related hearing loss, vitamin B-12, and folate in elderly women. *Am J Clin Nutr.* 1999 Mar;69(3):564–71. doi: 10.1093/ajcn/69.3.564. PMID: 10075346.

135. Lasisi AO, Fehintola FA, Lasisi TJ. The role of plasma melatonin and vitamins C and B12 in the development of idiopathic tinnitus in the elderly. *Ghana Med J.* 2012 Sep;46(3):152–7. PMID: 23661829; PMCID: PMC3645155.

136. Durga J, Verhoef P, Anteunis LJ, Schouten E, Kok FJ. Effects of folic acid supplementa-tion on hearing in older adults: A randomized, controlled trial. *Ann Intern Med.* 2007 Jan 2;146(1):1–9. doi: 10.7326/0003-4819-146-1-200701020-00003. PMID: 17200216.

137. Berkiten G, Yildirim G, Topaloglu I, Ugras H. Vitamin B12 levels in patients with tinni-tus and effectiveness of vitamin B12 treatment on hearing threshold and tinnitus. *B-ENT.* 2013;9(2):111–6. PMID: 23909117.

Nrf2 and Ocular Aging

Flavonoid and Nutraceuticals Use

6

Aaron L. Hilliard
Florida A&M University

Tanya D. Russell
University of Colorado Anschutz Medical Campus

Contents

DOI: 10.1201/9781003225225-6

INTRODUCTION

Aging is a leading cause of vision loss globally, directly resulting from numerous meta-bolic, nutritional, or environmental insults or an indirect development of ocular or sys-temic diseases [1–4]. An estimated 1 billion people worldwide have moderate to severe vision impairment or blindness due to age-related macular degeneration (AMD) (1.84 million), diabetic retinopathy (DR) (3.9 million), glaucoma (7.7 million), and cataracts (94 million) [5,6]. As aging is an inevitable process, and life expectancy continues to improve and increase the number of elderly individuals, finding improvements in mech-anisms to preserve sight from avoidable blindness is a primary focus of numerous global programs. Furthermore, vision health disparities continue to impact underrepresented ethnic groups in the United States.

Numerous studies indicate that these groups continue to have lower socioeco-nomic status and more significant burdens on health care access than the general population. Along with disproportionately being affected by cardiovascular disease, hypertension, diabetes, and cancer, Hispanic and African American patients experi-ence similar disparities in vision health. By 2040, 288 million people will be affected by AMD [7]. As socioeconomic status influences the overall prevalence of vision loss [8,9], this poses serious social and economic concerns among ethnic groups most affected.

Most type 1 diabetics and approximately 50% of people with type 2 diabetes become blind within 20 years of diabetes onset with delayed or non-treatment [10,11]. Numerous studies have demonstrated significant health disparities of DR among under-represented ethnic groups. Data from the National Health Interview indicate an ele-vated likelihood of DR among African American and Hispanic diabetics compared with whites (odds ratio of DR among blacks, 1.08; 95% CI: 0.70–1.67; odds ratio of DR among Hispanics, 1.3; 95% CI: 0.76–2.21) [10]. A study from the National Health and Nutrition Examination Survey III reported that African American and Hispanic diabetics aged 40 years and older had a higher prevalence of DR than white diabetics of the same age range [12]. The Multi-Ethnic Study of Atherosclerosis showed that the prevalence of DR was higher among African American (37%) and Hispanic (37%) dia-betic patients aged 45–85 years compared with similarly aged whites (25%) and Chinese (26%; $P=0.01$) diabetic patients [13].

African Americans and Hispanics are projected to account for 20% of glaucoma cases by 2050 [14], adding complexity to the myriad of barriers to access adequate care, education, and treatment as individuals in these populations become elders.

While studies of the prevalence of glaucoma in underrepresented patient populations are limited, the Baltimore Eye Survey in the 1990s was one of the first studies to report that African Americans had approximately 4–5 times the age-adjusted prevalence of glaucoma than that white patients [15]. Although older age is the primary risk factor for cataracts, there is evidence of an association between lower educational levels and increased rates of cataract development [16,17].

Access to and managing affordable medications is a significant concern for under-represented populations. Surgery has been a relatively successful treatment option for some age-related eye diseases, but not without problems. Surgery-associated complications may arise and unavoidably cause irreversible blindness [2,18]. Recent advances in non-surgical treatment options can lessen the impact of the progression of these diseases. However, many patients from underrepresented ethnic groups are diagnosed at advanced stages where effective treatments are no longer viable. Thus, there is an increased need to identify non-surgical, affordable therapeutics to treat and prevent age-related eye diseases.

Over 80% of the world's population relies upon traditional, natural plant-based systems of medicine such as nutraceuticals [18]. Nutraceuticals are functional foods comprised of many vitamins, antioxidants, and minerals that promote therapeutic benefits and protect against certain diseases [19]. Plant-derived polyphenols have gained attention as having beneficial nutritional properties and potent antioxidant therapeutic effects. In addition, plant-based polyphenol treatments may provide affordable, healthy options for underrepresented patient groups. Thus, the antioxidant properties of nutraceuticals such as polyphenols make them viable therapeutic agents in preventing and treating age-related eye diseases.

OXIDATIVE STRESS AND AGE-RELATED EYE DISEASES

Oxidative stress results from the imbalance between reactive oxygen species (ROS) production and the ability of antioxidants to detoxify the reactive intermediates [2,20,21]. It is an essential physiological regulator of normal cell cycle, migration, and cell death [2,22,23]. ROS are mainly short-lived and highly reactive and are induced through numerous intracellular pathways [2,24]. Oxidative stress and the decrease of antioxidant protection are two main contributors to the pathogenesis of age-related eye diseases. Recent studies have probed into the molecular details of oxidative stress involvement [2,18,21,25]. In particular, mechanisms of oxidative stress have been implicated in the activation of transcription factors such as nuclear factor (erythroid-derived 2)-like 2 (Nrf2) and Kelch-like erythroid cell-derived protein with CNC homology (ECH)-associated protein 1 (Keap1), which are both involved in the activation of cell survival and death processes [2,24] (Figure 6.1). Phase II antioxidants such as heme oxygenase one (HO-1) are regulated by the Nrf2, and overproduction of ROS leads to the suppression of Nrf2-dependent antioxidant protection [2,20,26].

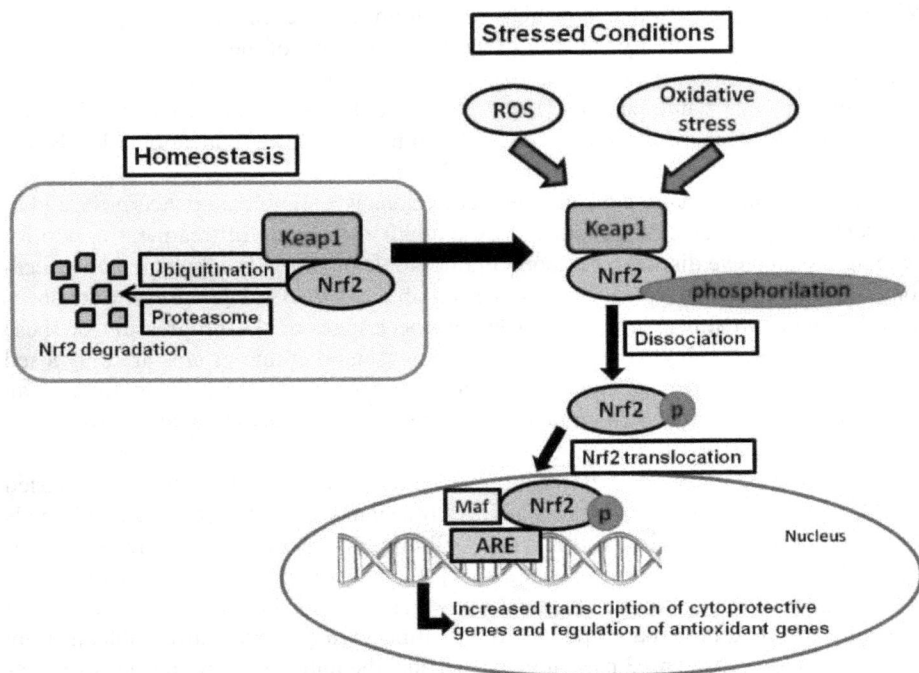

FIGURE 6.1 Keap1-Nrf2 system. The figure shows Nrf2 activation during stress conditions, which leads to the transcription of cytoprotective and antioxidant genes. Reprinted with permission from the author [24].

Oxidative Stress and Age-Related Macular Degeneration

AMD is a progressive degeneration of the underlying retinal pigment epithelium (RPE) and the retinal macula [4,27]. AMD is generally classified into early AMD, intermediate AMD, and advanced AMD [28–30]. Early AMD is characterized by small yellow or white spots known as drusen, pigment abnormalities, or increased retinal pigment deposits. Larger drusen are typically present in the intermediate AMD stage, with non-central geographic atrophy and mild vision perception impairments [28]. These attributes, along with mild vision impairments, may continue to progress over time to advanced AMD, eventually leading to blindness. Chronic oxidative stress and inflammation in the RPE are thought to play a vital role in the pathogenesis and progression of AMD. The RPE provides critical support to sustain the viability and function of the photoreceptors [31]. Its normal physiological processes are compromised during aging due to photo-oxidative stress, high oxygen tension, and excessive production and accumulation of ROS [4,28,31,32]. Elevated levels of ROS and subsequent oxidative stress and inflammatory responses lead to cell damage and apoptosis of RPE cells and photoreceptors, which contributes to retinal degeneration in AMD [4,28].

Oxidative Stress and Diabetic Retinopathy

DR results from inflammatory processes that damage blood vessels in the retina and is a significant complication of diabetes mellitus [4,33]. DR has been characterized as starting with alterations of the blood-retinal barrier permeability and vascular occlusion, leading to macular edema and tissue ischemia, then progressing to neovascular proliferation, increased ischemia, and detachment of the retina [33]. Recent studies have reported that oxidative stress plays a central role in the development and progression of DR. The diabetic retina contains high levels of ROS through numerous mechanisms, which ultimately contribute to retinal cell damage and DR pathogenesis [34,35]. ROS induces local hypoxia with upregulated mRNA expression levels of critical pro-apoptotic proteins, such as hypoxia-inducible factor 1 (HIF-1) and 50-adenosine monophosphate-activated protein kinase (AMPK) phosphorylation. Protein kinase C regulation by elevated oxidative and nitrosative stress has also been shown to contribute to ROS production, leading to DR pathogenic features in cell survival, growth, proliferation, migration, and apoptosis [33,34].

Oxidative Stress and Glaucoma

Glaucoma is a progressive optical neurodegenerative disease primarily affecting individuals older than 40 and is characterized by retinal ganglion cell (RGC) degeneration [36]. Elevated intraocular pressure (IOP) is also a common characteristic of glaucoma, a consequence of impaired aqueous humor drainage via the trabecular meshwork that leads to visual field defects and irreversible blindness due to RGC death [37–39]. Increased age is a risk factor for developing glaucoma and family history and belonging to susceptible ethnic groups [10,37,40]. Oxidative stress has been implicated in various stages of glaucomic pathogenesis. Both compromised blood flow in retinal vessels and elevated IOP lead to excessive amounts of ROS, which cause RGC death [38,41]. ROS may also stimulate apoptosis of endothelial cells that comprise the human trabecular meshwork, thus impairing the aqueous outflow pathway and increasing the IOP [4,37,42].

Oxidative Stress and Cataracts

Cataracts, opacification of the eye lens epithelia, are the leading cause of blindness worldwide. The human lens epithelium comprises the middle layer of the lens and a monolayer of metabolically active epithelial cells [2,24]. With aging, lens epithelial cells (LECs) migrate to the inner fibrous portion of the lens and transform into lens fibers, gradually compressing and forming nuclear opacity [2]. Oxidative stress may also lead to degradation and aggregation of the crystalline lens proteins, a b, and g, which comprise 90% of lens proteins, leading to opacity and cataract formation [1,2,18,24]. Glutathione, one of the most important antioxidants found in the lens, protects lens proteins against ROS such as hydrogen peroxide (H_2O_2), superoxide, and hydroxyl radicals in healthy lenses; reduced glutathione converts to its oxidized form when it reacts with ROS and is restored through the action of glutathione reductase (GSH) [18,25]. H_2O_2, a significant contributor of oxidative stress in the pathogenesis of cataracts, is generally eliminated by glutathione or through glutathione peroxidase and catalase action [18]. However, aging leads to a decrease in the activity of these protective mechanisms occurs, resulting in elevated H_2O_2 levels in the lens and ultimately LEC death and opacity [18,24].

Oxidative stress is also associated with DNA hypomethylation in the *Keap1* gene in cataracts. The loss of DNA methylation upregulates field 1 Keap1 gene expression; a demethylated *Keap1* promoter results in overexpression of *Keap1* and produces higher levels of Keap1 protein [1]. Higher level of Keap1 induces Nrf2 degradation by ubiquitin-mediated proteasomal degradation and ER-associated degradation, resulting in decreased Nrf2-dependent antioxidant protection and shifting the redox balance more toward lens oxidation [1,24,26,43–47]. Misfolded protein conformation then initiates the production of misfolded crystallin aggregation and ultimately cataract formation [1]. DNA hypomethylation in the *Keap1* promoter is close to 0% in lenses of younger individuals but is up to 40% and 50% in individuals older than 60 years of age [1,44,45]. A stress of 40%–50% loss of DNA methylation in elderly populations can increase to an average of 90% loss with cataractogenic stress in those who develop age-related cataracts, suggesting that the incidence of cataracts significantly increases with DNA hypomethylation [1,44,45].

Nrf2 AND AGE-RELATED EYE DISEASES

Nrf2 is the key controller of the redox homeostatic gene regulatory network, and the Nrf2-Keap1 complex is known as one of the main cellular defense mechanisms against oxidative stress [1,2]. Nrf2 regulates approximately 200–600 cytoprotective genes [1,48–54], serving as a vital nuclear transcriptional inducer [55] by binding to the antioxidant response element (ARE) in DNA promoters and controlling transcription of many antioxidant genes such as glutathione-S transferase, glutathione reductase, and thioredoxin [2,24,56,57]. To maintain homeostasis as an oxidative stress sensor, Keap1 serves as a primary Nrf2 inhibitor and regularly targets Nrf2 for ubiquitination and subsequent 26S proteasomal degradation to maintain basal levels of Nrf2 [2]. During unstressed conditions, Nrf2 is restricted to the cytoplasm by binding with Keap1 in a relatively rapid interaction, ensuring low basal levels of Nrf2 [1,58–60]. During stressed conditions (i.e., oxidative or endoplasmic reticulum stress), Nrf2 separates from Keap1, is phosphorylated, translocates into the nucleus, and induces ARE-controlled antioxidant gene transcription, ultimately initiating the detoxification of ROS through regulation of GSH [2,61]. Due to its ability to protect against oxidative stress, recent studies have focused attention on the potential role of Nrf2 as a therapeutic agent for age-related eye diseases.

Nrf2 and Age-Related Macular Degeneration

Due to its role as a critical regular of cellular oxidative stress, Nrf2 may be involved in AMD development. Zhao et al. developed a model for retinopathy using Nrf2-deficient mice. These mice also exhibited age-related pathologies similar to AMD, including drusen deposits, progressive RPE degeneration, and decreased electroretinography responses [31,62]. Lenox et al. demonstrated that increased activation of the unfolded protein response in aged retinas significantly decreased Nrf2 and one of its downstream targets, HO-1, resulting in increased proinflammatory markers such as RANTES [63,64]. Genetic mutations of Nrf2 have also been associated with a higher risk of AMD. Sliwinski et al. identified a mutation of Nrf2 at 25129A>C from DNA extracted from peripheral blood lymphocytes of wet and dry AMD patients, which increased the risk for AMD [63,65]. Collectively, these data indicate that the decline and impairment of Nrf2 seen in aging increase the probability of RPE damage due to oxidative stress, ultimately leading to AMD pathogenesis.

Nrf2 and Diabetic Retinopathy

Nrf2 is localized to many cell types, including numerous ocular cells, as a crucial regulator of cellular redox homeostasis. Using an immunohistochemical approach, Xu et al. demonstrated prominent Nrf2 localized to Muller cells, essential drivers of pro-inflammatory processes involved in DR progression [63,66]. This study also found a significant increase in retinal superoxide in diabetic Nrf2-deficient mice, supporting the notion that elevated glucose levels in diabetes decrease the protective effect of Nrf2 [66].

Nrf2 and Glaucoma

Nrf2 deletion mimics glaucoma pathogenesis in various models and ocular cell types. Patients with certain types of glaucoma show a 60%–70% reduction in total reactive antioxidant capacity, indicating a high susceptibility to damage from oxidative stress [67–69]. Himori et al. reported that optic nerve injury-induced RGC death was further aggravated by Nrf2 deletion [70]. Cheng et al. showed that Nrf2 expression is down-regulated in glaucomatous trabecular meshwork cells, and Nrf2 overexpression reduced apoptosis and restored cell viability [71]. Xu et al. developed Nrf2 knockout mice to study the role of Nrf2 in retinal neuroprotection from ischemia-reperfusion injury and demonstrated loss of Nrf2 activity and increased RGC loss [72]. A virus-mediated anti-oxidant gene therapy model showed that overexpression of Nrf2 effectively protected RGC from damage, degeneration, and cell death due to oxidative stress after acute nerve damage [73]. Taken together, these findings support the neuroprotective role of Nrf2 in protecting RGC and trabecular meshwork cells from oxidative stress and critical damage.

Nrf2 and Cataracts

Nrf2 has been implicated in protecting against oxidative stress in lens epithelia. Ma et al. observed that under H_2O_2-induced oxidative and ER stress, Nrf2 protects LECs with activating transcription factor 4 (ATF) and improves LEC morphology and viability

[74]. These results suggest that Nrf2 activation protects against H_2O_2-induced oxidative and ER stress in LECs, implicated in cataract formation and progression. Studies have shown significantly decreased Nrf2 gene and protein levels significantly increased Keap1 gene and protein levels, and highly elevated levels of DNA demethylation in the Keap1 promoter in cultured human LECs and aged human and diabetic cataractous lenses [2,44]. Gao et al. found DNA methylation of the *Keap1* promoter in healthy human lens and cultured LECs, suggesting that *Keap1* promoter demethylation is crucial for cataract formation [2,75]. *Keap1* promoter demethylation activates the expression of Keap1 protein, ultimately abolishing Nrf2 activity, which leads to an impaired Nrf2-dependent antioxidant system and cataract formation [2,75]. These results suggest using Nrf2 inducers as anti-cataract therapeutic compounds.

Numerous studies have also examined the potential therapeutic antioxidant and anti-inflammatory properties of Nrf2 inducers. Acetyl ester of the trimethylated amino acid L-carnitine (ALCAR) has been shown to prevent cataract formation by increasing Nrf2-regulated antioxidant proteins and decreasing ER stress-mediated proteins in homocysteine-treated cells [2,76]. Morin (3, 5, 7, 20, 40-pentahydroxyflavone) has been shown to increase the Nrf2 protein levels and stimulate the ERK-Nrf2 signaling pathway in human LECs, resulting in the upregulation of HO-1 and cytoprotective effects of Nrf2 against oxidative stress [2,77]. Plant-extracted isothiocyanate 1-isothiocyanate-4-methyl-sulfinyl butane (SFN) has also been shown as a potential anti-cataract therapeutic by increasing the activity of thioredoxin reductase (TrxR) in the mouse lens, which prevents against oxidative stress and prevents cataract formation when consumed [2]. The multi-target neuroprotective drug DL-3-n-butylphthalide (NBP) is widely used to treat ischemic stroke patients and decreases oxidative damage, increases mitochondrial function, reduces inflammation, and decreases neuronal apoptosis [2]. NBP has also been shown to increase the expression of Nrf2 in lenses of diabetic rats [2,78], and could potentially be a favorable anti-cataract therapeutic option. *Rosa laevigata Michx* (RLM) is another plant-based therapeutic option with antioxidant and free radical-scavenging capability. RLM has been examined in a model of diabetic cataracts by Liu et al. using an immortalized LEC line (SRA01/04) cultured with 5.5 mM high glucose [2,79]. RLM reduced the production of ROS and improved mitochondrial membrane potential via the stimulation of HO-1, an Nrf2-regulated gene, in hyperglycemic SRA01/04 cells, suggesting that the protective effects of RLM are controlled through the PI3K/serine-threonine kinase (AKT) and Nrf2/ARE signaling pathways [2,79].

POLYPHENOLS AS POTENTIAL THERAPIES FOR AGE-RELATED EYE DISEASES

Polyphenols have potent anti-inflammatory, anti-glycating, and antioxidant activity and are viable therapeutic options for age-related eye diseases. Polyphenols are the most abundant dietary antioxidants commonly found in fruits, vegetables, cereals, seeds, nuts, chocolate, coffee, tea, and wine [18]. With the growing interest in using food as

TABLE 6.1   Sources of polyphenols and their effect on eye diseases

POLYPHENOL	CHEMICAL STRUCTURE	DIETARY SOURCE	EFFECT ON EYE DISEASES
Resveratrol		Grapes, grape juice Wine Peanuts Cocoa Blueberries Bilberries Cranberries [80, 81]	Anti-oxidant effects on AMD pathogenesis [83, 84] Enhance oxidative markers in blood and retina in DR [80, 86] Anti-oxidative and anti-apoptotic roles in glaucoma [89] Prevent cataract formation [18, 24, 90-93]
Curcumin		Turmeric [94]	Protect cellular anti-oxidant properties in DR [94, 105-106] Suppress oxidative stress and prevent cataract formation [24, 95, 107-109]
Quercetin		Berries Apples Green tea Wine [28, 110, 111]	Protect against diabetes-induced retinal injuries [32, 112-114]
Epigallocatechin Gallate		Green tea [4]	Protect retinal neurons from high IOP in glaucoma [4, 120, 121] Anti-cataract properties [122-125]
Anthocyanins		Berries Cherries [33, 126, 127]	Prevent AMD [4, 130, 131] Prevent DR [132] Decrease IOP in glaucoma [134]

medicine, nutraceuticals made from polyphenols have gained attention in treating many chronic diseases. Recent studies have examined the therapeutic potential of several polyphenolic compounds on AMD, DR, glaucoma, and cataracts (Table 6.1).

Resveratrol

Resveratrol is a polyphenol found in grapes, red wine, grape juice, peanuts, cocoa, blueberries, bilberries, and cranberries [80,81]. Dietary resveratrol supplements from root extracts from Japanese knotweed, *Polygonum cuspidatum*, are also available. However, the safety and efficacy in preventing human diseases have yet to be fully determined [80]. Resveratrol displays anti-oxidative activity in vitro and in vivo to inhibit ROS and induce superoxide dismutase (SOD), catalase, and glutathione peroxidase 1 [82]. These properties suggest that resveratrol may be a beneficial treatment option for age-related eye diseases.

A limited number of studies have reported evidence of the anti-oxidative effects of resveratrol on AMD pathogenesis. Using an in vitro model of human RPE cells, King et al. showed that resveratrol prevents oxidative stress-induced and sodium iodate-induced apoptosis [83]. Studies have reported that resveratrol protects against cytotoxicity in human RPE by inhibiting levels of intracellular ROS via increasing SOD, glutathione peroxidase, and catalase activities [84].

Studies on human patients with AMD have also reported the benefits of resveratrol. Richer et al. reported the efficacy of Longevinex, a resveratrol dietary supplement, against AMD. They demonstrated enhanced eye structure and activity in three pants with AMD over a 2–3-year period [85].

Studies have provided evidence for resveratrol as a therapeutic option for DR. Resveratrol supplementation has been shown to significantly enhance oxidative markers in the blood and retina in diabetic rats [80,86]. Kim et al. reported that resveratrol treatment suppresses vessel leakage and pericyte loss in the retinas of diabetes-induced mice [87]. In a study investigating the ability of resveratrol to inhibit RPE cell inflammation caused by hyperglycemia, Losso et al. showed that resveratrol significantly inhibited the accumulation of proinflammatory markers such as VEGF, TGF-1, cyclo-oxygenase-2, interleukin-6, and interleukin-8 in a dose-dependent manner [88].

There is evidence that resveratrol provides anti-oxidative and anti-apoptotic roles in glaucoma.

Luna et al. reported the therapeutic effects of resveratrol in trabecular meshwork cells subjected to chronic oxidative stress [89]. Their study demonstrated that resveratrol decreased intracellular ROS production and inflammatory markers such as interleukin-1a, interleukin-6, interleukin-8, and endothelial-leukocyte adhesion molecule-1 [89]. Additionally, resveratrol could also play an anti-apoptotic role in preventing trabecular meshwork cell damage without detrimental effects on cell proliferation [89].

Resveratrol has also been shown to prevent cataract formation by suppressing apoptosis of LECs [18,24,90]. Higashi et al. showed that although resveratrol did not entirely prevent the appearance of diabetic cataracts, it did significantly delay the progression of cataracts [91]. Resveratrol was also shown to suppress increased levels of protein carbonyls, which were shown to be increased in diabetic rat lenses, suggesting that resveratrol delays the progression of diabetic cataracts by lessening oxidative damage to lens proteins [91]. Doganay et al. reported that resveratrol effectively suppressed sodium selenite-induced cataract development [92]. Zheng et al. showed that resveratrol inhibited p53-dependent apoptosis by activating sirtuin-1, thus reversing morphological damages caused by hydrogen peroxide and protecting LECs from oxidative stress via p53 pathway inhibition [93].

Curcumin

Curcumin is the water-insoluble, orange-colored pigment extracted from turmeric, the rhizome of *Curcuma longa* of the Zingiberaceae family [94]. Curcumin has been used in traditional Chinese and Ayurvedic herbal remedies for thousands of years to treat many diseases with its antioxidant and anti-inflammatory activity [95–101]. Turmeric, a well-known source of curcumin as a spice widely used in cooking, acts through various mechanisms that may scavenge ROS and reactive nitrogen species and control the activity of enzymes responsible for the neutralization of GSH, catalase, and SOD [95,102–104]. Turmeric may also inhibit enzymes that generate ROS, such as lipoxygenase/cyclooxygenase and xanthine hydrogenase/oxidase, thus exhibiting antioxidant properties [95,102].

The anti-inflammatory and antioxidant properties of curcumin have been studied as a potential therapeutic agent for DR. Experiments by Mrudula et al. demonstrated that a diet enriched with 0.01% curcumin, or 0.5% *Curcuma longa* for 8 weeks reduced VEGF expression in streptozocin-treated mice, and a 1 g of curcumin per kg of body-weight treatment over 16 weeks reduced levels of glutathione, SOD, catalase, TNF-α, and VEGF in the retina [105]. Kowluru and Kanwar reported that curcumin could either protect cellular antioxidant properties or downregulate interleukin-1β, VEGF, and NF-κB levels without inducing blood glucose levels in diabetic mice [94,106].

Curcumin has been examined in various cataract models, demonstrating its ability to suppress selenium-induced oxidative stress and delay cataract formation by inhibiting non-enzymatic antioxidant depletion in rat organ cultured lens [24,95,107]. Curcumin was also shown to slow the progression of diabetic cataracts by significantly decreasing GSH levels, preventing the alteration of protein carbonyls, glutathione peroxidase, and glucose-6-phosphate dehydrogenase (G6PD), thus preventing hyperglycemia-induced oxidative stress in rat lenses [95,108]. Cao et al. showed that curcumin attenuated selenite-induced cataract formation by reducing intracellular ROS production and protecting cells from oxidative damage [109].

Quercetin

Quercetin is a flavonoid found in berries, apples, green tea, and wine. Researchers have studied its potential as a therapeutic agent in reducing AMD occurrence and progression. It has been shown to increase the viability of ARPE-19 cells, a human RPE cell line, under H_2O_2-mediated oxidative stress by activating various cellular pro-survival mechanisms and decreasing proinflammatory cytokines interleukin-6 and interleukin-8 [28,110,111].

Quercetin has also been suggested as a treatment option for DR. It has been reported to exhibit protective action against diabetes-induced injuries in the retina by decreasing levels of ROS via attenuating high glucose-induced apoptosis and inflammation and proinflammatory molecules, MCP-1, and interleukin-6 [33,112–114]. Kumar et al. demonstrated that quercetin augmented antioxidant enzymes, GSH, SOD, and catalase and decreased TNF-a and interleukin-1 [113]. Additionally, Chen et al. found that quercetin downregulated MMP-9 and VEGF, critical proteins involved in retinal neovascularization [112].

Quercetin has been shown to protect against H_2O_2-induced cataracts and diabetes-induced retinal lesions [4,115]. Quercetin-3-D-galactoside (hyperoside) can inhibit oxidative stress by upregulating extracellular signal-regulated kinase (ERK) activity in hydrogen peroxide (H_2O_2)-treated human LECs; this increases Nrf2 expression and its antioxidant response [2,116]. Patil et al. found that quercetin was significantly effective in maintaining lens transparency and structural integrity of the glycation-induced cataractous lenses [117].

Epigallocatechin Gallate

Of the significant flavonoids present in green tea [(–)-epicatechin, (–)-epigallocatechin, (–)-epicatechin gallate, and (–)-epigallocatechin gallate] epigallocatechin gallate (EGCG), represents more than 50% of the polyphenols in green tea [4]. It has been shown to exhibit significant antioxidant properties by inhibiting ROS-generating enzymes [4]. Investigators have used both in vitro and in vivo models of age-related eye diseases to elucidate the antioxidant effects of the EGCG. Lee et al. showed that doses of EGCG at 20 and 40 mM inhibited vascular permeability, angiogenesis, and corneal neovascularization, implying a protective role of EGCG in AMD and DR [118]. Kumar et al. administered green tea supplements to diabetic rats and found increased GSH levels, SOD activities, and reduced VEGF and TNF-α values, suggesting EGCG protection of retinal vasculature and retinal endothelial cells from apoptosis [119].

Short-term EGCG supplementation with green tea leaf extract has shown favorable effects on the treatment of glaucoma by protecting retinal neurons from injuries sustained from high IOP [4,120,121]. In a double-blind, placebo-controlled study of 34 glaucoma patients (18 ocular hypertension patients and 16 open-angle glaucoma patients), EGCG showed favorable neuroprotective function noted by increased pattern electroretinogram amplitude in the open-angle glaucoma patients [121]. Zhang et al. reported that 25 mg/kg intraperitoneal or 5 µL of 200 µM intraocular administered EGCG protected retinal neurons from oxidative stress and ischemia/reperfusion [4,120].

Green tea leaf extracts and EGCG have also been associated with anti-cataract properties. Chaudhary et al. showed that tryptophan oxidation is involved in oxidative stress-mediated cataract formation and the inhibitory potential of EGCG [122–124]. Another more recent study by Chaudhury et al. investigated the fibrillar aggregation of human γB-crystallin with or without EGCG treatment using various techniques, including fluorescence and circular dichroism spectroscopy, and field emission scanning electron and high-resolution transmission electron microscopy [125]. In the presence of EGCG, a noticeable decrease in absorbance was seen, suggesting that EGCG can prevent aggregation [125]. Circular dichroism spectroscopy further monitored the secondary structural changes of γB-crystallin in the absence and presence of EGCG, with a native human γB-crystallin sample containing a mostly β-sheet secondary structure and much slighter decrease in absorption minimum at ~218 nm in the presence of EGCG suggesting that EGCG could protect protein aggregation [125]. In all, these studies indicate that EGCG prevents γB-crystallin fibrillar aggregation in stressed environments by preventing the formation of extended β-sheets [125]. These studies help further identify how to design EGCG nutraceuticals to combat cataract formation.

Anthocyanins

Berries and cherries contain high concentrations of anthocyanins, flavonoid compounds that provide natural blue, red, and purple pigmentations [33,126,127]. Anthocyanins have been shown to exhibit many beneficial attributes, including, but not limited to, antioxidant and anti-inflammatory activities, immune response regulation, and peroxidation [4,128,129]. Use of bilberry (*Vaccinium myrtillus*) extracts in human RPE cells has been shown to prevent AMD by inhibiting photooxidation of pyridinium bis-retinoid and neutralizing oxygen free radicals [4,130,131]. In vivo studies administering bilberry extract orally to streptozotocin-induced diabetic rats at a dose of 100 mg/kg for 6 weeks demonstrated prevention of DR [132], providing evidence of using a dietary bilberry supplement as a potential treatment option for AMD and DR. Song et al. reported that doses of 20, 40, and 80 mg/kg blueberry anthocyanins administered orally to streptozotocin-induced diabetic rats over 12 weeks protected retinal cells from oxidative stress and inflammation, potentially via Nrf2/HO-1 signaling [133]. Szumny et al. examined the effects of anthocyanins in dried cornelian cherries (*Cornus mas L.*) in New Zealand white rabbits aged between 6 and 12 months and showed a decrease in IOP [134], suggesting a therapeutic role of anthocyanins in glaucoma.

CONCLUSION

Aging, vision health disparities, and increased oxidative stress are the leading culprits of age-related eye diseases. The Nrf2/Keap1/ARE signaling pathway has been implicated as a significant cell defense mechanism against oxidative stresses [2,24]. Nrf2-dependent antioxidant protection by overproduction of ROS and/or DNA damage and subsequent demethylation of Keap1 is suppressed by chronic stress, which leads to Nrf2 loss and age-related eye disease development (Figure 6.2). Conventional treatment

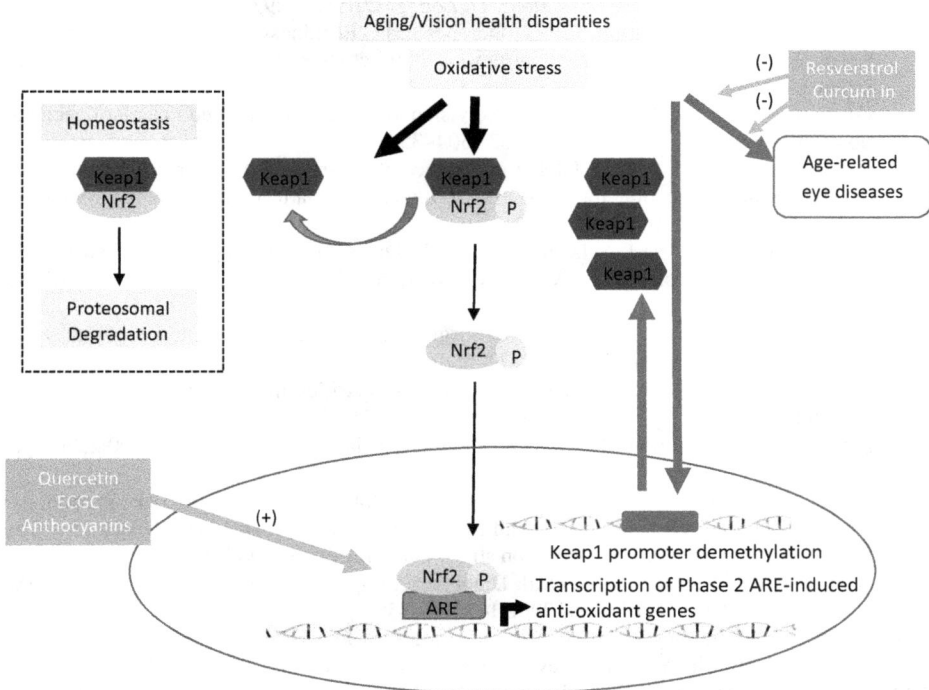

FIGURE 6.2 Effects of aging, oxidative stress, and Nrf2 activation on age-related eye diseases. Aging, vision health disparities, and oxidative stress induce or are involved in many age-related eye diseases. Polyphenols have been shown to exert protective effects and potentially prevent pathogenesis and progression of age-related macular degeneration, diabetic retinopathy, glaucoma, and cataracts.

options may be limited by accessibility and affordability and surgery-associated complications. Diet and/or healthy, plant-derived nutraceuticals may alleviate barriers as alternative treatment options for age-related eye disease. Numerous natural compounds containing polyphenols have been shown to target directly or indirectly the Nrf2/Keap1/ARE signaling pathway. Thus, dietary plans and/or supplements containing polyphenols could profoundly impact the treatment of age-related eye diseases.

REFERENCES

1. Periyasamy P, Shinohara T. Age-related cataracts: Role of unfolded protein response, Ca(2+) mobilization, epigenetic DNA modifications, and loss of Nrf2/Keap1 dependent cytoprotection. *Prog Retin Eye Res* 2017;60:1–19.
2. Liu XF, Hao JL, Xie T, et al. Nrf2 as a target for prevention of age-related and diabetic cataracts by against oxidative stress. *Aging Cell* 2017;16:934–942.
3. Harding J. Biochemistry epidemiology and pharmacology. *Cataract* 1991;195–217.
4. Bungau S, Abdel-Daim MM, Tit DM, et al. Health benefits of polyphenols and carotenoids in age-related eye diseases. *Oxid Med Cell Longev* 2019;2019:9783429.
5. World Health Organization. (2022, October 13). "Blindness and vision impairment." Retrieved from https://www.who.int/news-room/fact-sheets/detail/blindness-and-visual-impairment
6. Furtado JM, Jonas J, Peto T, et al. Global vision loss due to age-related macular degeneration. *Invest Ophthalmol Vis Sci* 2021;62:3504–3504.
7. Wong WL, Su X, Li X, et al. Global prevalence of age-related macular degeneration and disease burden projection for 2020 and 2040: A systematic review and meta-analysis. *Lancet Glob Health* 2014;2:e106–116.
8. Wang D, Jiang Y, He M, Scheetz J, Wang W. Disparities in the global burden of age-related macular degeneration: An analysis of trends from 1990 to 2015. *Curr Eye Res* 2019;44:657–663.
9. Wang W, Yan W, Fotis K, et al. Cataract surgical rate and socioeconomics: A global study. *Invest Ophthalmol Vis Sci* 2016;57:5872–5881.
10. Zambelli-Weiner A, Crews JE, Friedman DS. Disparities in adult vision health in the United States. *Am J Ophthalmol* 2012;154:S23–30.e21.
11. Fong DS, Aiello L, Gardner TW, et al. Retinopathy in diabetes. *Diabetes Care* 2004;27(Suppl 1):S84–87.
12. Harris MI, Klein R, Cowie CC, Rowland M, Byrd-Holt DD. Is the risk of diabetic retinopathy greater in non-Hispanic blacks and Mexican Americans than in non-Hispanic whites with type 2 diabetes? A US population study. *Diabetes Care* 1998;21:1230–1235.
13. Wong TY, Klein R, Islam FM, et al. Diabetic retinopathy in a multi-ethnic cohort in the United States. *Am J Ophthalmol* 2006;141:446–455.
14. Umfress AC, Brantley MA, Jr. Eye care disparities and health-related consequences in elderly patients with age-related eye disease. *Semin Ophthalmol* 2016;31:432–438.
15. Tielsch JM, Sommer A, Katz J, Royall RM, Quigley HA, Javitt J. Racial variations in the prevalence of primary open-angle glaucoma: The Baltimore Eye Survey. *JAMA* 1991;266:369–374.
16. Zhang X, Cotch MF, Ryskulova A, et al. Vision health disparities in the United States by race/ethnicity, education, and economic status: Findings from two nationally representative surveys. *Am J Ophthalmol* 2012;154:S53–62.e51.

17. West SK, Valmadrid CT. Epidemiology of risk factors for age-related cataracts. *Surv Ophthalmol* 1995;39:323–334.
18. Kaur A, Gupta V, Christopher AF, Malik MA, Bansal P. Nutraceuticals in the prevention of cataract – An evidence-based approach. *Saudi J Ophthalmol* 2017;31:30–37.
19. Rossino MG, Casini G. Nutraceuticals for the treatment of diabetic retinopathy. *Nutrients* 2019;11:771.
20. Kesic MJ, Simmons SO, Bauer R, Jaspers I. Nrf2 expression modifies influenza A entry and replication in nasal epithelial cells. *Free Radic Biol Med* 2011;51:444–453.
21. Babizhayev MA, Yegorov YE. Reactive oxygen species and the aging eye: Specific role of metabolically active mitochondria in maintaining lens function and in the initiation of the oxidation-induced maturity onset cataract – A novel platform of mitochondria-targeted antioxidants with broad therapeutic potential for redox regulation and detoxification of oxidants in eye diseases. *Am J Ther* 2016;23:e98–117.
22. Redza-Dutordoir M, Averill-Bates DA. Activation of apoptosis signalling pathways by reactive oxygen species. *Biochim Biophys Acta* 2016;1863:2977–2992.
23. Schumann C, Chan S, Khalimonchuk O, et al. Mechanistic nanotherapeutic approach based on siRNA-mediated DJ-1 protein suppression for platinum-resistant ovarian cancer. *Mol Pharm* 2016;13:2070–2083.
24. Hilliard A, Mendonca P, Russell TD, Soliman KFA. The protective effects of flavonoids in cataract formation through the activation of Nrf2 and the inhibition of MMP-9. *Nutrients* 2020;12:3651.
25. Truscott RJ. Age-related nuclear cataract: A lens transport problem. *Ophthalmic Res* 2000;32:185–194.
26. Elanchezhian R, Palsamy P, Madson CJ, et al. Low glucose under hypoxic conditions induces unfolded protein response and produces reactive oxygen species in lens epithelial cells. *Cell Death Dis* 2012;3:e301.
27. Datta S, Cano M, Ebrahimi K, Wang L, Handa JT. The impact of oxidative stress and inflammation on RPE degeneration in non-neovascular AMD. *Prog Retin Eye Res* 2017;60:201–218.
28. Parmar T, Ortega JT, Jastrzebska B. Retinoid analogs and polyphenols as potential therapeutics for age-related macular degeneration. *Exp Biol Med (Maywood)* 2020;245:1615–1625.
29. Mitchell P, Liew G, Gopinath B, Wong TY. Age-related macular degeneration. *Lancet* 2018;392:1147–1159.
30. Ferris FL, 3rd, Wilkinson CP, Bird A, et al. Clinical classification of age-related macular degeneration. *Ophthalmology* 2013;120:844–851.
31. Lambros ML, Plafker SM. Oxidative stress and the Nrf2 antioxidant transcription factor in age-related macular degeneration. *Adv Exp Med Biol* 2016;854:67–72.
32. Liguori I, Russo G, Curcio F, et al. Oxidative stress, aging, and diseases. *Clin Interv Aging* 2018;13:757–772.
33. Matos AL, Bruno DF, Ambrósio AF, Santos PF. The benefits of flavonoids in diabetic retinopathy. *Nutrients* 2020;12:3169.
34. Rodríguez ML, Pérez S, Mena-Mollá S, Desco MC, Ortega ÁL. Oxidative stress and microvascular alterations in diabetic retinopathy: Future therapies. *Oxid Med Cell Longev* 2019;2019:4940825.
35. Kowluru RA, Mishra M. Oxidative stress, mitochondrial damage and diabetic retinopathy. *Biochim Biophys Acta* 2015;1852:2474–2483.
36. Rocha LR, Nguyen Huu VA, Palomino La Torre C, et al. Early removal of senescent cells protects retinal ganglion cells loss in experimental ocular hypertension. *Aging Cell* 2020;19:e13089.
37. Ahmad A, Ahsan H. Biomarkers of inflammation and oxidative stress in ophthalmic disorders. *J Immunoassay Immunochem* 2020;41:257–271.

38. McMonnies C. Reactive oxygen species, oxidative stress, glaucoma, and hyperbaric oxygen therapy. *J Optom* 2018;11:3–9.
39. Nita M, Grzybowski A. The role of the reactive oxygen species and oxidative stress in the pathomechanism of the age-related ocular diseases and other pathologies of the anterior and posterior eye segments in adults. *Oxid Med Cell Longev* 2016;2016:3164734.
40. Coleman AL, Miglior S. Risk factors for glaucoma onset and progression. *Surv Ophthalmol* 2008;53(Suppl. 1):S3–10.
41. Kumar DM, Agarwal N. Oxidative stress in glaucoma: A burden of evidence. *J Glaucoma* 2007;16:334–343.
42. Sacca SC, Izzotti A. Oxidative stress and glaucoma: Injury in the anterior segment of the eye. *Prog Brain Res* 2008;173:385–407.
43. Elanchezhian R, Palsamy P, Madson CJ, Lynch DW, Shinohara T. Age-related cataracts: Homocysteine coupled endoplasmic reticulum stress and suppression of Nrf2-dependent antioxidant protection. *Chem Biol Interact* 2012;200:1–10.
44. Palsamy P, Ayaki M, Elanchezhian R, Shinohara T. Promoter demethylation of Keap1 gene in human diabetic cataractous lenses. *Biochem Biophys Res Commun* 2012;423:542–548.
45. Palsamy P, Bidasee KR, Ayaki M, Augusteyn RC, Chan JY, Shinohara T. Methylglyoxal induces endoplasmic reticulum stress and DNA demethylation in the Keap1 promoter of human lens epithelial cells and age-related cataracts. *Free Radic Biol Med* 2014;72:134–148.
46. Palsamy P, Bidasee KR, Shinohara T. Valproic acid suppresses Nrf2/Keap1 dependent antioxidant protection through induction of endoplasmic reticulum stress and Keap1 promoter DNA demethylation in human lens epithelial cells. *Exp Eye Res* 2014;121:26–34.
47. Palsamy P, Bidasee KR, Shinohara T. Selenite cataracts: Activation of endoplasmic reticulum stress and loss of Nrf2/Keap1-dependent stress protection. *Biochim Biophys Acta* 2014;1842:1794–1805.
48. Enomoto A, Itoh K, Nagayoshi E, et al. High sensitivity of Nrf2 knockout mice to acetaminophen hepatotoxicity associated with decreased expression of ARE-regulated drug-metabolizing enzymes and antioxidant genes. *Toxicol Sci* 2001;59:169–177.
49. Kwak MK, Kensler TW, Casero RA, Jr. Induction of phase 2 enzymes by serum oxidized polyamines through activation of Nrf2: Effect of the polyamine metabolite acrolein. *Biochem Biophys Res Commun* 2003;305:662–670.
50. Lee JM, Calkins MJ, Chan K, Kan YW, Johnson JA. Identification of the NF-E2-related factor-2-dependent genes conferring protection against oxidative stress in primary cortical astrocytes using oligonucleotide microarray analysis. *J Biol Chem* 2003;278:12029–12038.
51. Nguyen T, Huang HC, Pickett CB. Transcriptional regulation of the antioxidant response element: Activation by Nrf2 and repression by MafK. *J Biol Chem* 2000;275:15466–15473.
52. Thimmulappa RK, Mai KH, Srisuma S, Kensler TW, Yamamoto M, Biswal S. Identification of Nrf2-regulated genes induced by the chemopreventive agent sulforaphane by oligonucleotide microarray. *Cancer Res* 2002;62:5196–5203.
53. Venugopal R, Jaiswal AK. Nrf1 and Nrf2 positively and c-Fos and Fra1 negatively regulate the human antioxidant response element-mediated expression of NAD(P)H: Quinone oxidoreductase1 gene. *Proc Natl Acad Sci U S A* 1996;93:14960–14965.
54. Wild AC, Moinova HR, Mulcahy RT. Regulation of gamma-glutamylcysteine synthetase subunit gene expression by the transcription factor Nrf2. *J Biol Chem* 1999;274:33627–33636.
55. Cullinan SB, Diehl JA. PERK-dependent activation of Nrf2 contributes to redox homeostasis and cell survival following endoplasmic reticulum stress. *J Biol Chem* 2004;279:20108–20117.
56. Rushmore TH, Morton MR, Pickett CB. The antioxidant responsive element: Activation by oxidative stress and identification of the DNA consensus sequence required for functional activity. *J Biol Chem* 1991;266:11632–11639.

57. Yu S, Khor TO, Cheung KL, et al. Nrf2 expression is regulated by epigenetic mechanisms in prostate cancer of TRAMP mice. *PLoS One* 2010;5:e8579.
58. Hong F, Sekhar KR, Freeman ML, Liebler DC. Specific patterns of electrophile adduction trigger Keap1 ubiquitination and Nrf2 activation. *J Biol Chem* 2005;280:31768–31775.
59. Katoh Y, Iida K, Kang MI, et al. Evolutionary conserved N-terminal domain of Nrf2 is essential for the Keap1-mediated degradation of the protein by the proteasome. *Arch Biochem Biophys* 2005;433:342–350.
60. Kobayashi M, Yamamoto M. Nrf2-Keap1 regulation of cellular defense mechanisms against electrophiles and reactive oxygen species. *Adv Enzyme Regul* 2006;46:113–140.
61. Nakagami Y. Nrf2 is an attractive therapeutic target for retinal diseases. *Oxid Med Cell Longev* 2016;2016:7469326.
62. Zhao Z, Chen Y, Wang J, et al. Age-related retinopathy in NRF2-deficient mice. *PLoS One* 2011;6:e19456.
63. Batliwala S, Xavier C, Liu Y, Wu H, Pang IH. Involvement of Nrf2 in ocular diseases. *Oxid Med Cell Longev* 2017;2017:1703810.
64. Lenox AR, Bhootada Y, Gorbatyuk O, Fullard R, Gorbatyuk M. Unfolded protein response is activated in aged retinas. *Neurosci Lett* 2015;609:30–35.
65. Sliwinski T, Kolodziejska U, Szaflik JP, Blasiak J, Szaflik J. Association between the 25129A>C polymorphism of the nuclear respiratory factor 2 gene and age-related macular degeneration. *Klin Oczna* 2013;115:96–102.
66. Xu Z, Wei Y, Gong J, et al. NRF2 plays a protective role in diabetic retinopathy in mice. *Diabetologia* 2014;57:204–213.
67. Wang M, Li J, Zheng Y. The potential role of nuclear factor erythroid 2-related factor 2 (Nrf2) in glaucoma: A review. *Med Sci Monit* 2020;26:e921514.
68. Wang M, Zheng Y. Oxidative stress and antioxidants in the trabecular meshwork. *PeerJ* 2019;7:e8121.
69. Ferreira SM, Lerner SF, Brunzini R, Evelson PA, Llesuy SF. Oxidative stress markers in aqueous humor of glaucoma patients. *Am J Ophthalmol* 2004;137:62–69.
70. Himori N, Yamamoto K, Maruyama K, et al. Critical role of Nrf2 in oxidative stress-induced retinal ganglion cell death. *J Neurochem* 2013;127:669–680.
71. Cheng J, Liang J, Qi J. Role of nuclear factor (erythroid-derived 2)-like 2 in the age-resistant properties of the glaucoma trabecular meshwork. *Exp Ther Med* 2017;14:791–796.
72. Xu Z, Cho H, Hartsock MJ, et al. Neuroprotective role of Nrf2 for retinal ganglion cells in ischemia-reperfusion. *J Neurochem* 2015;133:233–241.
73. Xiong W, MacColl Garfinkel AE, Li Y, Benowitz LI, Cepko CL. NRF2 promotes neuronal survival in neurodegeneration and acute nerve damage. *J Clin Invest* 2015;125:1433–1445.
74. Ma TJ, Lan DH, He SZ, et al. Nrf2 protects human lens epithelial cells against H_2O_2-induced oxidative and ER stress: The ATF4 may be involved. *Exp Eye Res* 2018;169:28–37.
75. Gao Y, Yan Y, Huang T. Human age-related cataracts: Epigenetic suppression of the nuclear factor erythroid 2-related factor 2-mediated antioxidant system. *Mol Med Rep* 2015;11:1442–1447.
76. Elanchezhian R, Ramesh E, Sakthivel M, et al. Acetyl-L-carnitine prevents selenite-induced cataractogenesis in an experimental animal model. *Curr Eye Res* 2007;32:961–971.
77. Park JY, Kang KA, Kim KC, Cha JW, Kim EH, Hyun JW. Morin induces heme oxygenase-1 via ERK-Nrf2 signaling pathway. *J Cancer Prev* 2013;18:249–256.
78. Wang F, Ma J, Han F, et al. DL-3-n-butylphthalide delays the onset and progression of diabetic cataract by inhibiting oxidative stress in rat diabetic model. *Sci Rep* 2016;6:19396.
79. Liu Y, Luo W, Luo X, Yong Z, Zhong X. Effects of Rosa laevigata Michx extract on reactive oxygen species production and mitochondrial membrane potential in lens epithelial cells cultured under high glucose. *Int J Clin Exp Med* 2015;8:15759–15765.

80. Abu-Amero KK, Kondkar AA, Chalam KV. Resveratrol and ophthalmic diseases. *Nutrients* 2016;8:200.

81. Baur JA, Sinclair DA. Therapeutic potential of resveratrol: The in vivo evidence. *Nat Rev Drug Discov* 2006;5:493–506.

82. Xia N, Daiber A, Habermeier A, et al. Resveratrol reverses endothelial nitric-oxide synthase uncoupling in apolipoprotein E knockout mice. *J Pharmacol Exp Ther* 2010;335:149–154.

83. King RE, Kent KD, Bomser JA. Resveratrol reduces the oxidation and proliferation of human retinal pigment epithelial cells via extracellular signal-regulated kinase inhibition. *Chem Biol Interact* 2005;151:143–149.

84. Pintea A, Rugina D, Pop R, Bunea A, Socaciu C, Diehl HA. Antioxidant effect of trans-resveratrol in cultured human retinal pigment epithelial cells. *J Ocul Pharmacol Ther* 2011;27:315–321.

85. Richer S, Patel S, Sockanathan S, Ulanski LJ, 2nd, Miller L, Podella C. Resveratrol-based oral nutritional supplement produces long-term beneficial effects on the structure and visual function in human patients. *Nutrients* 2014;6:4404–4420.

86. Soufi FG, Mohammad-Nejad D, Ahmadieh H. Resveratrol improves diabetic retinopathy possibly through oxidative stress – Nuclear factor kappaB – Apoptosis pathway. *Pharmacol Rep* 2012;64:1505–1514.

87. Kim YH, Kim YS, Roh GS, Choi WS, Cho GJ. Resveratrol blocks diabetes-induced early vascular lesions and vascular endothelial growth factor induction in mouse retinas. *Acta Ophthalmol* 2012;90:e31–37.

88. Losso JN, Truax RE, Richard G. Trans-resveratrol inhibits hyperglycemia-induced inflammation and connexin downregulation in retinal pigment epithelial cells. *J Agric Food Chem* 2010;58:8246–8252.

89. Luna C, Li G, Liton PB, et al. Resveratrol prevents the expression of glaucoma markers induced by chronic oxidative stress in trabecular meshwork cells. *Food Chem Toxicol* 2009;47:198–204.

90. Tanaka J, Kadekaru T, Ogawa K, Hitoe S, Shimoda H, Hara H. Maqui berry (Aristotelia chilensis) and the constituent delphinidin glycoside inhibit photoreceptor cell death induced by visible light. *Food Chem* 2013;139:129–137.

91. Higashi Y, Higashi K, Mori A, Sakamoto K, Ishii K, Nakahara T. Anti-cataract effect of resveratrol in high-glucose-treated streptozotocin-induced diabetic rats. *Biol Pharm Bull* 2018;41:1586–1592.

92. Doganay S, Borazan M, Iraz M, Cigremis Y. The effect of resveratrol in experimental cataract model formed by sodium selenite. *Curr Eye Res* 2006;31:147–153.

93. Zheng T, Lu Y. SIRT1 protects human lens epithelial cells against oxidative stress by inhibiting p53-dependent apoptosis. *Curr Eye Res* 2016;41:1068–1075.

94. Pescosolido N, Giannotti R, Plateroti AM, Pascarella A, Nebbioso M. Curcumin: Therapeutical potential in ophthalmology. *Planta Med* 2014;80:249–254.

95. Radomska-Lesniewska DM, Osiecka-Iwan A, Hyc A, Gozdz A, Dabrowska AM, Skopinski P. Therapeutic potential of curcumin in eye diseases. *Cent Eur J Immunol* 2019;44:181–189.

96. Ammon HP, Wahl MA. Pharmacology of Curcuma longa. *Planta Med* 1991;57:1–7.

97. Tilak JC, Banerjee M, Mohan H, Devasagayam TP. Antioxidant availability of turmeric in relation to its medicinal and culinary uses. *Phytother Res* 2004;18:798–804.

98. Singh S, Aggarwal BB. Activation of transcription factor NF-kappa B is suppressed by curcumin (diferuloylmethane) [corrected]. *J Biol Chem* 1995;270:24995–25000.

99. Schaffer M, Schaffer PM, Zidan J, Bar Sela G. Curcuma as a functional food in the control of cancer and inflammation. *Curr Opin Clin Nutr Metab Care* 2011;14:588–597.

100. Aggarwal BB, Harikumar KB. Potential therapeutic effects of curcumin, the anti-inflammatory agent, against neurodegenerative, cardiovascular, pulmonary, metabolic, autoimmune and neoplastic diseases. *Int J Biochem Cell Biol* 2009;41:40–59.

101. Jurenka JS. Anti-inflammatory properties of curcumin, a major constituent of Curcuma longa: A review of preclinical and clinical research. *Altern Med Rev* 2009;14:141–153.
102. Lin YG, Kunnumakkara AB, Nair A, et al. Curcumin inhibits tumor growth and angiogenesis in ovarian carcinoma by targeting the nuclear factor-kappaB pathway. *Clin Cancer Res* 2007;13:3423–3430.
103. Marchiani A, Rozzo C, Fadda A, Delogu G, Ruzza P. Curcumin and curcumin-like molecules: From spice to drugs. *Curr Med Chem* 2014;21:204–222.
104. Menon VP, Sudheer AR. Antioxidant and anti-inflammatory properties of curcumin. *Adv Exp Med Biol* 2007;595:105–125.
105. Mrudula T, Suryanarayana P, Srinivas PN, Reddy GB. Effect of curcumin on hyperglycemia-induced vascular endothelial growth factor expression in streptozotocin-induced diabetic rat retina. *Biochem Biophys Res Commun* 2007;361:528–532.
106. Kowluru RA, Kanwar M. Effects of curcumin on retinal oxidative stress and inflammation in diabetes. *Nutr Metab (Lond)* 2007;4:8.
107. Manikandan R, Thiagarajan R, Beulaja S, et al. Anti-cataractogenic effect of curcumin and aminoguanidine against selenium-induced oxidative stress in the eye lens of Wistar rat pups: An in vitro study using the isolated lens. *Chem Biol Interact* 2009;181:202–209.
108. Suryanarayana P, Saraswat M, Mrudula T, Krishna TP, Krishnaswamy K, Reddy GB. Curcumin and turmeric delay streptozotocin-induced diabetic cataracts in rats. *Invest Ophthalmol Vis Sci* 2005;46:2092–2099.
109. Cao J, Wang T, Wang M. Investigation of the anti-cataractogenic mechanisms of curcumin through in vivo and in vitro studies. *BMC Ophthalmol* 2018;18:48.
110. Cao X, Liu M, Tuo J, Shen D, Chan CC. The effects of quercetin in cultured human RPE cells under oxidative stress and in Ccl2/Cx3cr1 double deficient mice. *Exp Eye Res* 2010;91:15–25.
111. Weng S, Mao L, Gong Y, Sun T, Gu Q. Role of quercetin in protecting ARPE19 cells against H_2O_2 induced injury via nuclear factor erythroid 2 like 2 pathway activation and endoplasmic reticulum stress inhibition. *Mol Med Rep* 2017;16:3461–3468.
112. Chen B, He T, Xing Y, Cao T. Effects of quercetin on the expression of MCP-1, MMP-9 and VEGF in rats with diabetic retinopathy. *Exp Ther Med* 2017;14:6022–6026.
113. Kumar B, Gupta SK, Nag TC, et al. Retinal neuroprotective effects of quercetin in streptozotocin-induced diabetic rats. *Exp Eye Res* 2014;125:193–202.
114. Wang X, Li H, Wang H, Shi J. Quercetin attenuates high glucose-induced injury in human retinal pigment epithelial cell line ARPE-19 by up-regulation of miR-29b. *J Biochem* 2020;167:495–502.
115. Sanderson J, McLauchlan WR, Williamson G. Quercetin inhibits hydrogen peroxide-induced oxidation of the rat lens. *Free Radic Biol Med* 1999;26:639–645.
116. Park JY, Han X, Piao MJ, et al. Hyperoside induces endogenous antioxidant system to alleviate oxidative stress. *J Cancer Prev* 2016;21:41–47.
117. Patil KK, Meshram RJ, Barage SH, Gacche RN. Dietary flavonoids inhibit the glycation of lens proteins: Implications in the management of diabetic cataract. *3 Biotech* 2019;9:47.
118. Lee HS, Jun JH, Jung EH, Koo BA, Kim YS. Epigallocatechin-3-gallate inhibits ocular neovascularization and vascular permeability in human retinal pigment epithelial and human retinal microvascular endothelial cells via suppression of MMP-9 and VEGF activation. *Molecules* 2014;19:12150–12172.
119. Kumar B, Gupta SK, Nag TC, Srivastava S, Saxena R. Green tea prevents hyperglycemia-induced retinal oxidative stress and inflammation in streptozotocin-induced diabetic rats. *Ophthalmic Res* 2012;47:103–108.
120. Zhang B, Safa R, Rusciano D, Osborne NN. Epigallocatechin gallate, an active ingredient from green tea, attenuates damaging influences to the retina caused by ischemia/reperfusion. *Brain Res* 2007;1159:40–53.

121. Falsini B, Marangoni D, Salgarello T, et al. Effect of epigallocatechin-gallate on inner retinal function in ocular hypertension and glaucoma: A short-term study by pattern electroretinogram. *Graefes Arch Clin Exp Ophthalmol* 2009;247:1223–1233.
122. Chaudhury S, Ghosh I, Saha G, Dasgupta S. EGCG Prevents tryptophan oxidation of cataractous ocular lens human γ-crystallin in the presence of H_2O_2. *Int J Biol Macromol* 2015;77:287–292.
123. Van Heyningen R. Fluorescent glucoside in the human lens. *Nature* 1971;230:393–394.
124. McNulty R, Wang H, Mathias RT, Ortwerth BJ, Truscott RJ, Bassnett S. Regulation of tissue oxygen levels in the mammalian lens. *J Physiol* 2004;559:883–898.
125. Chaudhury S, Dutta A, Bag S, Biswas P, Das AK, Dasgupta S. Probing the inhibitory potency of epigallocatechin gallate against human γB-crystallin aggregation: Spectroscopic, microscopic and simulation studies. *Spectrochim Acta A Mol Biomol Spectrosc* 2018;192:318–327.
126. Lin D, Xiao M, Zhao J, et al. An overview of plant phenolic compounds and their importance in human nutrition and management of type 2 diabetes. *Molecules* 2016;21:1374.
127. Khoo HE, Azlan A, Tang ST, Lim SM. Anthocyanidins and anthocyanins: Colored pigments as food, pharmaceutical ingredients, and the potential health benefits. *Food Nutr Res* 2017;61:1361779.
128. Sole P, Rigal D, Peyresblanques J. Effects of cyaninoside chloride and Heleniene on mesopic and scotopic vision in myopia and night blindness. *J Fr Ophtalmol* 1984;7:35–39.
129. Upadhyay S, Dixit M. Role of polyphenols and other phytochemicals on molecular signaling. *Oxid Med Cell Longev* 2015;2015:504253.
130. Jang YP, Zhou J, Nakanishi K, Sparrow JR. Anthocyanins protect against A2E photooxidation and membrane permeabilization in retinal pigment epithelial cells. *Photochem Photobiol* 2005;81:529–536.
131. Milbury PE, Graf B, Curran-Celentano JM, Blumberg JB. Bilberry (Vaccinium myrtillus) anthocyanins modulate heme oxygenase-1 and glutathione S-transferase-pi expression in ARPE-19 cells. *Invest Ophthalmol Vis Sci* 2007;48:2343–2349.
132. Kim J, Kim CS, Lee YM, Sohn E, Jo K, Kim JS. Vaccinium myrtillus extract prevents or delays the onset of diabetes-induced blood-retinal barrier breakdown. *Int J Food Sci Nutr* 2015;66:236–242.
133. Song Y, Huang L, Yu J. Effects of blueberry anthocyanins on retinal oxidative stress and inflammation in diabetes through Nrf2/HO-1 signaling. *J Neuroimmunol* 2016;301:1–6.
134. Szumny D, Sozanski T, Kucharska AZ, et al. Application of cornelian cherry iridoid-polyphenolic fraction and loganic acid to reduce intraocular pressure. *Evid Based Complement Alternat Med* 2015;2015:939402.

Role of Nrf2 in Obesity and Flavonoid Action

7

Seth Kwabena Amponsah
University of Ghana Medical School

Emmanuel Boadi Amoafo
North Dakota State University

Emmanuel Kwaku Ofori
University of Ghana Medical School

Contents

DOI: 10.1201/9781003225225-7

INTRODUCTION

Obesity, described as an excessive amount of body fat in an individual, is one of the most apparent yet most neglected public health issues that affect both resource-rich and resource-developing countries, according to the World Health Organization (WHO) [1]. Also, in a 2017 report, the WHO opinions nearly 2 billion people worldwide are overweight, with one-third of them being obese [2]. Obesity may not only be a challenge to the affected person, but related morbidity and mortality are also costly to society [3]. Furthermore, along with the rate of obesity-related health issues, obesity is predicted to rise in the next decades. Dysregulation in blood glucose and lipid metabolism, impairment in the rate of glucose disposal, and elevations in blood pressure are among the most common pathological conditions associated with excess deposition of fat. Generally, obesity can lead to chronic non-communicable diseases such as non-alcoholic fatty liver disease and type 2 diabetes (T2D), among others [3].

The most frequently accepted measure of obesity is a high body mass index (BMI). BMI is calculated as weight divided by height squared (kg/m^2). In actuarial research, the maximum limit for normal BMI in humans is 25 kg/m^2, with obesity delimited at a BMI>30 kg/m^2. BMIs between the aforementioned (normal and obese) are classified as "overweight." Obesity can be divided into three classes: BMI of 30–34.9 is deemed Class 1, BMI of 35–40 is deemed Class 2, and BMI>40 is regarded as Class 3 [4]. Nevertheless, BMI has several limitations as a defining metric because it does not distinguish between lean and fat mass or fat distribution nor take into account the heterogeneity of regional body fat deposition. According to recent studies, obesity-related risk factors depend on the regional distribution of fat depots in the body rather than on excess body weight [5]. As a result, abdominal fat is now well recognized as a significant risk factor for obesity-related disorders. In reality, visceral fat accumulation induces pro-oxidant and pro-inflammatory states [6].

Nuclear factor erythroid 2-related factor (Nrf2) is a basic leucine transcription factor that regulates cellular antioxidants, reduces inflammation, and helps maintain redox and metabolic balance [7,8]. As a result of its ability to regulate the expression of downstream target antioxidant proteins, Nrf2 has been extensively studied in several disorders, including insulin resistance [8,9]. In diseases characterized by chronic inflammation and reactive oxygen species (ROS) generation, Nrf2 activation has the tendency to decrease oxidative stress. However, chronic activation of Nrf2 could also result in metabolic derailments, which ultimately contribute to disease progression [10]. It is, thus, of great interest to investigate the potential protective functions of the Nrf2 pathway in obesity-related inflammation and oxidative injury [11].

Studies have linked flavonoid consumption to a lower risk of stroke, cardiovascular disease, asthma, and some types of cancer [12]. There is also evidence that dietary and herbal plant sources of flavonoids may offer potential benefits in the management of obesity and other metabolic disorders [13]. Under ordinary physiological and pathological conditions, flavonoids are effective alimentary phytochemicals that trigger the Nrf2 pathway [14], potentially offering therapeutic targets in obesity.

ADIPOGENESIS

Adipose tissue (AT) is a type of connective tissue that forms an insulating layer beneath the skin and helps to regulate body temperature. Additionally, AT serves as a structural component of the body, attaching the skin to the underlying tissue and cushioning body parts. The main component of AT is adipocytes. Adipocytes regulate energy balance by storing and mobilizing triacylglycerol. Additionally, adipocytes serve as endocrine and paracrine organs [15]. It is through a highly controlled process, adipogenesis, that adipocytes mature and become functional [16].

In the process of adipogenesis, fibroblasts are differentiated into mature and lipid-laden adipocytes that respond to insulin. In general, this process involves six distinct stages: mesenchymal precursors, committed preadipocytes, growth-arrested preadipocytes, mitotic clonal expansion, terminal differentiation, and mature adipocytes [15]. The stages of adipogenesis are summarized in Table 7.1. To successfully mature into adipocytes, preadipocytes undergo a series of morphological and genetic changes.

TABLE 7.1 Stages of adipogenesis and their characteristics

STAGES OF ADIPOGENESIS	NOTABLE CHARACTERISTICS
Mesenchymal precursor	• Proliferation • Capable of differentiating into multiple lineages
Committed preadipocyte	• Proliferation • Lineage commitment to adipocyte differentiation
Growth-arrested preadipocyte	• Fibroblast-like morphology • Contact inhibition results in a lack of proliferation
Mitotic clonal expansion	• Re-entry into the cell cycle due to hormonal stimulation • Multiple rounds of the division of cells (i.e., mitotic clonal expansion)
Terminal differentiation	• Cell-cycle arrest • Transcriptional activation of adipocyte genes (lipid and carbohydrate metabolism genes and adipokines)
Mature adipocyte	• High expression of adipocyte genes • Signet-ring morphology: large lipid droplet occupies the majority of cell volume

ADIPOGENESIS

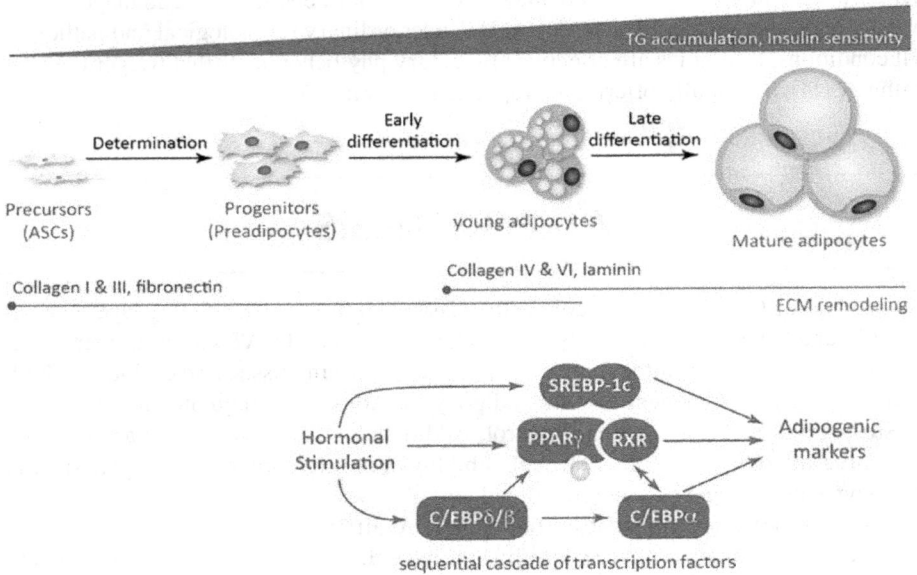

FIGURE 7.1 An illustration of how mesenchymal precursors control the process of adipogenesis.

During adipogenesis, cells are in constant communication with one another and with their surroundings. Several factors involved in adipogenesis have been identified, but many molecular details remain unknown.

According to the traditional paradigm, stem cells become preadipocytes when they lose their potential to differentiate into other mesenchymal lineages (such as myocyte, chondrocyte, or osteocyte) and become committed to the adipocyte lineage [17]. Preadipocytes undergo mitosis and serve as a stable source of adipocytes (Figure 7.1).

DETERMINATION

Determination of a cell occurs when it irreversibly commits to a path of differentiation. The principle of determination limits the developmental potential of a cell. Essentially, there are two types of determination: cells that can independently decide how to differentiate (said to be autonomous) and cells that depend on instructions from neighboring cells to determine how to differentiate (said to be interactive) [16].

A protein family called bone morphogenetic protein (BMP) may act as a signal to stimulate pluripotent stem cells to differentiate into adipocytes. These proteins are members of the transforming growth factor (TGF-) superfamily that act locally on cell surface receptors to activate transcription factors SMADs 1, 5, and 8 [18]. Cells that differentiate into adipocytes or other cell types from multipotent C3H10T1/2 or 2T3 can be stimulated by BMPs 2, 4, and 7 depending on the culture conditions and the expression of BMP receptors [19,20].

DIFFERENTIATION

The process of cell differentiation occurs when cells derived from a common ancestor become more differentiated in function and morphology from one another (Figure 7.1). Specific genes that determine the exact phenotype of adipocytes are expressed in chronological order throughout the differentiation process. Communications between individual cells and the extracellular environment are the two factors that affect differentiation [16].

The onset of adipogenesis involves sequential activation of transcription factors that result in lipid accumulation and insulin sensitivity. In addition, extracellular matrix remodeling occurs during adipogenesis [21,22].

PATHOPHYSIOLOGY OF OBESITY

AT is a large endocrine organ involved in triglyceride storage as well as the synthesis of numerous proteins and factors. When energy is needed, AT fat is released into circulation as free fatty acids (FFAs) that can be transported to the liver and muscle tissues for oxidation [23]. Several years ago, AT was considered only as a storage site for excess energy. However, advances in science over the last couple of decades have enhanced our understanding of AT as a complex endocrine organ with multiple functions. AT is made up of adipocytes, preadipocytes, immune cells, and endothelium. Several signaling molecules with endocrine functions are expressed and secreted by AT [24]. Leptin, adiponectin, interleukin-6 (IL-6), tumor necrosis factor cc (TNF-cc), complement components, plasminogen activator inhibitor-1, renin-angiotensin system proteins, and resistin are all examples of AT signaling molecules. Collectively, these signaling molecules are known as adipokines. These molecules are involved in the regulation of appetite, fuel metabolism, innate immune function, growth, and reproduction [25].

REACTIVE OXYGEN SPECIES AND OBESITY

Oxidative stress is a factor in diseases such as obesity, diabetes, heart disease, and atherosclerosis. In obesity, oxidative stress is linked with irregular adipokine production, which may lead to metabolic syndrome [26]. Under physiological and disease conditions, ROS can cause direct or indirect damage to organs. Even though adipocytes and preadipocytes have been identified as sources of pro-inflammatory cytokines (such as TNF-α, IL-1, and IL-6), the increase in obesity-related oxidative stress is most likely a consequence of elevated AT itself. Therefore, obesity is regarded as a state of chronic inflammation. Since these cytokines are effective stimulators of macrophages and ROS, a rise in cytokine levels could be related to an increase in oxidative stress [27].

Increased oxygen intake produces ROS due to excessive mitochondrial respiration and electron loss in the electron transport chain, culminating in the generation of superoxide radicals [28,29]. As a result of the pressure effects of fat cells, excess fat accumulation can cause cellular damage (e.g., non-alcoholic steatohepatitis). In turn, cellular damage increases cytokine production, such as TNF-α, which in turn increases lipid peroxidation in the tissues by generating ROS [29]. Diet may also play a role in the production of ROS during obesity. Diets high in fat may cause changes in oxygen metabolism. Oxidative reactions are sensitive to fatty deposits. Oxidative stress generated in lipid peroxidation may promote the development of atherosclerosis if the generation of these ROS surpasses the antioxidant potential of the cell [29].

INFLAMMATION AND OBESITY

Inflammation occurs as a result of an organism's reaction or response to an unwanted stimulus (physical, chemical, or biological). Usually, the response leads to the restoration of homeostasis. In response to an initial stimulus and subsequent responses, many cell types and mediators act together in coordination [30].

Aside from serving as the most important fat-storing organ, white AT is also the largest endocrine organ that secretes adipokines and cytokines. Several metabolic and physiological signaling cascades are affected by adipokines, including insulin signaling, glucose uptake, fatty acid oxidation, and many other metabolic and energy-producing processes [31].

Several cytokines play a role in regulating inflammation and resolution of inflammation, as well as adaptive and reparative angiogenesis. In obese individuals, the white AT may become inflamed because of the infiltration of immune cells into the stromal vascular fraction as well as the appearance of inflamed and dysfunctional adipocytes [32,33]. As adipocytes become inflamed, they release pro-inflammatory cytokines locally and systemically, which disrupt the normal function of ATs [33]. It is generally known that inflammation is an energy waster that enhances energy expenditure and reduces energy intake in direct and indirect ways. To increase energy expenditure, inflammatory cytokines, such as TNF-α, IL-1, and IL-6, bind to signaling receptors found in the central nervous system or other tissues. Moreover, these cytokines provide leptin-like effects that contribute to energy expenditure [34,35].

Adipocytes and resident immune cells still secrete inflammatory mediators, including chemokines and cytokines, during inflammation of adipocytes. AT inflammation shares several similar features with traditional inflammation, such as the infiltration of bone marrow–derived immune cells and the release of inflammatory mediators, including chemokines and cytokines. Inflamed white ATs are also capable of causing widespread systemic inflammation via the release of cytokines, even in apparently healthy people of normal weight [36].

INFLAMMATION AND OXIDATIVE STRESS IN OBESITY

In obesity, there are increases in the amount of FFAs, ROS, and reactive nitrogen species in the bloodstream. Obesity also leads to pro-inflammatory adipokine production, immunological activation, and chronic inflammation. Furthermore, leptin and insulin dysregulation in fat, muscle, and liver tissues occurs in obesity [37].

In obese people, blood provision to adipocytes may become insufficient as adipocytes expand rapidly, resulting in hypoxia [38–40]. Hypoxia is thought to be one of the vital catalysts to AT modification in obesity. Hypoxia also leads to AT destruction and inflammatory response [41]. Apart from driving a heightened pro-inflammatory response, the expansion of AT during obesity can cause an increase in free radical species, eventually leading to increased oxidative stress. Although the mechanisms underlying these processes are complex, there is a clear link between blood capillary narrowing (vessel rarefaction) and oxidative stress via ROS [42,43].

An imbalance between the generation and buildup of ROS in cells, as well as the ability to detoxify these reactive products, causes oxidative stress [44]. Oxidative stress, on the other hand, plays a key role in the etiology of obesity and the development of co-morbidities [45,46]. Oxidative stress may influence food intake by affecting hypothalamic neurons that regulate satiety and hunger [47,48].

Macrophages are chief inherent phagocytic cells found in almost all tissues and play important roles in both natural and acquired immunity. TNF, IL-1, IL-6, IL-8, and IL-12 are chemokines secreted by macrophages in reaction to provoking stimuli [49]. The quantity of macrophages in AT is closely associated with BMI and total body fat [50]. Obesity causes the release of pro-inflammatory chemokines such as TNF-α and IL-6 in AT [51–54]. TNF-α has been demonstrated to cause the generation of ROS, suggesting one of many plausible linkages in obesity-related oxidative stress and inflammation [55].

NUCLEAR FACTOR ERYTHROID 2-RELATED FACTOR

Nrf2 is a transcription factor that contains a basic leucine-zipper protein. One of the main functions of Nrf2 is to regulate cellular antioxidants. Nrf2 reduces inflammation by maintaining redox and metabolic balance [7,8]. Normal conditions result in Nrf2 being sequestered in the cytoplasm by association with the proteins: Keap1 and Cullin 3. Nrf2 is ubiquitinated by Cullin 3. In addition to being a substrate for Cullin 3, Keap1 aids Cullin 3 ubiquitination [56]. When a cell is under oxidative stress, Keap1 detects this and produces Nrf2, which then travels to the nucleus. In the nucleus, Nrf2 binds to the antioxidant response element (ARE) in the promoter region of genes that produce antioxidants, where it forms a complex with Maf and Jun proteins and initiates transcription [57]. With these actions, Nrf2 functions as a primary cellular defense against oxidative stress.

It is noteworthy that depending on the conditions and processes of disease, activation of Nrf2-ARE signaling can have either positive or detrimental effects [7]. For example, activation of Nrf2 may protect against oxidative stress in disorders involving chronic inflammation and the formation of ROS; nevertheless, sustained activation of Nrf2 causes metabolic alterations, which contribute to disease development [10]. Since obesity is associated with inflammation and oxidative stress, the Nrf2 pathway (Figure 7.2) is a possible protective role.

Figure 7.2 shows Nrf2 being linked to the Keap1 protein in the cytoplasm. Keap1 inhibits the signaling pathway of Nrf2. Nrf2 is ubiquitinated by Keap1 and then degraded by a proteasomal pathway. Oxidative stress, Nrf2 activators, or both can induce the Nrf2-Keap1 complex to dissociate, resulting in Nrf2 phosphorylation and eventual movement into the nucleus. Nrf2 then binds to the promoter regions of target genes (ARE) in the nucleus. This aids the transcriptional activation of antioxidants and detoxifying enzymes.

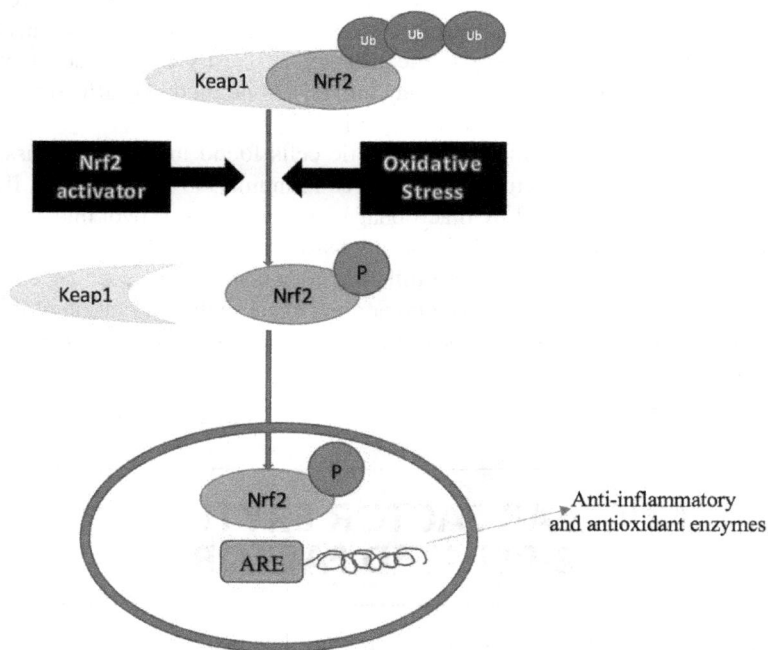

FIGURE 7.2   An illustration of the Nrf2 pathway.

ROLE OF Nrf2 PATHWAY IN ADIPOGENESIS

Adipocyte-like, multipotent, mesenchymal stem cells, which have been shown to express the platelet-derived growth factor receptor-α (PDGFRα) and/or PDGFRβ, restrict themselves to the adipocyte lineage without noticeable changes in morphology and then from preadipocytes. After committing, the cells undergo terminal differentiation, during which a subset of preadipocytes undergo growth arrest, accumulate lipid droplets, and mature into functional, insulin-responsive adipocytes [58,59]. An intricate network of transcription factors controls this complex adipogenic process, which coordinates the expression of hundreds of proteins responsible for establishing the mature adipocyte phenotype [60]. Peroxisome proliferator-activated receptor γ (PPARγ) and CCAAT/enhancer-binding protein α (C/EBPα), which together oversee terminal differentiation, play central roles in this process.

In light of the role ROS play in adipogenesis, as well as the antioxidant actions of Nrf2 as a master regulator of antioxidant gene expression, it would be reasonable to hypothesize that Nrf2 plays a role in redox-associated adipogenesis. Oxidative stress has been shown to promote Nrf2 recruitment to sterol regulatory element-binding proteins (SREBP1), leading to gene transcription and subsequent lipogenesis [61]. The Nrf2 protein directly impacts adipogenesis, as mice lacking Nrf2 showed inhibition of adipocyte differentiation, coupled with downregulation of PPARγ and C/EBPα expression after 12 weeks on a high-fat diet (HFD) [61]. By suppressing the activity of Nrf2, either chemically or genetically, 3T3-L1 preadipocytes, primary mouse embryonic fibroblasts, or human subcutaneous preadipocytes demonstrated impaired adipogenesis [62]. In contrast, activation of Nrf2 through knockdown of Kelch-like ECH-associated protein 1 (Keap1) enhanced adipogenic differentiation in 3T3-L1 preadipocytes [62].

Nrf2, ADIPOCYTE FUNCTION, AND METABOLISM

The white adipocyte tissue is the main physiologically responsive organ of insulin signaling and the main tissue for storing and transferring energy, which is essential for maintaining glucose and lipid homeostasis [63,64]. A diminished adipocyte function makes it difficult for FFAs in the blood to be stored, which contributes to insulin resistance and T2D [65]. Increased white adipocyte tissue mass and adipocyte size have been shown to be associated with reduced lipid storage ability, low-grade inflammation, inadequate vascularization, hypoxia, fibrosis, and macrophage infiltration. On the other hand, decreased adipogenesis causes insulin resistance as well as white adipocyte tissue dysfunction, for instance, in lipodystrophy [66]. As a result, functioning adipocytes are required for the homeostatic control of glucose and lipid metabolism in white adipocyte tissue, and Nrf2 has emerged as a prominent regulator in this complex process.

In addition to maintaining the shape of lipid droplets, increasing the storage of TAGs, and reducing the release of FFAs, Nrf2 can enhance the phosphorylation of lipolytic enzymes. During lipolysis, an adipocyte sequentially hydrolyzes one TAG molecule into three FFAs and one glycerol; the aforementioned process is catalyzed by lipases [67]. Furthermore, PPARγ protects against lipotoxicity by regulating the terminal differentiation of preadipocytes, adipocyte storage capacity, and lipid synthesis [68]. There is also evidence that Nrf2 activity is enhanced when Keap1 is knocked down, resulting in an increase in FFA in white adipocyte tissue [69].

ROLE OF Nrf2 PATHWAY IN OBESITY

The Nrf2 pathway plays a critical role in anti-inflammatory and antioxidant responses. Several studies have found an association between the Nrf2 pathway and obesity. In one study, an Nrf2 activator intermittently stimulated Nrf2 signaling, while in another, mice with Nrf2 knockout (KO) or Keap1 knockdown (KD) were genetically manipulated [70]. An Nrf2 KO mouse has no constitutive expression of Nrf2 and, therefore, is not able to produce cytoprotective genes under oxidative stress. Genetically engineered Keap1 KD mice, unlike Nrf2 KO mice, are intended for testing the effects of constitutive Nrf2 overexpression [71].

Effect of Nrf2 Gene Deletion on Obesity

The role of Nrf2 in a long-term obesity mouse model (180 days of HFD induced by 60 kcal % fat) has been studied by Chartoumpekiss and colleagues [70]. In their study, Nrf2-KO mice were partially protected against obesity-inducing HFDs. The results of another study revealed that Nrf2-disrupted mice under an HFD gained less weight than wild-type (WT) mice, as was also shown in a study of HFD-induced obese mice (60 kcal % fat) [72]. In another study, targeted Nrf2 KO in mice reduced the mass of AT and prevented weight gain when mice consumed HFD (41 kcal % fat) [62]. According to these studies, Nrf2 regulates blood glucose, body weight, and insulin sensitivity. It was found that systemic Nrf2 deficiency increased insulin resistance and protected against obesity [73,74], but target-specific KO of Nrf2 in myeloid cells or adipocytes did not successfully overcome these effects. This shows that Nrf2 may influence metabolic syndrome differently [75].

Role of Nrf2 Overexpression in Obesity

Genetically engineered Keap1 KD mice, unlike Nrf2 KO mice, are intended for testing the effects of constitutive Nrf2 overexpression [71]. Xu et al. discovered that Keap1-KO mice with genetically boosted Nrf2 activity had lower obesity and lipid buildup in white AT when fed an HFD (60 kcal % fat) [76]. Studies involving Keap1-KD or Nrf2-KO

TABLE 7.2   The role of Nrf2 in obesity

REGULATION OF NRF2	EFFECT ON NRF2 AND OBESITY	REFERENCES
Nrf2 KO mice	Nrf2↓ → obesity↓	[62]
Keap1-KD, Keap1-KD mice	Nrf2↑ → obesity↓	[76]
Nrf2 agonist: CDDO-imidazolide	Nrf2↑ → obesity↓	[72]
Nrf2 disrupted mice	Nrf2↓ → obesity↓	[72]
Nrf2-null mice, Keap1-KD mice	Nrf2↓ → obesity↔	[82]
Nrf2 agonist: Curcumin, resveratrol or ellagic acid	Nrf2↑ → obesity↓	[83]

Key: ↓, decrease; ↑, increase; ↔, unchanged.

mice demonstrated that Nrf2 prevents weight gain under HFD conditions. Long-term feeding of HFD to Keap1-KD mice, however, impaired insulin sensitivity and resulted in weight gain compared to WT mice [77], suggesting that prolonged constitutive Nrf2 activation might not be protective. Although Keap1-KD mice fed on a short-term HFD were protected from obesity, long-term HFD caused increased obesity and worsened insulin resistance in Keap1-KD mice. It is unclear why Keap1-KD animals administered HFD for the short term differed from Keap1-KD mice fed HFD over the long term.

Pharmacological Activators of Nrf2

Varied Nrf2 pharmacological activators have been investigated in HFD-induced obese mice models [78]. These activators include curcumin, sulforaphane, oltipraz, and 1-[2-cyano-3, 12-dioxooleana-1,9[11]-dien-28-oyl] imidazole (CDDO-imidazolide). The Nrf2 activators can induce Nrf2 expression in vitro and in vivo [72,76,78]. Shin and colleagues found that CDDO-imidazolide prevented weight gain, AT accumulation, and hepatic lipid accumulation during an HFD-induced experiment in mice [42].

Again, by activating Nrf2, oxidative stress associated with inflammation and endoplasmic reticulum stress, both of which contribute to insulin resistance, can be alleviated [79,80]. Another mechanism by which Nrf2 activators reduce obesity is by stimulating the AMP-activated protein kinase (AMPK) enzyme [81]. The role of Nrf2 in obesity under different conditions is summarized in Table 7.2.

FLAVONOIDS

Flavonoids get their name from the Latin word flavus, which means "yellow" [84]. More than 5,000 polyphenolic compounds have been described so far, and compounds in this group are still being identified. Flavonoids can be found in a wide range of foods, including seeds, nuts, fruits, vegetables, stems, and flowers.

Flavonoids have a distinct C6-C3-C6 structure at their most basic level. Flavonoids have two aromatic rings (also known as rings A and B) connected by a three-carbon chain, resulting in an oxygenated heterocycle (ring C) [84]. There are several types of flavonoids, including flavone, flavonol, flavanone, flavan-3-ol, isoflavone, and anthocyanin. Among these groups, flavonoids are differentiated by their substitutions of the A and B rings, as well as their different hydroxyls [85], as shown in Figure 7.3. Most of these flavonoids are obtained from dietary sources (Table 7.3).

Flavonoids are known to have anti-inflammatory [91], blood vessel relaxant [92], anticoagulant [93], cardioprotective [94], antidiabetic [95], chemoprotective [96], neuroprotective [97], and antidepressant properties [98]. Furthermore, existing evidence suggests that flavonoids derived from plant sources may be beneficial in obesity management [13,99]. Flavonoids may control an individual's appetite and limit food consumption, decrease intestinal fat absorption, and alter adipocyte differentiation, adipogenesis, lipolysis, 3-oxidation, and apoptosis. In addition, flavonoids increase non-shivering thermogenesis and cause obesity-induced dysbiosis of the gut microbiota [100].

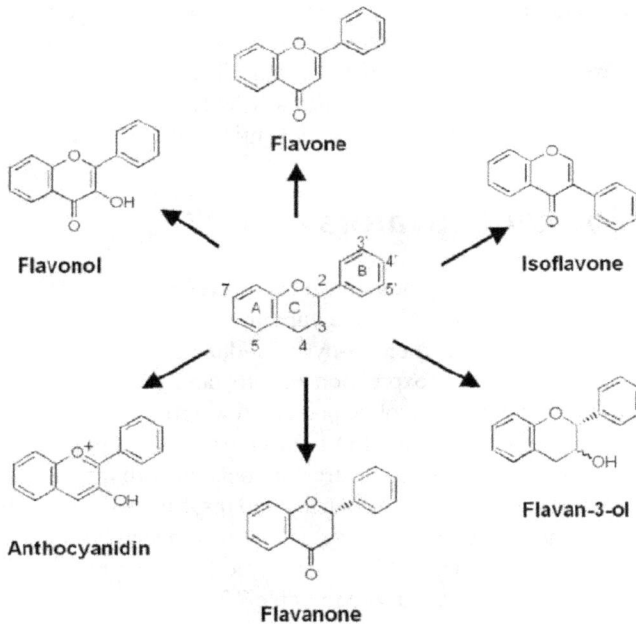

FIGURE 7.3   Chemical structures of some of the most important flavonoids.

TABLE 7.3   Flavonoids and their dietary sources

FLAVONOID	SUBGROUP	DIETARY SOURCES	REFERENCES
Quercetin	Flavonols	Vegetables, fruits, spices	[86]
Genistein	Isoflavone	Tofu, soyabean	[87]
Taxifolin	Flavanonol	Vinegar	[88]
Theaflavin	Catechins	Tea leaves, black tea	[89]
Peonidin	Anthocyanidin	Cranberries, blueberries, grapes	[90]

Role of Flavonoids in Nrf2 Signaling and Obesity

Under normal physiological and induced conditions, flavonoids are among the most effective dietary phytochemicals that activate the Nrf2/ARE pathway. In both in vitro and pre-clinical trials, flavones (apigenin, luteolin, and baicalin) have been reported to upregulate Nrf2 protein expression [14,101]. Flavanones (naringenin and hesperidin), flavonols (quercetin), and flavan-3-ols have all been found to upregulate the Nrf2 protein (epigallocatechin-3-gallate) [102].

Flavonoids activate the Nrf2/ARE pathway downstream of Nrf2 nuclear translocation. Flavanones (naringenin and hesperidin), flavones (baicalein, luteolin, baicalin, and chrysin), flavonols (quercetin and rutin), isoflavones, and anthocyanins (C3G) were found to overexpress antioxidant defense genes and phase 2 detoxification genes. At physiologically greater doses, baicalein has been found to upregulate the expression of downstream target genes in liver cells exposed to high glucose-induced oxidative stress [103,104]. By activating the Nrf2/ARE pathway, oxidative stress is greatly alleviated, and this has the tendency to reduce obesity.

CONCLUSION

Inflammation and oxidative stress are important in the etiology of obesity. Furthermore, oxidative stress may influence food intake by affecting hypothalamic neurons that regulate satiety and hunger. Several studies have investigated the effect of the Nrf2 pathway in obesity, with possible antioxidant and anti-inflammatory actions reported. Nrf2 activators have proven to be useful tools to ameliorate the progression of obesity. Furthermore, flavonoids, which are potent phytochemicals, have been shown to activate the Nrf2 pathway and could be possible agents in the management of obesity.

REFERENCES

1. Ulijaszek, S.J., Obesity: Preventing and managing the global epidemic. Report of a WHO consultation. WHO technical report series 894. pp. 252. (World Health Organization, Geneva, 2000.) SFr 56.00, ISBN 92-4-120894-5, paperback. *Journal of Biosocial Science*, 2003, 35(4): 624–625.
2. WHO, Obesity and overweight, 2017. http://www.who.int/mediacentre/factsheets/fs311/en/, Accessed: December 17, 2021.
3. Vasileva, L.V., A.S. Marchev, and M.I. Georgiev, Causes and solutions to "globesity": The new fa(s)t alarming global epidemic. *Food and Chemical Toxicology*, 2018, 121: 173–193.
4. Centers for Disease Control and Prevention, Defining adult overweight and obesity. Available at: www.cdc.gov/obesity/adult/defining.html. Assessed: December 18, 2021.
5. Després, J.P., et al., Regional distribution of body fat, plasma lipoproteins, and cardiovascular disease. *Arteriosclerosis (Dallas, Tex.)*, 1990, 10(4): 497–511.

6. Fernández-Sánchez, A., et al., Inflammation, oxidative stress, and obesity. *International Journal of Molecular Sciences*, 2011, 12(5): 3117–3132.
7. Li, R., Z. Jia, and Z. Hong, Regulation of Nrf2 signaling. *Reactive Oxygen Species*, 2019, 8: 312–322.
8. Tonelli, C., and C. Chio II, and D.A. Tuveson, Transcriptional regulation by Nrf2. *Antioxidants & Redox Signaling*, 2011, 29: 1727–1745.
9. Matzinger, M., K. Fischhuber, and E.H. Heiss, Activation of Nrf2 signaling by natural products-can it alleviates diabetes? *Biotechnology Advances*, 2018, 36(6): 1738–1767.
10. Dodson, M., et al., Modulating NRF2 in disease: Timing is everything. *Annual Review of Pharmacology and Toxicology*, 2019, 59(1): 555–575.
11. Hurrle, S., and W.H. Hsu, The etiology of oxidative stress in insulin resistance. *Biomedical Journal*, 2017, 40(5): 257–262.
12. Vernarelli, J.A., and J.D. Lambert, Flavonoid intake is inversely associated with obesity and C-reactive protein, a marker for inflammation, in US adults. *Nutrition & Diabetes*, 2017, 7(5): e276–e276.
13. Marranzano, M., et al., The association between dietary flavonoid intake and obesity in a cohort of adults living in the Mediterranean area. *International Journal of Food Sciences and Nutrition*, 2018, 69(8): 1020–1029.
14. Li, L., et al., Luteolin protects against diabetic cardiomyopathy by inhibiting NF-κB-mediated inflammation and activating the Nrf2-mediated antioxidant responses. *Phytomedicine (Stuttgart)*, 2019, 59: 152774–152774.
15. Lefterova, M.I., and M.A. Lazar, New developments in adipogenesis. *Trends in Endocrinology and Metabolism*, 2009, 20(3): 107–114.
16. Ali, A.T., et al., Adipocyte and adipogenesis. *European Journal of Cell Biology*, 2013, 92(6–7): 229–236.
17. Gregoire, F.M., C.M. Smas, and H.S. Sul, Understanding adipocyte differentiation. *Physiological Reviews*, 1998, 78(3): 783–809.
18. Zhang, Y., and R. Derynck, Regulation of Smad signalling by protein associations and signalling crosstalk. *Trends in Cell Biology*, 1999, 9(7): 274–279.
19. Chen, D., et al., Differential roles for bone morphogenetic protein (BMP) receptor type IB and IA in differentiation and specification of mesenchymal precursor cells to osteoblast and adipocyte lineages. *The Journal of Cell Biology*, 1998, 142(1): 295–305.
20. Butterwith, S.C., R.S. Wilkie, and M. Clinton, Treatment of pluripotential C3H 10T1/2 fibroblasts with bone morphogenetic protein-4 induces adipocyte commitment. *Biochemical Society Transactions*, 1996, 24(2): 163S–163S.
21. Roth, S., *Mechanisms of development*, edited by R.G. Ham and M.J. Veomett. St. Louis: C. V. Mosby, 1980: 262–263.
22. Bourgeois, C., et al., Specific biological features of adipose tissue, and their impact on HIV persistence. *Frontiers in Microbiology*, 2019, 10: 2837.
23. Apovian, C.M., Obesity: Definition, co-morbidities, causes, and burden. *The American Journal of Managed Care*, 2016, 22(7 Suppl): S176–S185.
24. Halberg, N.P., I.P. Wernstedt-Asterholm, and P.E.P. Scherer, The adipocyte as an endocrine cell. *Endocrinology and Metabolism Clinics of North America*, 2008, 37(3): 753–768.
25. Galic, S., J.S. Oakhill, and G.R. Steinberg, Adipose tissue as an endocrine organ. *Molecular and Cellular Endocrinology*, 2010, 316(2): 129–139.
26. Esposito, K., et al., Oxidative stress in the metabolic syndrome. *Journal of Endocrinological Investigation*, 2006, 29(9): 791–795.
27. Fonseca-Alaniz, M.H., et al., Adipose tissue as an endocrine organ: From theory to practice. *Journal of Pediatr (Rio J)*, 2007, 83(5 Suppl): S192–203.
28. Farshad, A., et al., Is obesity associated with increased plasma lipid peroxidation and oxidative stress in women? *Arya Atherosclerosis*, 2010, 2(4): 189–192.

29. Khan, N, Naz, L, and Y. Ghazala, An independent risk factor systemic oxidative stress. *Journal of Pharmaceutical Sciences*, 2006, 19(1): 62–69.
30. Qatanani, M., and M.A. Lazar, Mechanisms of obesity-associated insulin resistance: Many choices on the menu. *Genes & Development*, 2007, 21(12): 1443–1455.
31. Ahima, R.S., and M.A. Lazar, Adipokines and the peripheral and neural control of energy balance. *Molecular Endocrinology (Baltimore, Md.)*, 2008, 22(5): 1023–1031.
32. Hotamisligil, G.S., Inflammation, and metabolic disorders. *Nature (London)*, 2006, 444(7121): 860–867.
33. Hotamisligil, G.S., Inflammation, metaflammation, and immunometabolic disorders. *Nature (London)*, 2017, 542(7640): 177–185.
34. Anforth, H.R., et al., Biological activity and brain actions of recombinant rat interleukin-1alpha and interleukin-1beta. *European Cytokine Network*, 1998, 9(3): 279–288.
35. Jansson, J.-O., et al., Interleukin-6-deficient mice develop mature-onset obesity. *Nature Medicine*, 2002, 8(1): 75–79.
36. Oliveros, E., et al., The concept of normal weight obesity. *Progress in Cardiovascular Diseases*, 2014, 56(4): 426–433.
37. Sharma, R.S., et al., Experimental nonalcoholic steatohepatitis and liver fibrosis are ameliorated by pharmacologic activation of Nrf2 (NF-E2 p45-related factor 2). *Cellular and Molecular Gastroenterology and Hepatology*, 2018, 5(3): 367–398.
38. Blaak, E.E., et al., β-adrenergic stimulation and abdominal subcutaneous fat blood flow in lean, obese, and reduced-obese subjects. *Metabolism, Clinical and Experimental*, 1995, 44(2): 183–187.
39. Kabon, B., et al., Obesity decreases perioperative tissue oxygenation. *Anesthesiology (Philadelphia)*, 2004, 100(2): 274–280.
40. Trayhurn, P., Hypoxia and adipose tissue function and dysfunction in obesity. *Physiological Reviews*, 2013, 93(1): 1–21.
41. Ellulu, M.S., et al., Obesity and inflammation: The linking mechanism and the complications. *Archives of Medical Science*, 2017, 13(4): 851–863.
42. Okada, S., et al., Adipose tissue-specific dysregulation of angiotensinogen by oxidative stress in obesity. *Metabolism, Clinical and Experimental*, 2010, 59(9): 1241–1251.
43. Hajjar, D.P., and A.M. Gotto, Biological relevance of inflammation and oxidative stress in the pathogenesis of arterial diseases. *The American Journal of Pathology*, 2013, 182(5): 1474–1481.
44. Pizzino, G., et al., Oxidative stress: Harms and benefits for human health. *Oxidative Medicine and Cellular Longevity*, 2017, 2017: 8416763-13.
45. Savini, I., et al., Obesity-associated oxidative stress: Strategies finalized to improve redox state. *International Journal of Molecular Sciences*, 2013, 14(5): 10497–10538.
46. Manna, P., and S.K. Jain, Obesity, oxidative stress, adipose tissue dysfunction, and the associated health risks: Causes and therapeutic strategies. *Metabolic Syndrome and Related Disorders*, 2015: 423–444.
47. Horvath, T.L., Z.B. Andrews, and S. Diano, Fuel utilization by hypothalamic neurons: Roles for ROS. *Trends in Endocrinology and Metabolism*, 2008, 20(2): 78–87.
48. Sies, H., Oxidative stress: A concept in redox biology and medicine. *Redox Biology*, 2015, 4(C): 180–183.
49. Arango Duque, G., and A. Descoteaux, Macrophage cytokines: Involvement in immunity and infectious diseases. *Frontiers in Immunology*, 2014, 5: 491–491.
50. Subramanian, V., and A.W. Ferrante, Jr, Obesity, inflammation, and macrophages. *Nestlé Nutrition Institute Workshop Series: Pediatric Program*, 2009.
51. Morris, D.L., K. Singer, and C.N. Lumeng, Adipose tissue macrophages: Phenotypic plasticity and diversity in lean and obese states. *Current Opinion in Clinical Nutrition and Metabolic Care*, 2011, 14(4): 341–346.

52. Kratz, M., et al., Metabolic dysfunction drives a mechanistically distinct pro-inflammatory phenotype in adipose tissue macrophages. *Cell Metabolism*, 2014, 20(4): 614–625.

53. Hotamisligil, G.S., Inflammatory pathways, and insulin action. *International Journal of Obesity*, 2003, 27(S3): S53–S55.

54. Xu, H., et al., Chronic inflammation in fat plays a crucial role in the development of obesity-related insulin resistance. *The Journal of Clinical Investigation*, 2003, 112(12): 1821–1830.

55. Marseglia, L., et al., Oxidative stress in obesity: A critical component in human diseases. *International Journal of Molecular Sciences*, 2014, 16(1): 378–400.

56. Itoh, K., et al., Keap1 represses nuclear activation of antioxidant responsive elements by Nrf2 through binding to the amino-terminal Neh2 domain. *Genes & Development*, 1999, 13(1): 76–86.

57. Itoh, K., et al., An Nrf2/small Maf heterodimer mediates the induction of phase II detoxifying enzyme genes through antioxidant response elements. *Biochemical and Biophysical Research Communications*, 1997, 236(2): 313–322.

58. Farmer, S.R., Transcriptional control of adipocyte formation. *Cell Metabolism*, 2006, 4(4): 263–273.

59. Rosen, E.D., and O.A. MacDougald, Adipocyte differentiation from the inside out. *Nature Reviews. Molecular Cell Biology*, 2006, 7(12): 885–896.

60. Vishvanath, L., and R.K. Gupta, Contribution of adipogenesis to healthy adipose tissue expansion in obesity. *The Journal of Clinical Investigation*, 2019, 129(10): 4022–4031.

61. Sun, X., et al., Nuclear factor E2-related factor 2 mediates oxidative stress-induced lipid accumulation in adipocytes by increasing adipogenesis and decreasing lipolysis. *Antioxidants & Redox Signaling*, 2020, 32(3): 173–192.

62. Pi, J., et al., Deficiency in the nuclear factor E2-related factor-2 transcription factor results in impaired adipogenesis and protects against diet-induced obesity. *The Journal of Biological Chemistry*, 2010, 285(12): 9292–9300.

63. Kim, D.-H., et al., Rapid and weight-independent improvement of glucose tolerance induced by a peptide designed to elicit apoptosis in adipose tissue endothelium. *Diabetes (New York, N.Y.)*, 2012, 61(9): 2299–2310.

64. Zhu, W., et al., Endoplasmic reticulum stress may be involved in insulin resistance and lipid metabolism disorders of the white adipose tissues induced by high-fat diet containing industrial trans-fatty acids. *Diabetes, Metabolic Syndrome and Obesity*, 2019, 12: 1625–1638.

65. Kloting, N., and M. Bluher, Adipocyte dysfunction, inflammation and metabolic syndrome. *Reviews in Endocrine & Metabolic Disorders*, 2014, 15(4): 277–287.

66. Scherer, P.E., The many secret lives of adipocytes: Implications for diabetes. *Diabetologia*, 2018, 62(2): 223–232.

67. Wang, C., et al., The effect and mechanism of TLR9/KLF4 in FFA-induced adipocyte inflammation. *Mediators of Inflammation*, 2018, 2018: 6313484-10.

68. Medina-Gomez, G., S. Gray, and A. Vidal-Puig, Adipogenesis and lipotoxicity: Role of peroxisome proliferator-activated receptor-gamma (PPARgamma) and PPARgammacoactivator-1 (PGC1). *Public Health Nutrition*, 2007, 10(10A): 1132.

69. Xu, J., et al., Keap1-knockdown decreases fasting-induced fatty liver via altered lipid metabolism and decreased fatty acid mobilization from adipose tissue. *PLoS One*, 2013, 8(11): e79841–e79841.

70. Chartoumpekis, D.V., et al., Nrf2 represses FGF21 during long-term high-fat diet-induced obesity in mice. *Diabetes (New York, N.Y.)*, 2011, 60(10): 2465–2473.

71. Li, S., et al., The role of the Nrf2 signaling in obesity and insulin resistance. *International Journal of Molecular Sciences*, 2020, 21(18): 6973.

72. Shin, S., et al., Role of Nrf2 in preventing high-fat diet-induced obesity by synthetic triterpenoid CDDO-imidazolide. *European Journal of Pharmacology*, 2009, 620(1): 138–144.

73. Meher, A.K., et al., Nrf2 deficiency in myeloid cells is not sufficient to protect mice from HFD-induced adipose tissue inflammation and insulin resistance. *Free Radical Biology & Medicine*, 2012, 52(9): 1708–1715.
74. Peng, X.U.E., et al., Adipose deficiency of Nrf2 in ob/ob mice results in severe metabolic syndrome. *Diabetes (New York, N.Y.)*, 2013, 62(3): 845–854.
75. Gaikwad, A., et al., In vivo role of NAD(P)H: Quinone oxidoreductase 1 (NQO1) in the regulation of intracellular redox state and accumulation of abdominal adipose tissue. *The Journal of Biological Chemistry*, 2001, 276(25): 22559–22564.
76. Jialin, X.U., et al., Enhanced Nrf2 activity worsens insulin resistance, impairs lipid accumulation in adipose tissue, and increases hepatic steatosis in leptin-deficient mice. *Diabetes (New York, N.Y.)*, 2012, 61(12): 3208–3218.
77. More, V.R., et al., Keap1 knockdown increases markers of metabolic syndrome after long-term high fat diet feeding. *Free Radical Biology & Medicine*, 2013, 61: 85–94.
78. Yu, Z., et al., Oltipraz upregulates the nuclear respiratory factor 2 alpha subunit (NRF2) antioxidant system and prevents insulin resistance and obesity induced by a high-fat diet in C57BL/6J mice. *Diabetologia*, 2010, 54(4): 922–934.
79. Jung, U.J., and M.-S. Choi, Obesity and its metabolic complications: The role of adipokines and the relationship between obesity, inflammation, insulin resistance, dyslipidemia and non-alcoholic fatty liver disease. *International Journal of Molecular Sciences*, 2014, 15(4): 6184–6223.
80. Zhang, W., et al., ER stress potentiates insulin resistance through PERK-mediated FOXO phosphorylation. *Genes & Development*, 2013, 27(4): 441–449.
81. Choi, K.-M., et al., Sulforaphane attenuates obesity by inhibiting adipogenesis and activating the AMPK pathway in obese mice. *The Journal of Nutritional Biochemistry*, 2014, 25(2): 201–207.
82. Collins, A.R., et al., Myeloid deletion of nuclear factor erythroid 2-related factor 2 increases atherosclerosis and liver injury. *Arteriosclerosis, Thrombosis, and Vascular Biology*, 2012, 32(12): 2839–2846.
83. He, H.-J., et al., Curcumin attenuates Nrf2 signaling defect, oxidative stress in muscle and glucose intolerance in high fat diet-fed mice. *World Journal of Diabetes*, 2012, 3(5): 94–104.
84. Havsteen, B.H., The biochemistry and medical significance of the flavonoids. *Pharmacology & Therapeutics (Oxford)*, 2002, 96(2): 67–202.
85. Kawser Hossain, M., et al., Molecular mechanisms of the anti-obesity and anti-diabetic properties of flavonoids. *International Journal of Molecular Sciences*, 2016, 17(4): 569–569.
86. Hertog, M.G.L., P.C.H. Hollman, and B. van de Putte, Content of potentially anticarcinogenic flavonoids of tea infusions, wines, and fruit juices. *Journal of Agricultural and Food Chemistry*, 1993, 41(8): 1242–1246.
87. Thompson, L.U., et al., Phytoestrogen content of foods consumed in Canada, including isoflavones, lignans, and coumestan. *Nutrition and Cancer*, 2006, 54(2): 184–201.
88. Cerezo, A.B., et al., Effect of wood on the phenolic profile and sensory properties of wine vinegars during ageing. *Journal of Food Composition and Analysis*, 2010, 23(2): 175–184.
89. Leung, L.K., et al., Theaflavins in black tea and catechins in green tea are equally effective antioxidants. *Journal of Nutrition*, 2001, 131(9): 2248–2251.
90. Truong, V.D., et al., Characterization of anthocyanins and anthocyanidins in purple-fleshed sweet potatoes by HPLC-DAD/ESI-MS/MS. *Journal of Agricultural and Food Chemistry*, 2010, 58(1): 404–410.
91. Ribeiro, D., et al., Pro-inflammatory pathways: The modulation by flavonoids. *Medicinal Research Reviews*, 2015, 35(5): 877–936.

92. Almeida Rezende, B., et al., Vascular effects of flavonoids. *Current Medicinal Chemistry*, 2016, 23(1): 87–102.

93. Mira, A., W. Alkhiary, and K. Shimizu, Antiplatelet and anticoagulant activities of angelica shikokiana extract and its isolated compounds. *Clinical and Applied Thrombosis/Hemostasis*, 2017, 23(1): 91–99.

94. Wang, C.-Z., et al., Botanical flavonoids on coronary heart disease. *The American Journal of Chinese Medicine*, 2011, 39(4): 661–671.

95. Proença, C., et al., α-Glucosidase inhibition by flavonoids: An in vitro and in silico structure-activity relationship study. *Journal of Enzyme Inhibition and Medicinal Chemistry*, 2017, 32(1): 1216–1228.

96. Amawi, H., C.R. Ashby, and A.K. Tiwari, Cancer chemoprevention through dietary flavonoids: What's limiting? *Ai Zheng*, 2017, 36(10): 455–467.

97. Frandsen, J.R., and P. Narayanasamy, Neuroprotection through flavonoid: Enhancement of the glyoxalase pathway. *Redox Biology*, 2018, 14: 465–473.

98. Khan, H., et al., Current standing of plant-derived flavonoids as an antidepressant. *Food and Chemical Toxicology*, 2018, 119: 176–188.

99. Song, D., et al., The modulatory effect and the mechanism of flavonoids on obesity. *Journal of Food Biochemistry*, 2019, 43(8): e12954-n/a.

100. Rufino, A.T., et al., Flavonoids as antiobesity agents: A review. *Medicinal Research Reviews*, 2021, 41(1): 556–585.

101. Zhang, H.-B., et al., Baicalin reduces early brain injury after subarachnoid hemorrhage in rats. *Chinese Journal of Integrative Medicine*, 2020, 26(7): 510–518.

102. Schadich, E., et al., Effects of ginger phenylpropanoids and quercetin on Nrf2-ARE pathway in human BJ fibroblasts and HaCaT keratinocytes. *Biomed Research International*, 2016, 2016: 2173275-6.

103. Tian, S., et al., Pharmacokinetic study of baicalein after oral administration in monkeys. *Fitoterapia*, 2012, 83(3): 532–540.

104. Dong, Y., et al., Baicalein alleviates liver oxidative stress and apoptosis induced by high-level glucose through the activation of the PERK/Nrf2 signaling pathway. *Molecules (Basel, Switzerland)*, 2020, 25(3): 599.

Flavonoids Activation of Nrf2 and Osteoporosis

8

Samia S. Messeha and Karam F. A. Soliman
Florida A&M University

Contents

DOI: 10.1201/9781003225225-8

INTRODUCTION

Aging is a complicated process influenced by genetic and environmental variables that may be described as the gradual loss of an organism's optimal function until death [1]. Osteoporosis (OP) is an age-related skeletal disorder defined by low bone mass and micro-architectural degeneration of bone structure, which leads to bone fragility and increases fracture risk and mortality rate [2]. OP is ubiquitous in the elderly and post-menopausal women. However, other causes such as lifestyle systemic disease—such as diabetes, hypothyroidism, and long-term drug therapy—are also considered risk factors of OP. In the United States, about 10 million are diagnosed with OP, in addition to almost 34 million at risk [3]. OP has a significant impact on the quality of life due to pain, dis-ability, depression, and expected fractures such as hip, vertebra, and wrist fractures [4]. Yet, hip fracture is the most common among older people of both sexes, which signifi-cantly reduces the quality of life and increases mortality rate [5]. Osteoporotic fractures (OFs) increase the risk of various chronic diseases, including cancer and cardiovascular diseases [6]. Women are more vulnerable to OF than men since, at age 50 years, 50% of women vs. 20% of men are expected to have an OF in their remaining lifetime [3]. Hence, hospital admission is required for patients with OF, particularly hip fractures [7]. Once hospitalized, these patients start suffering from additional complications such as thrombosis, urinary tract infections, and pneumonia. Thus, treating OP and preventing fractures is critical for improving patient health and managing hospital costs. Therefore, this disease poses a considerable demand on the healthcare system since the number of patients diagnosed each year increases vigorously [3].

Over the last three decades, innovations in pharmacological OP therapy have evolved promising drugs for preventing excessive bone resorption and promoting bone growth [3]. Moreover, there is an increased number of untreated patients either because they are not receiving the treatments at all or not taking their medicines [8]. Furthermore, challenges such as infrequent adverse effects and poor long-term efficacy of currently available antiresorptive medications lead to the OP treatment gap [9].

Modulation of gene expression and stimulation of crucial proteins have emerged as a promising approach in managing age-related disorders [10]. There is a strong belief that aging is closely associated with unbalanced oxidant/antioxidant, impaired nuclear factor erythroid-derived 2-like 2 (Nrf2) signaling, and phase 2 response [11].

Flavonoids are a large family of polyphenolic compounds abundantly found in our daily consumed plants. Besides safety, flavonoids are characterized by various biological properties, mainly the antioxidant role that reduces various diseases and enhances human health [12]. These properties encouraged evaluation of its anti-osteo-porotic potential in clinical trials [4].

BONE FORMATION

A distinct composition characterizes bone to maintain the body's posture and protect the internal organs [13]. The bone is composed mainly of proteins—such as collagenous and non-collagenous—and inorganic ions for enhancing its functions. Bone also harbors fat and various types of minerals such as calcium, magnesium, phosphate, bicarbonate, and sodium. These minerals are found at a homeostatic level under normal physiological conditions and in the presence of various regulators such as parathyroid hormone, vitamin D, calcitonin, and other cellular elements [13–15]. Both adipocytes and osteoblasts cells are segregated from mesenchymal stem cells (MSCs) in the bone marrow. Moreover, the decrease in osteogenesis and adipogenesis increase contribute significantly to age-related OP [16]. Bone contains four different cell types: osteoblasts, bone lining cells, osteocytes, and osteoclasts [17,18]. These cells are classified according to various criteria such as their origin, location, and specific function [17,19].

OSTEOBLASTS

Osteoblasts, the bone-forming cells, originated from MSCs and play an essential role in the bone-forming process [20]. The mechanism of MSC-osteoblastic differentiation is complicated and precisely controlled, as demonstrated by Bellavia et al. [4,21] (Figure 8.1). Typically, two families of the growth factors are involved in osteoblasts differentiation: a portmanteau of Wingless and integration 1 (Wnt) family and bone morphogenetic proteins (BMPs) [22,23]. The significant function of the canonical Wnt signaling in bone development is well recognized [24]. Out of the 19 members of the Wnt family, Wnt10b has gained particular attention in bone formation. Wnt10b is activated in the bone marrow by osteoblast precursors [25]. The transgenic overexpression of the Wnt10b in MSC leads to increased bone density, enhanced osteoblast-induced bone development (osteoblastogenesis), as well as stimulating osteoblast functions [26]. The growth factors BMPs are members of the transforming growth factor-beta (TGF-β) superfamily that present an essential factor in the skeletogenesis mechanism [27,28]. The mechanism of MSC-osteoblast differentiation is also regulated by two main transcription factors: stimulatory transcription factors and inhibitory transcription factors (ITFs) [23]. These stimulatory genes include β-catenin, runt-related 2 (Runx2), Osterix (Osx), smads, enhancer-binding protein, and others [20,29]. Meanwhile, Runx2 has gained substantial attention in osteoblastogenesis [23]. The fact that BMPs are controlling the

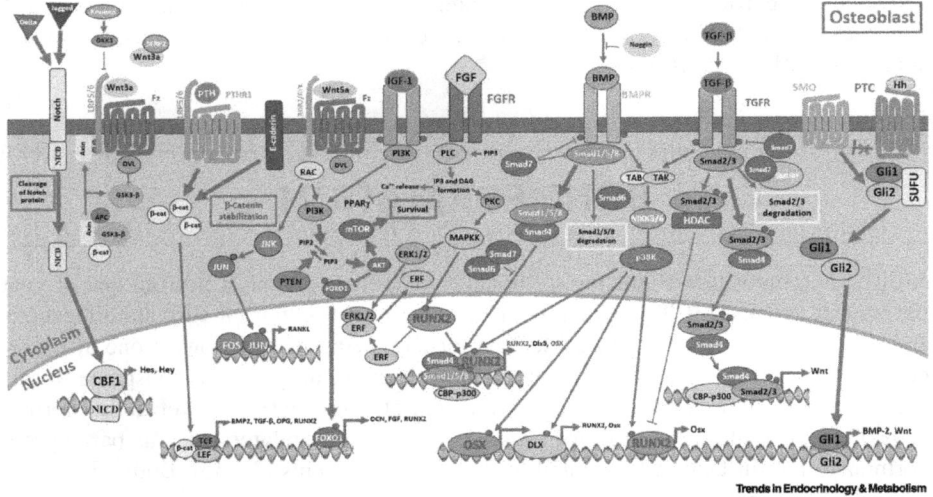

FIGURE 8.1   Different signaling pathways mediating osteoblast formation as expressed by Bellavia et al. [4,21].

expression of Osx and Runx2 [30] proposed BMPs as highly potent stimulators of mesenchymal precursor cell differentiation into osteoblasts [31]. Furthermore, the promising outcome of using BMP members in some human orthopedic surgery [32] and the enhanced healing rate without an invasive secondary surgery [33]. On the other hand, the ITF peroxisome proliferator-activated receptor γ (PPARγ) and TWIST are well-known inhibitors of Runx2 and β-catenin [34,35]. Osteoblast differentiation is also controlled by several factors, including microRNAs (miRNA), fibroblast growth factors (FGFs), and connexin 43 [36–39]. FGF knockout showed decreased bone density [38] through autocrine mechanism [40]. Likewise, connexin 43 mutagenesis is linked to skeletal malformation [41]. Members of miRNAs are showing dual functions during osteoblastogenesis. They act as positive regulators by activating Wnt signaling pathway or negative regulators by inhibiting Runx2 [42,43]. The secretion of bone matrix proteins is essential during the transition of preosteoblasts to mature osteoblasts. At the same time, the mechanism of bone matrix synthesis is established by osteoblasts through two major steps, including deposition of organic matrix and mineralization [22].

BONE LINING CELLS

Bone lining cells are inactive osteoblasts adjacent to the bone surfaces [44]. This cell type controls bone resorption by preventing direct contact between osteoclasts and bone matrix. The essential functions performed by the bone lining cells include osteoclast differentiation in addition to the production of osteoprotegerin (OPG) and the receptor activator of nuclear factor-kappa-B ligand (RANKL) [45,46]. During the bone remodeling cycle, the bone lining and other bone cells are essential components of the basic multicellular unit [47].

OSTEOCYTES

Osteocytes are the most long-lived and abundant bone cells, accounting for more than 90% of all bone cells [48,49]. Meanwhile, bone lining cells, osteoblasts, and osteoclasts are adjacent to the bone surface; osteocyte cells are found inside the bone [17,19]. This type of bone cell is commonly released from mature osteoblasts captured inside the canaliculi of the bone matrix since they are produced but no longer contribute to bone production [48]. Osteocytogenesis is characterized by four stages: osteoid-osteocyte, preosteocyte, young osteocyte, and mature osteocyte [48]. Osteocytes have demonstrated crucial functions [49], whereas they orchestrate the process of bone remodeling by controlling osteoclast activities [50] and mediate osteocyte apoptosis during bone resorption [51–54].

OSTEOCLASTS

The multinucleated osteoclast bone cells are developed from the mononuclear hematopoietic stem cell described by Bellavia et al. [4,21] (Figure 8.2). Osteoclast-controlled

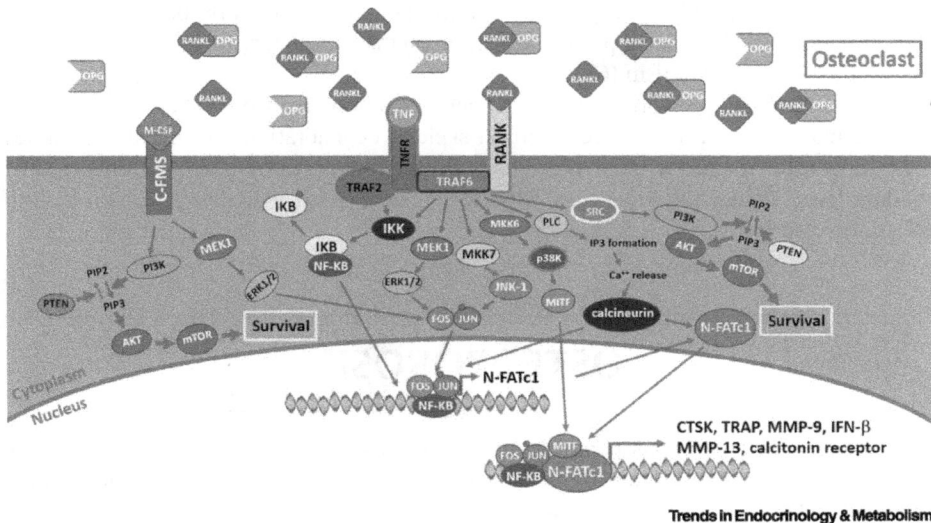

FIGURE 8.2 Different signaling pathways mediating osteoclast differentiation as expressed by Bellavia et al. [4,21].

bone resorption (osteoclastogenesis) is influenced by many factors such as the macrophage colony-stimulating factor (M-CSF), Receptor Activator of Nuclear Factor ĸ B (RANK) ligand (RANKL), and stromal cells [55,56]. Simultaneously, these factors activate essential transcription factors in osteoclasts [56,57]. Meanwhile, a humoral tumor necrosis factor (TNF) receptor family protein OPG, released by a wide range of cells, is a crucial factor that inhibits the process of osteoclastogenesis [58–60]. Besides their primary function as bone-resorbing cells, osteoclasts also mediate the production of cytokines that regulate the activity of other cells such as osteoblasts and hematopoietic stem cell niches [61]. Significantly, OP and other bone illnesses are associated with an abnormal increase in osteoclast production and activity, in which bone resorption exceeds bone formation, leading to decreased bone density and increased bone fractures [22,62].

BONE REMODELING/METABOLISM

Bone metabolism appears continuously throughout a lifespan and is precisely controlled through two main processes: modeling and remodeling [63,64]. In bone modeling, the shape of existing bones is modified to a new bone to adapt to external stimuli. Meanwhile, bone remodeling is essential for removing old bone tissue and replacing it with new bone tissue, which is necessary for bone homeostasis [65]. Osteoblasts and osteocytes are essential cells for bone modeling and remodeling [66]. Initially, osteocytes trigger osteoblasts to release RANKL which promotes the development of osteoclasts [67]. RANKL-activated osteoclasts subsequently coordinate with osteoblasts to eliminate old bone and replace it with a new one through bone matrix deposition and mineralization [65,67,68]. Receptors for vitamin D, estrogen, parathyroid hormone, and parathyroid hormone–related protein are found on the cell surface of osteoblasts and are involved in bone metabolism [67].

Increased bone resorption and poor bone formation are two mechanisms involved in bone mass loss and micro-architectural skeletal degeneration. Furthermore, studies have shown that the redox imbalance has a significant impact on bone, with lower antioxidant levels enhancing bone resorption, whereas reduced oxidative stress protecting OP in the elderly [69,70].

OSTEOPOROSIS

Bone undergoes continuous turnover to sustain its strength and integrity [71]. OP is a progressive metabolic bone disease that causes decreased bone mass and micro-architectural degeneration of bone structure, which progress to bone fragility, increased fracture risk, and mortality rate [2]. Furthermore, OP can lead to other serious complications such as Alzheimer's and cardiovascular diseases [72]. Two main criteria are involved in OP disorder: the decreased osteoblast differentiation (osteoblastogenesis) accompanied by a reduced bone deposition and the increased osteoclast differentiation (osteoclastogenesis) leading to excessive bone resorption. Nevertheless, OP occurs when the osteoclastogenesis rate exceeds osteoblastogenesis [21].

Various factors, including physiological aging, post-menopause hormonal changes, genetic alterations, and pathological symptom-related medication can all lead to OP, which is characterized by a decrease in bone remodeling and imbalance between bone formation and bone resorption [13,70].

Epigenetic alterations are evolving as a novel mechanism in the pathogenesis of OP [73–75]. Also, the development of OP is closely linked to many hematopoietic and immune agents in the bone microenvironment [76,77]. Epigenetic alterations such as DNA methylation, non-coding RNA, and histone modifications are used as markers of bone loss in aged people [13]. DNA methylation is the primary epigenetic mutation of gene transcription [75,78]. Moreover, recent research has found that adequate physical exercise can help control DNA methylation in many pathological and physiological circumstances, such as aging [79,80]. In animal models, demethylating agents have demonstrated therapeutic advantages against OP [81,82]. Unfortunately, long-term administration of antidemethylating agents in patients led to severe side effects in some individuals [83]. Furthermore, inheritable alteration in some genes is significantly implicated in skeletal aging and OP [84]. Therefore, altered expressions of osteoblastic genes, including RUNX2, Wnt10b, RANKL, osteocalcin (OCN), OSX, SOST, and OPG, were previously found in patients with OP [85].

Oxidative stress is a sequel of an imbalance between oxidants production and elimination through various protective mechanisms, including antioxidants [86,87]. There is a simultaneous association between oxidative stress and OP. Many risk factors for OP, such as hypertension, diabetes mellitus, and smoking, are closely associated with elevated oxidative stress [88,89]. Oxidative stress triggered by reactive oxygen species (ROS) can adversely impact bone homeostasis and skeletal fragility [90,91]. Indeed, the two concomitant events, weak oxidative stress responses and low distributing antioxidants, are related to decreased bone mineral density. This redox imbalance is a substantial risk factor for OP [92–97].

On the contrary, the transcription factor Nrf2 is essential for the induction of cytoprotective genes-linked oxidative stress and bone homeostasis; meanwhile, the accumulation of ROS is a major cause of bone loss in the elderly [98,99]. Treating ovariectomized rats with antioxidants has shown protection against oxidative stress through Nrf2 activation-linked suppression of ROS levels. Hence, the notion of Nrf2 activation is a promising therapeutic approach in supporting bone health and reducing OP [100,101].

Physiological aging is frequently associated with various co-morbidities, with OP being one of the most prevalent [102]. Aging is always accompanied by multiple changes, including a substantial deterioration in osteoblasts proliferation, increased osteoblast and osteocytes apoptosis [103,104], elevated osteoblast senescence [105], defective osteoprogenitors [106], and subsequent increase in bone marrow adipogenesis [107]. Indeed, the reverse relationship between bone mass and bone marrow adipose tissue is found in old age [13].

Cessation of ovarian function and consequent estrogen deficiency is a typical sign of menopause [108]. Estrogen and its receptors α and β are essential mediators in maintaining bone homeostasis as evidenced by bone loss and OP at decreased estrogen-mediated menopause [109,110]. Usually, OP affects elderly postmenopausal women, but it can also affect younger women when their sex hormones are lost because of disease therapies or spontaneous early menopause [111,112]. As demonstrated by various studies, estrogen controls bone homeostasis through mechanisms such as inhibiting apoptosis in osteoblasts and osteocytes [113–115] and regulating bone resorption. In contrast, estrogen suppresses osteoclast differentiation and triggers osteoclast apoptosis [109,116–118]. The mechanism utilized by estrogen to inhibit osteoclastogenesis is achieved by either repressing the expression of osteoclast-associated RANKL or enhancing the production of OPG, a common decoy receptor of RANK [119–123]. Furthermore, estrogen reduces osteoclast formation by attenuating the expression of various osteoclastogenic cytokines, including TNF-α/β, IL-1, IL-6, IL-11, and M-CSF [124,125]. Estrogen deficiency can also lead to bone loss by diminishing the antioxidant level in osteoclasts [126]. Indeed, osteoporotic postmenopausal women showed reduced levels of antioxidant enzymes and higher plasma levels of malondialdehyde (MDA), the most commonly used lipid peroxidation indicator and oxidative stress biomarker [127]. In vivo investigations using ovariectomized rats have demonstrated that OP can delay callus formation and expand the fracture healing period [128].

Synthetic glucocorticoids such as dexamethasone are typically used for treating various autoimmune and inflammatory diseases [129]. Chronic treatment with these drugs is closely associated with varying degrees of skeletal disorder, eventually leading to glucocorticoid-linked osteoporosis (GLOP) and osteonecrosis [130,131]. Osteoblast apoptosis is also one of the anticipated adverse health effects of dexamethasone treatment, leading to oxidative stress elevation, accumulation of ROS, and impaired mitochondrial membrane potential [132–134]. GLOP therapeutic drugs might limit excessive bone resorption; however, it does not restore bone mass or bone microstructure, ultimately decreasing bone turnover [134]. The transcription factor Nrf2 is downregulated in various oxidative stress-related diseases [135]. ROS accumulation triggers GLOP development [136], and the upregulation of Nrf2 can significantly reduce oxidative stress [137], emphasizing the importance of Nrf2 as a promising therapeutic agent for GLOP. Indeed, reducing Nrf2 expression and ROS degrading enzyme superoxide dismutase (SOD) was accompanied by a substantial bone loss in OVAX rats compared with the control [69,100,127,128]. These findings indicate the significant role of Nrf2 in osteoprotection [138].

Nrf2 AND BONE FORMATION

The transcription factor Nrf2 is typically expressed in the cytosol; however, its low expression is maintained by its inhibitor Kelch-like Enoyl-CoA Hydratase (ECH)-associated protein 1 (Keap1) [139]. This inactive form of Nrf2 is expressed in most cells, including osteoblasts, osteoclasts, and osteocytes. The transcript pathway Nrf2 is regulated mainly by three distinct pathways, including keap1, phosphatidylinositol 3-kinase (PI3K)/Ak strain transforming (Akt) pathway, and epigenetics [140]. However, c-Jun N-terminal kinase (JNK) and mitogen-activated protein kinase (MAPK) signaling are also involved in Nrf2 upregulation [141]. Upon exposure to various stress, the stimulated Nrf2 detached from its inhibitor Keap1 and migrates to the cell nucleus, where it transactivates several downstream detoxifications and antioxidant enzymes [142,143], including SOD, catalase, and glutathione peroxidase [65,144]. Therefore, this signaling pathway has shown an essential role in bone formation (Figure 8.3) and during fracture healing [101].

Nrf2 deficiencies and the consequent reduction of antioxidative stress are closely associated with increased vulnerability to OP [69,145]. In contrast, enhancing Nrf2 expression through various activators is considered a protective mechanism against OP [138,146]. Epigenetic downregulation of Nrf2 could also lead to OP initiation and progression [71].

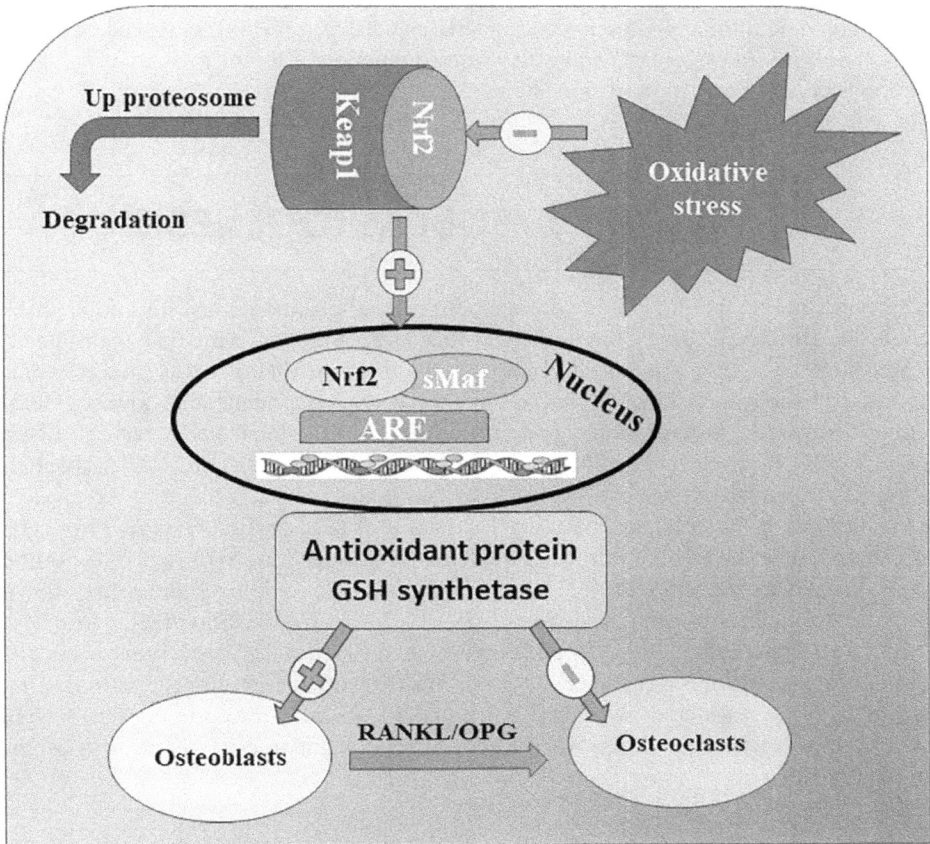

FIGURE 8.3   The role of the Nrf2 signaling pathway in bone formation.

Nrf2 AND BONE HOMEOSTASIS

The Nrf2 signaling pathway has emerged as an integral approach regulating oxidative stress-mediated bone homeostasis [65,147]. Nrf2 regulates various cytoprotective genes against oxidative stress and chemical offenses [65]. In contrast, ROS originates from hormone imbalance, aging, and other sources which are implicated in bone fragility [148]. In both osteoblast progenitor cells and osteoclast precursors, Nrf2 deficiency causes a rise in intracellular ROS levels as well as a failure in the production of some antioxidant enzymes and glutathione [149,150]. Furthermore, osteoblasts produce various antioxidants to protect against ROS [151,152]. A balanced expression between oxidants and antioxidants is an essential mechanism in maintaining the normal function of osteoblast and osteoclast [153]. Analogous to this fact, increased osteoclastic activity, along with decreased osteoblastic activity in postmenopausal OP, might be linked to an imbalance between oxidant and antioxidant levels [154]. Nrf2 deficiency increases radiation-stimulated bone loss [150], impairs the balance between bone formation and resorption, and ultimately lowers the bone mass and strength [147], as revealed in Nrf2 knockout mice. In osteoblasts and osteoclasts, regulation of Keap1-mediated Nrf2 activation is crucial for sustaining bone homeostasis [101]

Nrf2 AND OSTEOBLASTOGENESIS

The transcription factor Nrf2 is necessary for normal postnatal bone formation [155]. Evidence from Nrf2 deficiency indicated that mice with this deficiency exhibited a lower bone mass than the control. In this study, the bone disorder was interpreted as increased bone resorption and reduced bone formation, as evidenced by lower mineral appositional rate. It deteriorated bone formation in the lumbar vertebrae and distal femurs [147]. The relevance of Nrf2 in osteoblast differentiation and activity is debatable; however, various factors are involved, such as age, sex, genetic make-up, and physiological vs. pathological status. Also, the role of Nrf2 in osteoblast ancestor cells is influenced by the level of intracellular ROS [150]. Indeed, in Nrf2-deficient stromal cells, an elevated level of ROS [150] accompanied with oxidative stress has shown an inhibitory effect in osteoblastogenesis [92,156]. The transcription factor Runx2 is also a well-known regulator of bone formation and function [157]. Moreover, a previous study has shown the role of Nrf2 as an inhibitor of osteoblastogenesis [65]. This suggestion was validated in MC3T3-E1 osteoblastic cells where upregulated Nrf2 showed a potential to suppress Runx2 and induced negative consequences in osteoblasts [99,158].

Nrf2 AND OSTEOCLASTOGENESIS

Nrf2 signaling pathway is involved in osteoclast differentiation and activity (Figure 8.4). However, RANKL released by osteoblasts is the primary inducer of osteoclast formation. Low Nrf2/Keap1 ratio associated with RANKL exposure leads to a repression of Nrf2-dependent enzymes, supporting ROS signaling [65]. Activated Nrf2 boosts RANKL-mediated elevation of antioxidant enzymes and ultimately suppresses the process of osteoclast differentiation [65]. Nrf2 deletion decreases antioxidant enzymes and promotes intracellular ROS in osteoclasts, stimulating osteoclast differentiation and activity [149,159,160]. The transcription factor Nrf2 is also necessary for maintaining the average bone resorption rate, the mechanism regulated by the actin ring [68]. According to this pathway, Nrf2 deficiency stimulates RANKL trigger-actin ring formation and bone resorption [149]. The activity of Nrf2 in the osteoclast precursor cells was also proven by its interaction with the nuclear factor of activated T-cells, cytoplasmic 1 (NFATc1), and the crucial regulator of osteoclast differentiation [99,161].

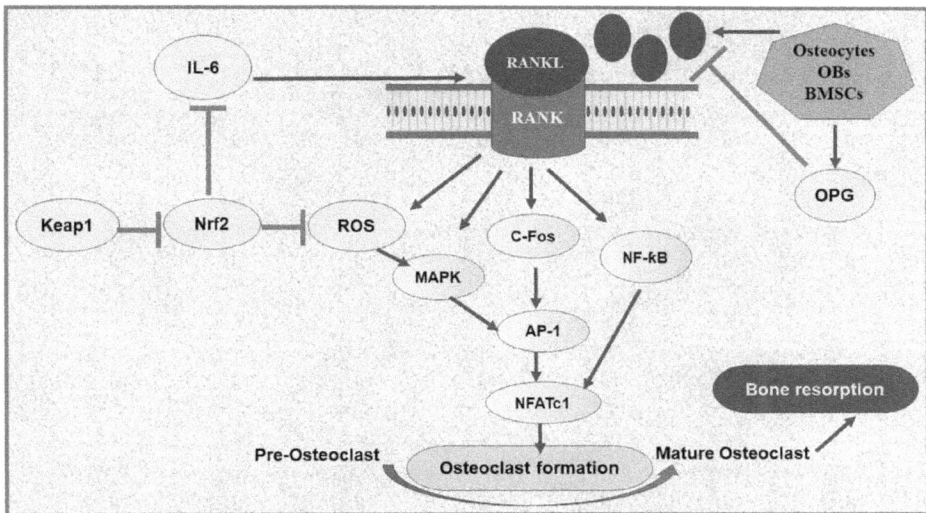

FIGURE 8.4 The role of RANK/RANKL signaling in osteoclasts differentiation. The diagram also shows the potential of Nrf2 in reducing osteoclastogenesis by inhibiting ROS formation.

Nrf2 AND FRACTURE HEALING MECHANISM

The vital role of Nrf2 in controlling bone cell formation can also be manifested during fracture healing [65], as evidenced by the upregulated Nrf2 expression during this mechanism [162]. This notion was endorsed by Lippross et al. [162], who demonstrated the slow bone healing process in Nrf2-deficient mice compared with the control and hypothesized the reduction in vascular endothelial growth factor as the underlying mechanism [162]. Under normal physiological condition, the transcriptional factor Nrf2 protect various body organs against different disease [163] by regulating the expression of antioxidant and detoxifying enzymes [101,164,165]. Similarly, Nrf2 was also found to activate stem cells during tissue regeneration [101]. ROS are excessively produced at the early stage of bone regeneration and under inflammatory conditions [166]. Knowingly, ROS negatively impacts bone homeostasis and fracture healing by hindering the differentiation of the anabolic cells (osteoblasts, osteocytes, and chondrocytes, while stimulating osteoclasts, the catabolic cells [160,167–171]. Indeed, the production of ROS is implicated in cell injury through damaging various proteins, nuclear acids, and lipid peroxidation, which leads to the production of MDA, the typical marker of oxidative stress [166,172]. Nrf2 signaling can also promote fracture healing (Figure 8.5) by inducing antioxidants to protect bone cells from ROS-mediated harmful effects and thus facilitate bone homeostasis [101].

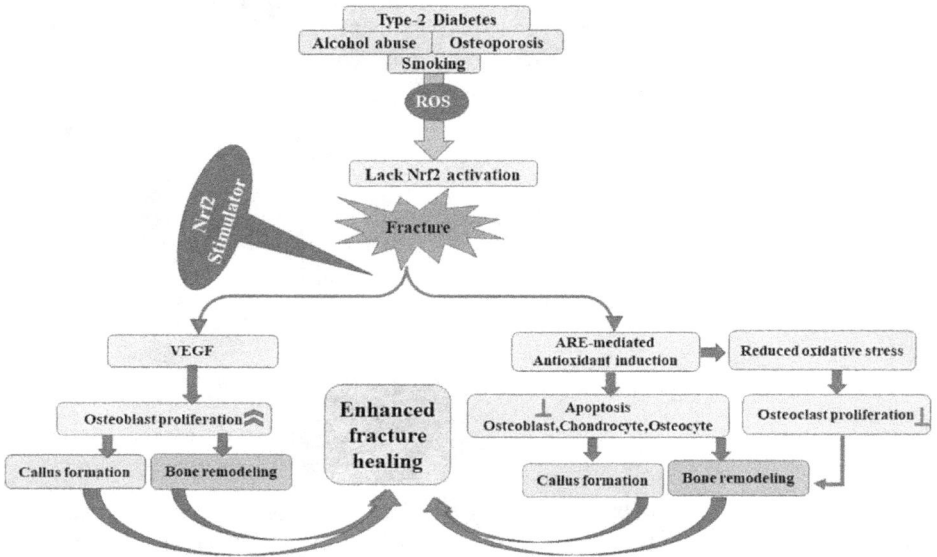

FIGURE 8.5 The role of the Nrf2 signaling pathway in the fracture healing process by inhibiting ROS formation.

TRADITIONAL OSTEOPOROSIS TREATMENT

A high prevalence of bone loss-linked diseases, mainly OP, is commonly found in the elderly population [6]. Intervention is highly recommended to evaluate and treat OP in those who have undergone a fragility fracture [173]. Moreover, the need for therapy increases as the likelihood of another fracture increases [174], which is most likely more severe in the post-fracture phase [175–177]. The health system has introduced numerous criteria in managing OP, including advanced interventions and diagnosis and fracture risk assessment. Also, several studies reveal that a minority of men and women at high fracture risk still receive treatment [178–184]. Currently, antiresorptive and ana-bolic drugs are the standard treatment options for OP. Antiresorptive agents—such as anti-RANKL antibodies, hormone-replacement therapy, bisphosphonates, raloxifene, selective estrogen-receptor modulators—and/or anabolic agents such as anabolic as low doses of antisclerostin antibodies and teriparatide can stimulate new bone development and enhance bone density [185,186]. Unfortunately, long-term use of these drugs might lead to various adverse health effects such as cancer, stroke, and heart diseases [185,187]. These obstacles advocated the need for alternative medicinal drugs and dietary supple-ments for bone health management and promotion. Natural compounds with power-ful bone-conserving properties and minor side effects could be proposed as alternative approaches to overcome the limitations of conventional medicines [188].

FLAVONOID AND OSTEOPOROSIS TREATMENT

Flavonoids are a distinct group of natural compounds abundantly found in our daily consumed food such as vegetables, fruits, cereal, wine, and tea [189,190]. Innovated technology has enhanced the extraction and identification of great numbers of natural flavonoids that reached over 5,000 compounds [191,192]. Generally, flavonoids can be categorized into three main sub-groups, including the iso-flavonoids (also known as phytoestrogens), the bioflavonoids, and the neoflavanoids [193]. However, these sub-groups are varied in their chemical structure and biological activity [12]. The extracted flavonoids have been emerged as prospective therapeutic candidates in different fields, particularly in pharmaceutical industries and healthcare purposes [194]. Indeed, inves-tigating the mechanism of actions for flavonoids have shown the potential of these natural compound to be used as antitumor, antioxidant, anti-inflammatory, antiresorp-tive effects, antiviral, in addition to its free radical scavenging abilities and the sig-nificant role in treating cardiovascular diseases [194,195]. Flavonoid is an alternative anti-osteoporotic drug since traditional hormone therapy leads to serious adverse side effects [196].

Interestingly, most of the studied flavonoids exhibited a tremendous antioxidant activity, which increases osteoblast proliferation, but decreases osteoclast differentiation.

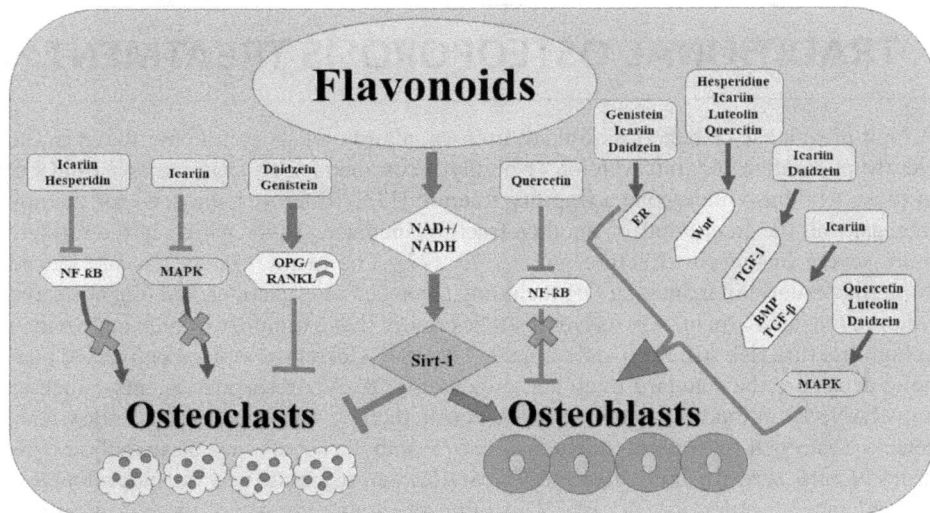

FIGURE 8.6   The impact of flavonoids on different signaling pathways that mediate osteo-blast proliferation and osteoblastic differentiation.

Indeed, these flavonoids showed a potential to regulate miRNA expression, DNA methylation, and histone (de)acetylation, as mentioned above. The precise mechanism of flavonoids involves SIRT-1 activation that is mediated by nicotinamide adenine dinucleotide + hydrogen (NAD+/NADH) ratio [4].

Various flavonoids such as quercetin, daidzein, kaempferol, genistein, etc. have shown substantial anti-osteoporotic effects [4] (Figure 8.6), and they have been employed in treating bone loss and fracture associated postmenopausal OP [197–199]. Soy isoflavones also revealed promising antiresorptive action by inhibiting osteoclasts and promoting osteoblast differentiation [200]. Numerous plant-derived antioxidants can stimulate the Nrf2 pathway and protect cells against oxidative stress damage [201]. Also, various flavonoids have shown a potential to upregulate MAPK cascade, which is directly involved in the activation of the Nrf2/antioxidant responsive element (ARE) pathway [141].

QUERCETIN

Quercetin is a natural dietary flavonoid found in vegetables and fruits. Out of the 5,000 members of flavonoids, quercetin stands as the most important and extensively studied flavonoid [188]. Myriads of researches shed light on the pharmaceutical properties of quercetin, for example, its anti-inflammatory [202], neuroprotective [203], anti-carcinogenic [204], antioxidative [202], cardioprotective [205], and immunomodulatory [202], in addition to its bone-conserving properties [188]. In China, quercetin was recommended in treating OP due to its significant antioxidant property [190].

Indeed, quercetin has exhibited various mechanisms for bone protection, including the regulation of RANK/RANKL/OPG by inhibiting RANKL-mediated osteoclast differentiation [206]. Quercetin regulates MAPK signaling pathways, the Nrf2 signaling pathway motivator that mediates osteoblast proliferation and osteoclast differentiation [188]. Furthermore, this compound can inhibit osteoblast's apoptosis while triggering apoptosis in osteoclasts [16]. The antioxidative role of quercetin is highly appreciated, as revealed by the substantial reduction in the intracellular ROS in osteoblast cells [207,208] after treating with quercetin. As mentioned above, the multidisciplinary transcription factor Nrf2 is involved in various cellular aspects [101,188,206]. In addition, it interacts with other signaling pathways such as extracellular signal-regulated kinase (ERK) and nuclear factor-kappa B (NF-κB). Activation of ERK signal pathway promoting the separation of Nrf2 from Keap1 [209]. Consequently, the activated Nrf2 hinders the expression of NF-κB through upregulating antioxidants and heme oxygenase-1 (HO-1) expression [210]. Stimulating the primary human osteoblasts with quercetin increased phosphorylation of both Nrf2 and MAPK signaling pathway and protect the cells against toxic reaction of oxidative stress [190]. In contrast, the expression of NF-κB p65 was significantly downregulated in osteoblast cells, following treatment with quercetin [211]. Quercetin also augments the expression of Nrf2 and its downstream genes: HO-1, NAD(P)H:glutathione peroxidase 3 (GPx3), catalase (CAT), and NAD(P)H quinone dehydrogenase 1 (NQO-1) [190,212]. Other signaling pathways such as apoptotic, canonical Wnt/b-catenin, OPG, BMP, and TGF-β are regulated by quercetin to maintain bone homeostasis [188].

GENISTEIN

Genistein is an iso-flavonoid phytoestrogen found in unprocessed soybeans and exhibiting estrogenic and anti-estrogenic behaviors [213,214]. Various in vivo and in vitro studies shed light on genistein's significant effect in treating bone disorders. These properties include a better bone mass [215], suppressing the osteogenesis inhibitor tumor necrosis factor-alpha (TNF-α) [216], preventing osteoclastogenesis and OP [217], and promoting osteoblastic differentiation through upregulating p38 MAPK-RUNX2 signaling pathway [218]. Genistein was previously found to induce an anti-inflammatory effect by activating Nrf2/HO-1 pathway [219]. The compound showed potential to attenuate RANKL-induced osteoclast differentiation by inhibiting NADPH oxidase 1-induced increase in ROS levels. Genistein also scavenges ROS through Nrf2-mediated initiation of phase II antioxidant enzymes, such as HO-1 and SOD [220,221]. Upregulation of ERK1/2 and protein kinase C (PKC) signaling pathways is considered another mechanism utilized by genistein to protect cells against oxidative stress and increase Nrf2 mRNA and protein expression [221]. Previous in vivo and in vitro studies by Li et al. demonstrated the ability of genistein to increase the mRNA expression of the typical osteogenic markers RUNX2, OPG, alkaline phosphatase (ALP), BMP-2, OCN, and estrogen receptor (ER) α/β, and meanwhile, osteoclast-linked markers RANKL, c-Fos, and NFATc1 were downregulated [222–224].

KAEMPFEROL

The natural bioflavonoid kaempferol and its derivatives are abundantly found in vegetables and fruits. Kaempferol has managed numerous diseases, including bone disease [225]. Previous studies have suggested the potential of kaempferol to alter the differentiation of bone marrow MSCs through increasing osteogenesis while decreasing adipogenesis [226,227]. Kaempferol also showed a significant role in bone formation by augmenting the expression of various downstream proteins promoting the mammalian target of rapamycin (mTOR) signaling pathway, suggesting its contribution to osteogenesis [228]. Previous studies have considered TNF-α as a crucial factor in OP due to its ability to upregulate both the NF-κB pathway and RANKL-induced differentiation of osteoclasts.

Moreover, TNF-α enhances bone resorption meanwhile, inhibits bone formation. Fortunately, kaempferol was found to attenuate these mechanisms [229–231]. Extensive studies have also shown kaempferol's ability to manage various disorders through upregulating Nrf2/HO-1 and Akt/Nrf2/HO-1 signaling [232–237]. The mechanisms might be linked to the reduction in NF-κB [233] and TNF-mediated apoptosis in osteoblastic cells [77]. Kaempferol exhibited a potential to activate ERK and MAPK signaling pathways, which mediated the activation of the Nrf2/ARE pathway, the defensive mechanism against oxidative stress [141,238]. Transcription factors of several genes, including RUNX2, which enhance bone mineralization [238], as well as other bone differentiation markers such as osteonectin (ON), collagen type I alpha 1 (COL1A1), OCN, and OSX [239] are also augmented by kaempferol.

MYRICETIN

Myricetin is a member of the flavonol subclass, mainly found in medicinal plants, tea, fruits, and vegetables [240,241]. Myricetin possesses various properties, including anticancer, antioxidant, anti-inflammatory, antiallergic, antimicrobial properties, and its ability to protect osteogenesis and inhibit osteoclasts differentiation [242]. Myricetin was previously found to target the RANK/RANKL pathway to inhibit F-actin ring formation and repress osteoclastogenic markers such as calcitonin receptor (CTR), tartrate-resistant acid phosphatase (TRAP), cathepsin K (CTSK), c-Fos, nuclear factor of activated T-cells c1 (NFATc1), and Atp6v0d2 (v-ATPase d2). Inhibition of the common pro-inflammatory cytokines and inflammatory mediators—such as TNF-a, inducible nitric oxide synthase (iNOS), interleukin-1B (IL-1β), prostaglandin-E2 (PGE-2), cyclooxygenase-2 (COX-2), and interleukin-6 (IL-6)—suppresses the NF-κB pathway responsible for osteoclast differentiation and bone resorption is also another mechanism utilized by myricetin [243]. As revealed by previous studies, repression of the NF-κB pathway is mediated by the activation of Nrf2/HO-1 and possibly the PI3K/AKT pathway [244]. Furthermore, myricetin was classified as an inhibitor of the mRNA expression level of various osteoclastogenic markers such as NFATc-1, c-FOS, TRAP, and CTSK [245]. In contrast, upregulated expression of osteogenic markers, including RUNX, OCN, COL-1, and ALP, was exhibited by myricetin [245].

ICARIIN

Icariin is a pharmaceutical component found in the herbaceous plant *Epimedium pubescens* [224,246]. This flavonoid is used to treat various diseases, including cardiovascular diseases, neurological disorders, and rheumatoid, and manage different bone diseases such as OP [247,248]. Icariin showed exciting properties, including the ability to inhibit osteoclast differentiation produced by RANKL and M-CSF and suppress bone resorption through triggering apoptosis of osteoclasts [224]. The expression of MAPK, as well as NF-κB activation, was also utilized by icariin to inhibit RANKL-induced osteoclastogenesis and bone resorption [249]. Extensive studies have also revealed the potential of icariin to enhance bone health through upregulating the expression of the typical osteogenic markers such as OCN, RUNX2, ALP, and bone sialoprotein (BSP) [250,251]. At the same time, icariin increases the proliferation rate and mineralization of osteoblasts by elevating the level of ALP and nitric oxide (NO), the common inhibitor of bone resorption [252]. Besides, icariin upregulates the expression of BMP-2/SMAD, and NO enhances RUNX2 transcription, thereby maintaining bone homeostasis. Furthermore, icariin acts as a radical scavenging candidate by decreasing ROS by activating Nrf2— to enhance the antioxidative stress activity and suppress NF-κB [246]—or through upregulating glutathione via the PI3K/Akt/Nrf2 pathway [253]. Indeed, a reduction of the ROS level, lipopolysaccharide (LPS)-induced osteoclast differentiation, the pro-inflammatory cytokines (IL-6 and TNF-α), and PGE-2 were also exhibited by icariin, and ultimately decreased bone resorption [254]. Suppressing the expression of caspase-3 was also established by icariin to inhibit osteoblast apoptosis by [252].

LUTEOLIN

The flavonoid luteolin is found in various herbal extracts and is used for many medicinal purposes [16]. Consistent with other flavonoids, luteolin has shown many medicinal properties. Previous studies have demonstrated the ability of luteolin to inhibit RANKL-induced osteoclast differentiation, downregulate the expression of osteoclast-linked genes, abolish oxidative stress markers, suppress bone resorption, and prevent bone loss [255,256]. On the other side, previous in vivo studies revealed the ability of luteolin to trigger osteoblastic activity and increase ALP and collagen production [257]. Furthermore, significant inhibition of crucial pro-inflammatory cytokines through inhibition of phosphorylated NF-κB as well as a decrease in ROS production was also exhibited by luteolin [258].

HESPERIDIN

Hesperidin is a member of the flavonoid subgroup, known as flavanones. It is found mainly in citrus fruits [259]. This compound has a considerable role in maintaining bone health [260]. Hesperidin was also found to increase the expression of ALP and OCN through upregulating OSX and RUNX2, which in turn involved in MAPK and BMP signaling pathways as well as Nrf2 stimulation [141]. Hesperidin might induce the induction of Nrf2 by activating Wnt/b-catenin and PI3K/AKT signaling pathways [140,261]. Inhibition of bone resorption and NF-κB-induced osteoclast differentiation was profoundly demonstrated by hesperidin [262].

APIGENIN

Apigenin belongs to the subgroup flavone, and it is abundantly found in various fruits and vegetables [16]. Apigenin has shown an intervention role in avoiding bone loss [263], mainly by upregulating antioxidant enzymes and glutathione peroxidase, which counteract ROS production. Various genes mediating osteoblasts differentiation such as OPG, ALP, BSP, osteopontin (OPN), OCN, OSX, and BMPs were also augmented by the compound, while IL-6 and NO were abolished [263]. JNK and p38 MAPK signaling pathways play an essential role during apigenin-triggered osteogenesis [263]. In LPS-stimulated macrophage cells, apigenin significantly inhibited collagenase, COX-2, NO [264], TNF-α, IL-6, and IL-1β [265]. Hence, this mechanism, accompanied by the ability of the compound to inhibit NF-κB, suggested the vital role of apigenin in treating OP [266].

DAIDZEIN

The phytoestrogen daidzein is a major compound in soy products. As a distinguished property, this isoflavonoid can bind to ERα/β and substitute estrogen replacement therapy [267]. Daizen enhances the differentiation and proliferation of osteoblast cells. Moreover, the treated cells showed a noticeable increase in OCN synthesis, ALP activity, and BMP-2 [268], which augment SMAD 1/5/8 phosphorylation, and ultimately increase the expression of various genes such as ALP, RUN-X2, COL-1, and OSX, the typical marker of osteogenesis [269]. Furthermore, the compound exhibited increased RUNX2 expression and OPG production, accompanied by a reduction of RANKL [270]. Treating OVAX mice with daidzein showed a substantial decrease in the osteoclastogenesis inducers, ROS, and TNF-α [271] as well as NF-κB signaling [272]. Moreover, treating osteoblast-like MG-63 cells with daidzein demonstrated elevated levels of COL-1 and ALP caused an incredible elevation in the levels of ALP and COL-1, as well as inhibited cisplatin-mediated apoptosis by enhancing PI3K/AKT and ER-involved MEK/ERK pathways [273].

OTHER FLAVONOIDS

Fisetin is a natural flavonoid found in *Rhus succedanea* that exhibited an ability to inhibit bone resorption and osteoclast differentiation. This flavonoid is blocking RANKL-stimulated ROS production by activating Nrf2-mediated the induction of many antioxidative enzymes, including HO-1, glutathione-S-transferase (GST), NQO-1, and glutamate-cysteine ligase (GCL) [274].

The natural flavonoid alpinumisoflavone derived from *Derris Ariocarpus* was previously found to protect against glucocorticoid-induced OP in rat models. Data from this study highlighted the potential of alpinumisoflavone to inhibit ROS expression, whereas upregulating the Nrf2 pathway and its downstream molecules NQO-1 and HO-1, which might reverse the osteoporotic effect of glucocorticoid [275].

The flavonoid neobavaisoflavone, extracted from the traditional Chinese medicinal plant *Psoralea corylifolia* L, revealed various pharmacological activities, including anticancer, antibacterial, and anti-osteoporotic effects [276]. In OVAX mice, neobavaisoflavone induced a profound inhibition in osteoclastogenesis and reduced bone loss [277]. Recently, neobavaisoflavone was found to protect osteoblasts against dexamethasone-generated oxidative stress by activating the colorectal neoplasia differentially expressed (CRNDE)-mediated Nrf2/HO-1/NQO1 signaling pathway [278].

Anthocyanin compounds exist in natural plants and possess promising bioactive properties [279]. Previous studies demonstrated the antioxidant mechanism of these compounds by upregulating Nrf2/HO-1 expression; meanwhile, the production of ROS and other inflammatory factors was inhibited [280].

In conclusion, OP is a critical health issue in aging populations. Progression of this disorder leads to profound implications such as fractures, which create adverse consequences on mobility, quality of life, and tremendous economic burden on the health system. The currently used OP treatment options include antiresorptive and/or anabolic agents. However, long-term administration is associated with severe adverse health effects [188]. This fact limited their uses and urged the searching for other alternatives. The extracted flavonoids have emerged as a prospective safe therapeutic option in different fields, particularly in pharmaceutical industries and healthcare purposes. The specific antioxidant properties of these flavonoids have nominated these natural compounds as a safe alternative to the current use of drugs. As declared by many studies, these bioactive compounds have shown the potential to enhance bone formation and decrease bone resorption. On the other hand, recent studies have shed light on the importance of the Nrf2 signaling pathway, which emerged as an integral approach in regulating oxidative stress-mediated bone homeostasis. Therefore, it is worthy to speculate the pharmacological upregulation of Nrf2 that might hold promise in maintaining bone health and treating different bone disorders, including OP and the associated bone fracture [101].

ABBREVIATION

AKT	AK strain transforming
ALP	Alkaline phosphatase
ARE	Antioxidant responsive element
BMPs	Bone morphogenetic proteins
BSP	Bone sialoprotein
CAT	Catalase
COL1A1	Collagen type I alpha 1
COX-2	Cyclooxygenase-2
CRNDE	Colorectal neoplasia differentially expressed
CTR	Calcitonin receptor
CTSK	Cathepsin K
ER	Estrogen receptor
ERK	Extracellular signal-regulated kinases
FGFs	Fibroblast growth factors
GCL	Glutamate-cysteine ligase
GLOP	Glucocorticoid-linked osteoporosis
GPx3	Glutathione peroxidase 3
GST	Glutathione-S-transferase
HO-1	Heme oxygenase-1
IL-1β	Interleukin-1B
IL-6	Interleukin-6
iNOS	Inducible nitric oxide synthase
ITFs	Inhibitory transcription factors
JNK	c-Jun N-terminal kinase
Keap1	Kelch-like Enoyl-CoA Hydratase (ECH)-associated protein 1
LPS	Lipopolysaccharide
MAPK	Mitogen-activated protein kinase
MAR	Mineral appositional rate
M-CSF	Macrophage colony-stimulating factor
MDA	Malondialdehyde
miRNA	MicroRNA
MSC	Mesenchymal stem cell
mTOR	Mammalian target of rapamycin
NAD	Nicotinamide adenine dinucleotide
NAD+/NADH	Nicotinamide adenine dinucleotide + hydrogen
NFATc1	Nuclear factor of activated T-cells, cytoplasmic 1

NF-κB	Nuclear factor-kappa B
NO	Nitric oxide
(NQO-1)	NAD(P)H quinone dehydrogenase 1
Nrf2	Nuclear factor erythroid-derived 2-like 2
OCN	Osteocalcin
OF	Osteoporotic fractures
OP	Osteoporosis
OPG	Osteoprotegerin
OPN	Osteopontin
OVAX	Ovariectomized
PGE-2	Prosteoglandin-E2
PI3K	Phosphatidylinositol 3-kinase
PPARγ	ITF peroxisome proliferator-activated receptor γ
RANK	Receptor activator of nuclear factor-kappa B
RANKL	Receptor activator of nuclear factor-kappa-B ligand
ROS	Reactive oxygen species
Runx2	Runt-related 2
SOD	Superoxide dismutase
TGF-β	Transforming growth factor-beta
TNF	Tumor necrosis factor
TRAP	Tartrate-resistant acid phosphatase
v-ATPase d2	Atp6v0d2
Wnt	Wingless and integration 1

REFERENCES

1. Cai, H.; Cong, W.N.; Ji, S.; Rothman, S.; Maudsley, S.; Martin, B. Metabolic dysfunction in Alzheimer's disease and related neurodegenerative disorders. *Curr Alzheimer Res* 2012, 9, 5–17. doi: 10.2174/156720512799015064.

2. Giannoudis, P.; Tzioupis, C.; Almalki, T.; Buckley, R. Fracture healing in osteoporotic fractures: Is it really different? A basic science perspective. *Injury* 2007, 38(Suppl. 1), S90–S99. doi: 10.1016/j.injury.2007.02.014.

3. Ayub, N.; Faraj, M.; Ghatan, S.; Reijers, J.A.A.; Napoli, N.; Oei, L. The treatment gap in osteoporosis. *J Clin Med* 2021, 10, 3002. doi: 10.3390/jcm10133002.

4. Bellavia, D.; Dimarco, E.; Costa, V.; Carina, V.; De Luca, A.; Raimondi, L.; Fini, M.; Gentile, C.; Caradonna, F.; Giavaresi, G. Flavonoids in bone erosive diseases: Perspectives in osteoporosis treatment. *Trends Endocrinol Metab* 2021, 32, 76–94. doi: 10.1016/j.tem.2020.11.007.

5. Stone, K.L.; Seeley, D.G.; Lui, L.Y.; Cauley, J.A.; Ensrud, K.; Browner, W.S.; Nevitt, M.C.; Cummings, S.R. BMD at multiple sites and risk of fracture of multiple types: Long-term results from the study of osteoporotic fractures. *J Bone Miner Res* 2003, 18, 1947–1954. doi: 10.1359/jbmr.2003.18.11.1947.

6. Castelo-Branco, C. Management of osteoporosis: An overview. *Drugs Aging* 1998, 12(Suppl. 1), 25–32. doi: 10.2165/00002512-199812001-00004.

7. Weycker, D.; Li, X.; Barron, R.; Bornheimer, R.; Chandler, D. Hospitalizations for osteoporosis-related fractures: Economic costs and clinical outcomes. *Bone Rep* 2016, 5, 186–191. doi: 10.1016/j.bonr.2016.07.005.
8. Khosla, S.; Shane, E. A crisis in the treatment of osteoporosis. *J Bone Miner Res* 2016, 31, 1485–1487. doi: 10.1002/jbmr.2888.
9. Kanis, J.A.; Svedbom, A.; Harvey, N.; McCloskey, E.V. The osteoporosis treatment gap. *J Bone Miner Res* 2014, 29, 1926–1928. doi: 10.1002/jbmr.2301.
10. Moskot, M.; Jakóbkiewicz-Banecka, J.; Kloska, A.; Smolińska, E.; Mozolewski, P.; Malinowska, M.; Rychłowski, M.; Banecki, B.; Węgrzyn, G.; Gabig-Cimińska, M. Modulation of expression of genes involved in glycosaminoglycan metabolism and lysosome biogenesis by flavonoids. *Sci Rep* 2015, 5, 9378. doi: 10.1038/srep09378.
11. Suzuki, T.; Yamamoto, M. Molecular basis of the Keap1-Nrf2 system. *Free Radic Biol Med* 2015, 88, 93–100. doi: 10.1016/j.freeradbiomed.2015.06.006.
12. Kumar, S.; Pandey, A.K. Chemistry and biological activities of flavonoids: An overview. *ScientificWorldJournal* 2013, 2013, 162750. doi: 10.1155/2013/162750.
13. Chandra, A.; Rajawat, J. Skeletal aging, and osteoporosis: Mechanisms and therapeutics. *Int J Mol Sci* 2021, 22, 553. doi: 10.3390/ijms22073553.
14. Almeida, M.; Han, L.; Martin-Millan, M.; Plotkin, L.I.; Stewart, S.A.; Roberson, P.K.; Kousteni, S.; O'Brien, C.A.; Bellido, T.; Parfitt, A.M., et al. Skeletal involution by age-associated oxidative stress and its acceleration by loss of sex steroids. *J Biol Chem* 2007, 282, 27285–27297. doi: 10.1074/jbc.M702810200.
15. Canalis, E. Update in new anabolic therapies for osteoporosis. *J Clin Endocrinol Metab* 2010, 95, 1496–1504. doi: 10.1210/jc.2009-2677.
16. Ramesh, P.; Jagadeesan, R.; Sekaran, S.; Dhanasekaran, A.; Vimalraj, S. Flavonoids: Classification, function, and molecular mechanisms involved in bone remodelling. *Front Endocrinol (Lausanne)* 2021, 12, 779638. doi: 10.3389/fendo.2021.779638.
17. Buckwalter, J.A.; Glimcher, M.J.; Cooper, R.R.; Recker, R. Bone biology. I: Structure, blood supply, cells, matrix, and mineralization. *Instr Course Lect* 1996, 45, 371–386.
18. Marks, S.C., Jr.; Popoff, S.N. Bone cell biology: The regulation of development, structure, and function in the skeleton. *Am J Anat* 1988, 183, 1–44. doi: 10.1002/aja.1001830102.
19. Ducy, P.; Schinke, T.; Karsenty, G. The osteoblast: A sophisticated fibroblast under central surveillance. *Science* 2000, 289, 1501–1504. doi: 10.1126/science.289.5484.1501.
20. Capulli, M.; Paone, R.; Rucci, N. Osteoblast and osteocyte: Games without frontiers. *Arch Biochem Biophys* 2014, 561, 3–12. doi: 10.1016/j.abb.2014.05.003.
21. Bellavia, D.; De Luca, A.; Carina, V.; Costa, V.; Raimondi, L.; Salamanna, F.; Alessandro, R.; Fini, M.; Giavaresi, G. Deregulated miRNAs in bone health: Epigenetic roles in osteoporosis. *Bone* 2019, 122, 52–75. doi: 10.1016/j.bone.2019.02.013.
22. Florencio-Silva, R.; Sasso, G.R.; Sasso-Cerri, E.; Simões, M.J.; Cerri, P.S. Biology of bone tissue: Structure, function, and factors that influence bone cells. *Biomed Res Int* 2015, 2015, 421746. doi: 10.1155/2015/421746.
23. Fakhry, M.; Hamade, E.; Badran, B.; Buchet, R.; Magne, D. Molecular mechanisms of mesenchymal stem cell differentiation towards osteoblasts. *World J Stem Cells* 2013, 5, 136–148. doi: 10.4252/wjsc.v5.i4.136.
24. Day, T.F.; Guo, X.; Garrett-Beal, L.; Yang, Y. Wnt/beta-catenin signaling in mesenchymal progenitors controls osteoblast and chondrocyte differentiation during vertebrate skeletogenesis. *Dev Cell* 2005, 8, 739–750. doi: 10.1016/j.devcel.2005.03.016.
25. Andrade, A.C.; Nilsson, O.; Barnes, K.M.; Baron, J. Wnt gene expression in the post-natal growth plate: Regulation with chondrocyte differentiation. *Bone* 2007, 40, 1361–1369. doi: 10.1016/j.bone.2007.01.005.
26. Zhong, Z.; Zylstra-Diegel, C.R.; Schumacher, C.A.; Baker, J.J.; Carpenter, A.C.; Rao, S.; Yao, W.; Guan, M.; Helms, J.A.; Lane, N.E., et al. Wntless functions in mature osteoblasts to regulate bone mass. *Proc Natl Acad Sci U S A* 2012, 109, E2197–E2204. doi: 10.1073/pnas.1120407109.

27. Li, X.; Cao, X. BMP signaling and skeletogenesis. *Ann N Y Acad Sci* 2006, 1068, 26–40. doi: 10.1196/annals.1346.006.
28. Canalis, E.; Economides, A.N.; Gazzerro, E. Bone morphogenetic proteins, their antagonists, and the skeleton. *Endocr Rev* 2003, 24, 218–235. doi: 10.1210/er.2002-0023.
29. Ducy, P.; Zhang, R.; Geoffroy, V.; Ridall, A.L.; Karsenty, G. Osf2/Cbfa1: A transcriptional activator of osteoblast differentiation. *Cell* 1997, 89, 747–754. doi: 10.1016/s0092-8674(00)80257-3.
30. Zaidi, M. Skeletal remodeling in health and disease. *Nat Med* 2007, 13, 791–801. doi: 10.1038/nm1593.
31. Yamaguchi, A.; Ishizuya, T.; Kintou, N.; Wada, Y.; Katagiri, T.; Wozney, J.M.; Rosen, V.; Yoshiki, S. Effects of BMP-2, BMP-4, and BMP-6 on osteoblastic differentiation of bone marrow-derived stromal cell lines, ST2 and MC3T3-G2/PA6. *Biochem Biophys Res Commun* 1996, 220, 366–371. doi: 10.1006/bbrc.1996.0411.
32. Agarwal, R.; Williams, K.; Umscheid, C.A.; Welch, W.C. Osteoinductive bone graft substitutes for lumbar fusion: A systematic review. *J Neurosurg Spine* 2009, 11, 729–740. doi: 10.3171/2009.6.Spine08669.
33. Garrison, K.R.; Shemilt, I.; Donell, S.; Ryder, J.J.; Mugford, M.; Harvey, I.; Song, F.; Alt, V. Bone morphogenetic protein (BMP) for fracture healing in adults. *Cochrane Database Syst Rev* 2010, 2010, CD006950. doi: 10.1002/14651858.CD006950.pub2.
34. Jeon, M.J.; Kim, J.A.; Kwon, S.H.; Kim, S.W.; Park, K.S.; Park, S.W.; Kim, S.Y.; Shin, C.S. Activation of peroxisome proliferator-activated receptor-gamma inhibits the Runx2-mediated transcription of osteocalcin in osteoblasts. *J Biol Chem* 2003, 278, 23270–23277. doi: 10.1074/jbc.M211610200.
35. Krause, U.; Harris, S.; Green, A.; Ylostalo, J.; Zeitouni, S.; Lee, N.; Gregory, C.A. Pharmaceutical modulation of canonical Wnt signaling in multipotent stromal cells for improved osteoinductive therapy. *Proc Natl Acad Sci U S A* 2010, 107, 4147–4152. doi: 10.1073/pnas.0914360107.
36. Buo, A.M.; Stains, J.P. Gap junctional regulation of signal transduction in bone cells. *FEBS Lett* 2014, 588, 1315–1321. doi: 10.1016/j.febslet.2014.01.025.
37. Kapinas, K.; Kessler, C.; Ricks, T.; Gronowicz, G.; Delany, A.M. MiR-29 modulates Wnt signaling in human osteoblasts through a positive feedback loop. *J Biol Chem* 2010, 285, 25221–25231. doi: 10.1074/jbc.M110.116137.
38. Montero, A.; Okada, Y.; Tomita, M.; Ito, M.; Tsurukami, H.; Nakamura, T.; Doetschman, T.; Coffin, J.D.; Hurley, M.M. Disruption of the fibroblast growth factor-2 gene results in decreased bone mass and bone formation. *J Clin Invest* 2000, 105, 1085–1093. doi: 10.1172/jci8641.
39. Zhang, Y.; Xie, R.L.; Croce, C.M.; Stein, J.L.; Lian, J.B.; van Wijnen, A.J.; Stein, G.S. A program of microRNAs controls osteogenic lineage progression by targeting transcription factor Runx2. *Proc Natl Acad Sci U S A* 2011, 108, 9863–9868. doi: 10.1073/pnas.1018493108.
40. Hamidouche, Z.; Fromigué, O.; Nuber, U.; Vaudin, P.; Pages, J.C.; Ebert, R.; Jakob, F.; Miraoui, H.; Marie, P.J. Autocrine fibroblast growth factor 18 mediates dexamethasone-induced osteogenic differentiation of murine mesenchymal stem cells. *J Cell Physiol* 2010, 224, 509–515. doi: 10.1002/jcp.22152.
41. Flenniken, A.M.; Osborne, L.R.; Anderson, N.; Ciliberti, N.; Fleming, C.; Gittens, J.E.; Gong, X.Q.; Kelsey, L.B.; Lounsbury, C.; Moreno, L., et al. A GJa1 missense mutation in a mouse model of oculodentodigital dysplasia. *Development* 2005, 132, 4375–4386. doi: 10.1242/dev.02011.
42. Li, Z.; Hassan, M.Q.; Volinia, S.; van Wijnen, A.J.; Stein, J.L.; Croce, C.M.; Lian, J.B.; Stein, G.S. A microRNA signature for a BMP2-induced osteoblast lineage commitment program. *Proc Natl Acad Sci U S A* 2008, 105, 13906–13911. doi: 10.1073/pnas.0804438105.
43. Zhang, J.; Tu, Q.; Bonewald, L.F.; He, X.; Stein, G.; Lian, J.; Chen, J. Effects of miR-335-5p in modulating osteogenic differentiation by specifically downregulating Wnt antagonist DKK1. *J Bone Miner Res* 2011, 26, 1953–1963. doi: 10.1002/jbmr.377.

44. Miller, S.C.; de Saint-Georges, L.; Bowman, B.M.; Jee, W.S. Bone lining cells: Structure and function. *Scanning Microsc* 1989, 3, 953–960; discussion 960–951.

45. Andersen, T.L.; Sondergaard, T.E.; Skorzynska, K.E.; Dagnaes-Hansen, F.; Plesner, T.L.; Hauge, E.M.; Plesner, T.; Delaisse, J.M. A physical mechanism for coupling bone resorption and formation in adult human bone. *Am J Pathol* 2009, 174, 239–247. doi: 10.2353/ajpath.2009.080627.

46. Mosley, J.R. Osteoporosis and bone functional adaptation: Mechanobiological regulation of bone architecture in growing and adult bone, a review. *J Rehabil Res Dev* 2000, 37, 189–199.

47. Everts, V.; Delaissé, J.M.; Korper, W.; Jansen, D.C.; Tigchelaar-Gutter, W.; Saftig, P.; Beertsen, W. The bone lining cell: Its role in cleaning Howship's lacunae and initiating bone formation. *J Bone Miner Res* 2002, 17, 77–90. doi: 10.1359/jbmr.2002.17.1.77.

48. Franz-Odendaal, T.A.; Hall, B.K.; Witten, P.E. Buried alive: How osteoblasts become osteocytes. *Dev Dyn* 2006, 235, 176–190. doi: 10.1002/dvdy.20603.

49. Bonewald, L.F. The amazing osteocyte. *J Bone Miner Res* 2011, 26, 229–238. doi: 10.1002/jbmr.320.

50. Bonewald, L.F. Osteocytes as dynamic multifunctional cells. *Ann N Y Acad Sci* 2007, 1116, 281–290. doi: 10.1196/annals.1402.018.

51. Noble, B.S.; Stevens, H.; Loveridge, N.; Reeve, J. Identification of apoptotic changes in osteocytes in normal and pathological human bone. *Bone* 1997, 20, 273–282. doi: 10.1016/s8756-3282(96)00365-1.

52. Aguirre, J.I.; Plotkin, L.I.; Stewart, S.A.; Weinstein, R.S.; Parfitt, A.M.; Manolagas, S.C.; Bellido, T. Osteocyte apoptosis is induced by weightlessness in mice and precedes osteoclast recruitment and bone loss. *J Bone Miner Res* 2006, 21, 605–615. doi: 10.1359/jbmr.060107.

53. Plotkin, L.I. Apoptotic osteocytes and the control of targeted bone resorption. *Curr Osteoporos Rep* 2014, 12, 121–126. doi: 10.1007/s11914-014-0194-3.

54. Liu, S.; Fan, Y.; Chen, A.; Jalali, A.; Minami, K.; Ogawa, K.; Nakshatri, H.; Li, B.Y.; Yokota, H. Osteocyte-driven downregulation of snail restrains effects of Drd2 inhibitors on mammary tumor cells. *Cancer Res* 2018, 78, 3865–3876. doi: 10.1158/0008-5472.Can-18-0056.

55. Crockett, J.C.; Mellis, D.J.; Scott, D.I.; Helfrich, M.H. New knowledge on critical osteoclast formation and activation pathways from the study of rare genetic diseases of osteoclasts: Focus on the RANK/RANKL axis. *Osteoporos Int* 2011, 22, 1–20. doi: 10.1007/s00198-010-1272-8.

56. Boyce, B.F.; Hughes, D.E.; Wright, K.R.; Xing, L.; Dai, A. Recent advances in bone biology provide insight into the pathogenesis of bone diseases. *Lab Invest* 1999, 79, 83–94.

57. Yavropoulou, M.P.; Yovos, J.G. Osteoclastogenesis – Current knowledge and future perspectives. *J Musculoskelet Neuronal Interact* 2008, 8, 204–216.

58. Boyce, B.F.; Xing, L. Functions of RANKL/RANK/OPG in bone modeling and remodeling. *Arch Biochem Biophys* 2008, 473, 139–146. doi: 10.1016/j.abb.2008.03.018.

59. Longhini, R.; de Oliveira, P.A.; de Souza Faloni, A.P.; Sasso-Cerri, E.; Cerri, P.S. Increased apoptosis in osteoclasts and decreased RANKL immunoexpression in periodontium of cimetidine-treated rats. *J Anat* 2013, 222, 239–247. doi: 10.1111/joa.12011.

60. Longhini, R.; Aparecida de Oliveira, P.; Sasso-Cerri, E.; Cerri, P.S. Cimetidine reduces alveolar bone loss in induced periodontitis in rat molars. *J Periodontol* 2014, 85, 1115–1125. doi: 10.1902/jop.2013.130453.

61. Charles, J.F.; Aliprantis, A.O. Osteoclasts: More than 'bone eaters'. *Trends Mol Med* 2014, 20, 449–459. doi: 10.1016/j.molmed.2014.06.001.

62. Feng, X.; McDonald, J.M. Disorders of bone remodeling. *Annu Rev Pathol* 2011, 6, 121–145. doi: 10.1146/annurev-pathol-011110-130203.

63. Frost, H.M. Skeletal structural adaptations to mechanical usage (SATMU): 2. Redefining Wolff's law: The remodeling problem. *Anat Rec* 1990, 226, 414–422. doi: 10.1002/ar.1092260403.
64. Frost, H.M. Skeletal structural adaptations to mechanical usage (SATMU): 1. Redefining Wolff's law: The bone modeling problem. *Anat Rec* 1990, 226, 403–413. doi: 10.1002/ar.1092260402.
65. Sun, Y.X.; Xu, A.H.; Yang, Y.; Li, J. Role of Nrf2 in bone metabolism. *J Biomed Sci* 2015, 22, 101. doi: 10.1186/s12929-015-0212-5.
66. Crockett, J.C.; Rogers, M.J.; Coxon, F.P.; Hocking, L.J.; Helfrich, M.H. Bone remodeling at a glance. *J Cell Sci* 2011, 124, 991–998. doi: 10.1242/jcs.063032.
67. Teitelbaum, S.L. Bone resorption by osteoclasts. *Science* 2000, 289, 1504–1508. doi: 10.1126/science.289.5484.1504.
68. Robling, A.G. The interaction of biological factors with mechanical signals in bone adaptation: Recent developments. *Curr Osteoporos Rep* 2012, 10, 126–131. doi: 10.1007/s11914-012-0099-y.
69. Ibáñez, L.; Ferrándiz, M.L.; Brines, R.; Guede, D.; Cuadrado, A.; Alcaraz, M.J. Effects of Nrf2 deficiency on bone microarchitecture in an experimental model of osteoporosis. *Oxid Med Cell Longev* 2014, 2014, 726590. doi: 10.1155/2014/726590.
70. Raisz, L.G. Pathogenesis of osteoporosis: Concepts, conflicts, and prospects. *J Clin Invest* 2005, 115, 3318–3325. doi: 10.1172/jci27071.
71. Chen, X.; Zhu, X.; Wei, A.; Chen, F.; Gao, Q.; Lu, K.; Jiang, Q.; Cao, W. Nrf2 epigenetic derepression induced by running exercise protects against osteoporosis. *Bone Res* 2021, 9, 15. doi: 10.1038/s41413-020-00128-8.
72. Wen, K.; Fang, X.; Yang, J.; Yao, Y.; Nandakumar, K.S.; Salem, M.L.; Cheng, K. Recent research on flavonoids and their biomedical applications. *Curr Med Chem* 2021, 28, 1042–1066. doi: 10.2174/0929867327666200713184138.
73. Marini, F.; Cianferotti, L.; Brandi, M.L. Epigenetic mechanisms in bone biology and osteoporosis: Can they drive therapeutic choices? *Int J Mol Sci* 2016, 17, 1329. doi: 10.3390/ijms17081329.
74. Vrtačnik, P.; Marc, J.; Ostanek, B. Epigenetic mechanisms in bone. *Clin Chem Lab Med* 2014, 52, 589–608. doi: 10.1515/cclm-2013-0770.
75. Letarouilly, J.G.; Broux, O.; Clabaut, A. New insights into the epigenetics of osteoporosis. *Genomics* 2019, 111, 793–798. doi: 10.1016/j.ygeno.2018.05.001.
76. Yu, B.; Wang, C.Y. Osteoporosis: The result of an 'aged' bone microenvironment. *Trends Mol Med* 2016, 22, 641–644. doi: 10.1016/j.molmed.2016.06.002.
77. Wang, N.; Xin, H.; Xu, P.; Yu, Z.; Shou, D. Erxian decoction attenuates TNF-α induced osteoblast apoptosis by modulating the Akt/Nrf2/HO-1 signaling pathway. *Front Pharmacol* 2019, 10, 988. doi: 10.3389/fphar.2019.00988.
78. Reppe, S.; Lien, T.G.; Hsu, Y.H.; Gautvik, V.T.; Olstad, O.K.; Yu, R.; Bakke, H.G.; Lyle, R.; Kringen, M.K.; Glad, I.K., et al. Distinct DNA methylation profiles in bone and blood of osteoporotic and healthy postmenopausal women. *Epigenetics* 2017, 12, 674–687. doi: 10.1080/15592294.2017.1345832.
79. Ferioli, M.; Zauli, G.; Maiorano, P.; Milani, D.; Mirandola, P.; Neri, L.M. Role of physical exercise in the regulation of epigenetic mechanisms in inflammation, cancer, neurodegenerative diseases, and the aging process. *J Cell Physiol* 2019. doi: 10.1002/jcp.28304.
80. Barrès, R.; Yan, J.; Egan, B.; Treebak, J.T.; Rasmussen, M.; Fritz, T.; Caidahl, K.; Krook, A.; O'Gorman, D.J.; Zierath, J.R. Acute exercise remodels promoter methylation in human skeletal muscle. *Cell Metab* 2012, 15, 405–411. doi: 10.1016/j.cmet.2012.01.001.
81. Agrawal, K.; Das, V.; Vyas, P.; Hajdúch, M. Nucleosidic DNA demethylating epigenetic drugs - A comprehensive review from discovery to clinic. *Pharmacol Ther* 2018, 188, 45–79. doi: 10.1016/j.pharmthera.2018.02.006.

82. Guan, H.; Mi, B.; Li, Y.; Wu, W.; Tan, P.; Fang, Z.; Li, J.; Zhang, Y.; Li, F. Decitabine represses osteoclastogenesis through inhibition of RANK and NF-κB. *Cell Signal* 2015, 27, 969–977. doi: 10.1016/j.cellsig.2015.02.006.

83. Martyn-St James, M.; Carroll, S. A meta-analysis of impact exercise on postmenopausal bone loss: The case for mixed loading exercise programs. *Br J Sports Med* 2009, 43, 898–908. doi: 10.1136/bjsm.2008.052704.

84. Duncan, E.L. Gene testing in everyday clinical use: Lessons from the bone clinic. *J Endocr Soc* 2021, 5, bvaa200. doi: 10.1210/jendso/bvaa200.

85. Patsch, J.M.; Kohler, T.; Berzlanovich, A.; Muschitz, C.; Bieglmayr, C.; Roschger, P.; Resch, H.; Pietschmann, P. Trabecular bone microstructure and local gene expression in iliac crest biopsies of men with idiopathic osteoporosis. *J Bone Miner Res* 2011, 26, 1584–1592. doi: 10.1002/jbmr.344.

86. Ji, L.L.; Yeo, D. Oxidative stress: An evolving definition. *Fac Rev* 2021, 10, 13. doi: 10.12703/r/10-13.

87. Sies, H. Oxidative stress: Concept and some practical aspects. *Antioxidants (Basel)* 2020, 9, 852. doi: 10.3390/antiox9090852.

88. Salim, A.; Nacamuli, R.P.; Morgan, E.F.; Giaccia, A.J.; Longaker, M.T. Transient changes in oxygen tension inhibit osteogenic differentiation and Runx2 expression in osteoblasts. *J Biol Chem* 2004, 279, 40007–40016. doi: 10.1074/jbc.M403715200.

89. Arnett, T.R.; Gibbons, D.C.; Utting, J.C.; Orriss, I.R.; Hoebertz, A.; Rosendaal, M.; Meghji, S. Hypoxia is a major stimulator of osteoclast formation and bone resorption. *J Cell Physiol* 2003, 196, 2–8. doi: 10.1002/jcp.10321.

90. Callaway, D.A.; Jiang, J.X. Reactive oxygen species and oxidative stress in osteoclastogenesis, skeletal aging and bone diseases. *J Bone Miner Metab* 2015, 33, 359–370. doi: 10.1007/s00774-015-0656-4.

91. Weitzmann, M.N.; Pacifici, R. Estrogen deficiency and bone loss: An inflammatory tale. *J Clin Invest* 2006, 116, 1186–1194. doi: 10.1172/jci28550.

92. Bai, X.C.; Lu, D.; Bai, J.; Zheng, H.; Ke, Z.Y.; Li, X.M.; Luo, S.Q. Oxidative stress inhibits osteoblastic differentiation of bone cells by ERK and NF-kappaB. *Biochem Biophys Res Commun* 2004, 314, 197–207. doi: 10.1016/j.bbrc.2003.12.073.

93. Nojiri, H.; Saita, Y.; Morikawa, D.; Kobayashi, K.; Tsuda, C.; Miyazaki, T.; Saito, M.; Marumo, K.; Yonezawa, I.; Kaneko, K., et al. Cytoplasmic superoxide causes bone fragility owing to low-turnover osteoporosis and impaired collagen cross-linking. *J Bone Miner Res* 2011, 26, 2682–2694. doi: 10.1002/jbmr.489.

94. Manolagas, S.C. From estrogen-centric to aging and oxidative stress: A revised perspective of the pathogenesis of osteoporosis. *Endocr Rev* 2010, 31, 266–300. doi: 10.1210/er.2009-0024.

95. Pfeilschifter, J. Role of cytokines in postmenopausal bone loss. *Curr Osteoporos Rep* 2003, 1, 53–58. doi: 10.1007/s11914-003-0009-4.

96. Forte, G.I.; Scola, L.; Bellavia, D.; Vaccarino, L.; Sanacore, M.; Sisino, G.; Scazzone, C.; Caruso, C.; Barbieri, R.; Lio, D. Characterization of two alternative interleukin(IL)-10 5'UTR mRNA sequences, induced by lipopolysaccharide (LPS) stimulation of peripheral blood mononuclear cells. *Mol Immunol* 2009, 46, 2161–2166. doi: 10.1016/j.molimm.2009.04.034.

97. Caradonna, F.; Cruciata, I.; Schifano, I.; La Rosa, C.; Naselli, F.; Chiarelli, R.; Perrone, A.; Gentile, C. Methylation of cytokines gene promoters in IL-1β-treated human intestinal epithelial cells. *Inflamm Res* 2018, 67, 327–337. doi: 10.1007/s00011-017-1124-5.

98. Pellegrini, G.G.; Cregor, M.; McAndrews, K.; Morales, C.C.; McCabe, L.D.; McCabe, G.P.; Peacock, M.; Burr, D.; Weaver, C.; Bellido, T. Nrf2 regulates mass accrual and the antioxidant endogenous response in bone differently depending on the sex and age. *PLoS One* 2017, 12, e0171161. doi: 10.1371/journal.pone.0171161.

99. Park, C.K.; Lee, Y.; Kim, K.H.; Lee, Z.H.; Joo, M.; Kim, H.H. Nrf2 is a novel regulator of bone acquisition. *Bone* 2014, 63, 36–46. doi: 10.1016/j.bone.2014.01.025.

100. Li, H.; Huang, C.; Zhu, J.; Gao, K.; Fang, J.; Li, H. Lutein suppresses oxidative stress and inflammation by Nrf2 activation in an osteoporosis rat model. *Med Sci Monit* 2018, 24, 5071–5075. doi: 10.12659/msm.908699.

101. Kubo, Y.; Wruck, C.J.; Fragoulis, A.; Drescher, W.; Pape, H.C.; Lichte, P.; Fischer, H.; Tohidnezhad, M.; Hildebrand, F.; Pufe, T., et al. Role of Nrf2 in fracture healing: Clinical aspects of oxidative stress. *Calcif Tissue Int* 2019, 105, 341–352. doi: 10.1007/s00223-019-00576-3.

102. Tang, Y.; Wu, X.; Lei, W.; Pang, L.; Wan, C.; Shi, Z.; Zhao, L.; Nagy, T.R.; Peng, X.; Hu, J., et al. TGF-beta1-induced migration of bone mesenchymal stem cells couples bone resorption with formation. *Nat Med* 2009, 15, 757–765. doi: 10.1038/nm.1979.

103. Jilka, R.L.; Almeida, M.; Ambrogini, E.; Han, L.; Roberson, P.K.; Weinstein, R.S.; Manolagas, S.C. Decreased oxidative stress and greater bone anabolism in the aged, when compared to the young, murine skeleton with parathyroid hormone administration. *Aging Cell* 2010, 9, 851–867. doi: 10.1111/j.1474-9726.2010.00616.x.

104. Abdallah, B.M.; Haack-Sørensen, M.; Fink, T.; Kassem, M. Inhibition of osteoblast differentiation but not adipocyte differentiation of mesenchymal stem cells by sera obtained from aged females. *Bone* 2006, 39, 181–188. doi: 10.1016/j.bone.2005.12.082.

105. Farr, J.N.; Fraser, D.G.; Wang, H.; Jaehn, K.; Ogrodnik, M.B.; Weivoda, M.M.; Drake, M.T.; Tchkonia, T.; LeBrasseur, N.K.; Kirkland, J.L. et al. Identification of senescent cells in the bone microenvironment. *J Bone Miner Res* 2016, 31, 1920–1929. doi: 10.1002/jbmr.2892.

106. Kassem, M.; Marie, P.J. Senescence-associated intrinsic mechanisms of osteoblast dysfunctions. *Aging Cell* 2011, 10, 191–197. doi: 10.1111/j.1474-9726.2011.00669.x.

107. Singh, L.; Brennan, T.A.; Russell, E.; Kim, J.H.; Chen, Q.; Brad Johnson, F.; Pignolo, R.J. Aging alters bone-fat reciprocity by shifting in vivo mesenchymal precursor cell fate towards an adipogenic lineage. *Bone* 2016, 85, 29–36. doi: 10.1016/j.bone.2016.01.014.

108. Riggs, B.L.; Khosla, S.; Melton, L.J., 3rd. A unitary model for involutional osteoporosis: Estrogen deficiency causes both types I and type II osteoporosis in postmenopausal women and contributes to bone loss in aging men. *J Bone Miner Res* 1998, 13, 763–773. doi: 10.1359/jbmr.1998.13.5.763.

109. Khosla, S.; Oursler, M.J.; Monroe, D.G. Estrogen and the skeleton. *Trends Endocrinol Metab* 2012, 23, 576–581. doi: 10.1016/j.tem.2012.03.008.

110. Oursler, M.J.; Osdoby, P.; Pyfferoen, J.; Riggs, B.L.; Spelsberg, T.C. Avian osteoclasts as estrogen target cells. *Proc Natl Acad Sci U S A* 1991, 88, 6613–6617. doi: 10.1073/pnas.88.15.6613.

111. Ström, O.; Borgström, F.; Kanis, J.A.; Compston, J.; Cooper, C.; McCloskey, E.V.; Jönsson, B. Osteoporosis: Burden, health care provision and opportunities in the EU: A report prepared in collaboration with the International Osteoporosis Foundation (IOF) and the European Federation of Pharmaceutical Industry Associations (EFPIA). *Arch Osteoporos* 2011, 6, 59–155. doi: 10.1007/s11657-011-0060-1.

112. Machura, P.; Grymowicz, M.; Rudnicka, E.; Pięta, W.; Calik-Ksepka, A.; Skórska, J.; Smolarczyk, R. Premature ovarian insufficiency - hormone replacement therapy and management of long-term consequences. *Prz Menopauzalny* 2018, 17, 135–138. doi: 10.5114/pm.2018.78559.

113. Tomkinson, A.; Reeve, J.; Shaw, R.W.; Noble, B.S. The death of osteocytes via apoptosis accompanies estrogen withdrawal in human bone. *J Clin Endocrinol Metab* 1997, 82, 3128–3135. doi: 10.1210/jcem.82.9.4200.

114. Kousteni, S.; Chen, J.R.; Bellido, T.; Han, L.; Ali, A.A.; O'Brien, C.A.; Plotkin, L.; Fu, Q.; Mancino, A.T.; Wen, Y. et al. Reversal of bone loss in mice by nongenotropic signaling of sex steroids. *Science* 2002, 298, 843–846. doi: 10.1126/science.1074935.

115. Emerton, K.B.; Hu, B.; Woo, A.A.; Sinofsky, A.; Hernandez, C.; Majeska, R.J.; Jepsen, K.J.; Schaffler, M.B. Osteocyte apoptosis and control of bone resorption following ovariectomy in mice. *Bone* 2010, 46, 577–583. doi: 10.1016/j.bone.2009.11.006.

116. Faloni, A.P.; Sasso-Cerri, E.; Katchburian, E.; Cerri, P.S. Decrease in the number and apoptosis of alveolar bone osteoclasts in estrogen-treated rats. *J Periodontal Res* 2007, 42, 193–201. doi: 10.1111/j.1600-0765.2006.00932.x.

117. Faloni, A.P.; Sasso-Cerri, E.; Rocha, F.R.; Katchburian, E.; Cerri, P.S. Structural and functional changes in the alveolar bone osteoclasts of estrogen-treated rats. *J Anat* 2012, 220, 77–85. doi: 10.1111/j.1469-7580.2011.01449.x.

118. Hughes, D.E.; Dai, A.; Tiffee, J.C.; Li, H.H.; Mundy, G.R.; Boyce, B.F. Estrogen promotes apoptosis of murine osteoclasts mediated by TGF-beta. *Nat Med* 1996, 2, 1132–1136. doi: 10.1038/nm1096-1132.

119. Phan, T.C.; Xu, J.; Zheng, M.H. Interaction between osteoblast and osteoclast: Impact in bone disease. *Histol Histopathol* 2004, 19, 1325–1344. doi: 10.14670/hh-19.1325.

120. Li, M.; Xu, D. Antiresorptive activity of osteoprotegerin requires an intact heparan sulfate-binding site. *Proc Natl Acad Sci U S A* 2020, 117, 17187–17194. doi: 10.1073/pnas.2005859117.

121. Kawamoto, S.; Ejiri, S.; Nagaoka, E.; Ozawa, H. Effects of oestrogen deficiency on osteoclastogenesis in the rat periodontium. *Arch Oral Biol* 2002, 47, 67–73. doi: 10.1016/s0003-9969(01)00086-3.

122. Eghbali-Fatourechi, G.; Khosla, S.; Sanyal, A.; Boyle, W.J.; Lacey, D.L.; Riggs, B.L. Role of RANK ligand in mediating increased bone resorption in early postmenopausal women. *J Clin Invest* 2003, 111, 1221–1230. doi: 10.1172/jci17215.

123. Robinson, L.J.; Yaroslavskiy, B.B.; Griswold, R.D.; Zadorozny, E.V.; Guo, L.; Tourkova, I.L.; Blair, H.C. Estrogen inhibits RANKL-stimulated osteoclastic differentiation of human monocytes through estrogen and RANKL-regulated interaction of estrogen receptor-alpha with BCAR1 and Traf6. *Exp Cell Res* 2009, 315, 1287–1301. doi: 10.1016/j.yexcr.2009.01.014.

124. Pacifici, R. Estrogen, cytokines, and pathogenesis of postmenopausal osteoporosis. *J Bone Miner Res* 1996, 11, 1043–1051. doi: 10.1002/jbmr.5650110802.

125. Cenci, S.; Weitzmann, M.N.; Roggia, C.; Namba, N.; Novack, D.; Woodring, J.; Pacifici, R. Estrogen deficiency induces bone loss by enhancing T-cell production of TNF-alpha. *J Clin Invest* 2000, 106, 1229–1237. doi: 10.1172/jci11066.

126. Lean, J.M.; Davies, J.T.; Fuller, K.; Jagger, C.J.; Kirstein, B.; Partington, G.A.; Urry, Z.L.; Chambers, T.J. A crucial role for thiol antioxidants in estrogen-deficiency bone loss. *J Clin Invest* 2003, 112, 915–923. doi: 10.1172/jci18859.

127. Muthusami, S.; Ramachandran, I.; Muthusamy, B.; Vasudevan, G.; Prabhu, V.; Subramaniam, V.; Jagadeesan, A.; Narasimhan, S. Ovariectomy induces oxidative stress and impairs bone antioxidant system in adult rats. *Clin Chim Acta* 2005, 360, 81–86. doi: 10.1016/j.cccn.2005.04.014.

128. Shuid, A.N.; Mohamad, S.; Muhammad, N.; Fadzilah, F.M.; Mokhtar, S.A.; Mohamed, N.; Soelaiman, I.N. Effects of α-tocopherol on the early phase of osteoporotic fracture healing. *J Orthop Res* 2011, 29, 1732–1738. doi: 10.1002/jor.21452.

129. Schäcke, H.; Döcke, W.D.; Asadullah, K. Mechanisms involved in the side effects of glucocorticoids. *Pharmacol Ther* 2002, 96, 23–43. doi: 10.1016/s0163-7258(02)00297-8.

130. Han, D.; Gu, X.; Gao, J.; Wang, Z.; Liu, G.; Barkema, H.W.; Han, B. Chlorogenic acid promotes the Nrf2/HO-1 anti-oxidative pathway by activating p21(Waf1/Cip1) to resist dexamethasone-induced apoptosis in osteoblastic cells. *Free Radic Biol Med* 2019, 137, 1–12. doi: 10.1016/j.freeradbiomed.2019.04.014.

131. Xu, W.N.; Zheng, H.L.; Yang, R.Z.; Jiang, L.S.; Jiang, S.D. HIF-1α regulates glucocorticoid-induced osteoporosis through PDK1/AKT/mTOR signaling pathway. *Front Endocrinol (Lausanne)* 2019, 10, 922. doi: 10.3389/fendo.2019.00922.

132. Li, H.; Qian, W.; Weng, X.; Wu, Z.; Li, H.; Zhuang, Q.; Feng, B.; Bian, Y. Glucocorticoid receptor and sequential P53 activation by dexamethasone mediates apoptosis and cell cycle arrest of osteoblastic MC3T3-E1 cells. *PLoS One* 2012, 7, e37030. doi: 10.1371/journal. pone.0037030.

133. Zhen, Y.F.; Wang, G.D.; Zhu, L.Q.; Tan, S.P.; Zhang, F.Y.; Zhou, X.Z.; Wang, X.D. P53 dependent mitochondrial permeability transition pore opening is required for dexamethasone-induced death of osteoblasts. *J Cell Physiol* 2014, 229, 1475–1483. doi: 10.1002/ jcp.24589.

134. Chen, L.; Hu, S.L.; Xie, J.; Yan, D.Y.; Weng, S.J.; Tang, J.H.; Wang, B.Z.; Xie, Z.J.; Wu, Z.Y.; Yang, L. Proanthocyanidins-mediated Nrf2 activation ameliorates glucocorticoid-induced oxidative stress and mitochondrial dysfunction in osteoblasts. *Oxid Med Cell Longev* 2020, 2020, 9102012. doi: 10.1155/2020/9102012.

135. Kumar, H.; Kim, I.S.; More, S.V.; Kim, B.W.; Choi, D.K. Natural product-derived pharmacological modulators of Nrf2/ARE pathway for chronic diseases. *Nat Prod Rep* 2014, 31, 109–139. doi: 10.1039/c3np70065h.

136. Bhogal, R.H.; Weston, C.J.; Curbishley, S.M.; Adams, D.H.; Afford, S.C. Autophagy: A cytoprotective mechanism which prevents primary human hepatocyte apoptosis during oxidative stress. *Autophagy* 2012, 8, 545–558. doi: 10.4161/auto.19012.

137. Zhao, C.; Gillette, D.D.; Li, X.; Zhang, Z.; Wen, H. Nuclear factor E2-related factor-2 (Nrf2) is required for NLRP3 and AIM2 inflammasome activation. *J Biol Chem* 2014, 289, 17020–17029. doi: 10.1074/jbc.M114.563114.

138. Sun, X.; Xie, Z.; Hu, B.; Zhang, B.; Ma, Y.; Pan, X.; Huang, H.; Wang, J.; Zhao, X.; Jie, Z. et al. The Nrf2 activator RTA-408 attenuates osteoclastogenesis by inhibiting STING dependent NF-κb signaling. *Redox Biol* 2020, 28, 101309. doi: 10.1016/j.redox.2019.101309.

139. Kensler, T.W.; Wakabayashi, N.; Biswal, S. Cell survival responses to environmental stresses via the Keap1-Nrf2-ARE pathway. *Annu Rev Pharmacol Toxicol* 2007, 47, 89–116. doi: 10.1146/annurev.pharmtox.46.120604.141046.

140. Zhou, S.; Jin, J.; Bai, T.; Sachleben, L.R., Jr.; Cai, L.; Zheng, Y. Potential drugs which activate nuclear factor E2-related factor 2 signaling to prevent diabetic cardiovascular complications: A focus on fumaric acid esters. *Life Sci* 2015, 134, 56–62. doi: 10.1016/j.lfs.2015.05.015.

141. Cimino, F.; Speciale, A.; Anwar, S.; Canali, R.; Ricciardi, E.; Virgili, F.; Trombetta, D.; Saija, A. Anthocyanins protect human endothelial cells from mild hyperoxia damage through modulation of Nrf2 pathway. *Genes Nutr* 2013, 8, 391–399. doi: 10.1007/ s12263-012-0324-4.

142. Guo, Y.; Yu, S.; Zhang, C.; Kong, A.N. Epigenetic regulation of Keap1-Nrf2 signaling. *Free Radic Biol Med* 2015, 88, 337–349. doi: 10.1016/j.freeradbiomed.2015.06.013.

143. Aspera-Werz, R.H.; Ehnert, S.; Heid, D.; Zhu, S.; Chen, T.; Braun, B.; Sreekumar, V.; Arnscheidt, C.; Nussler, A.K. Nicotine and cotinine inhibit catalase and glutathione reductase activity contributing to the impaired osteogenesis of SCP-1 cells exposed to cigarette smoke. *Oxid Med Cell Longev* 2018, 2018, 3172480. doi: 10.1155/2018/3172480.

144. Kansanen, E.; Kuosmanen, S.M.; Leinonen, H.; Levonen, A.L. The Keap1-Nrf2 pathway: Mechanisms of activation and dysregulation in cancer. *Redox Biol* 2013, 1, 45–49. doi: 10.1016/j.redox.2012.10.001.

145. Sykiotis, G.P.; Habeos, I.G.; Samuelson, A.V.; Bohmann, D. The role of the antioxidant and longevity-promoting Nrf2 pathway in metabolic regulation. *Curr Opin Clin Nutr Metab Care* 2011, 14, 41–48. doi: 10.1097/MCO.0b013e32834136f2.

146. Sun, X.; Zhang, B.; Pan, X.; Huang, H.; Xie, Z.; Ma, Y.; Hu, B.; Wang, J.; Chen, Z.; Shi, P. Octyl itaconate inhibits osteoclastogenesis by suppressing Hrd1 and activating Nrf2 signaling. *Faseb J* 2019, 33, 12929–12940. doi: 10.1096/fj.201900887RR.

147. Sun, Y.X.; Li, L.; Corry, K.A.; Zhang, P.; Yang, Y.; Himes, E.; Mihuti, C.L.; Nelson, C.; Dai, G.; Li, J. Deletion of Nrf2 reduces skeletal mechanical properties and decreases load-driven bone formation. *Bone* 2015, 74, 1–9. doi: 10.1016/j.bone.2014.12.066.

148. Terpos, E.; Ntanasis-Stathopoulos, I.; Dimopoulos, M.A. Myeloma bone disease: From biology findings to treatment approaches. *Blood* 2019, 133, 1534–1539. doi: 10.1182/blood-2018-11-852459.

149. Hyeon, S.; Lee, H.; Yang, Y.; Jeong, W. Nrf2 deficiency induces oxidative stress and promotes RANKL-induced osteoclast differentiation. *Free Radic Biol Med* 2013, 65, 789–799. doi: 10.1016/j.freeradbiomed.2013.08.005.

150. Rana, T.; Schultz, M.A.; Freeman, M.L.; Biswas, S. Loss of Nrf2 accelerates ionizing radiation-induced bone loss by upregulating RANKL. *Free Radic Biol Med* 2012, 53, 2298–2307. doi: 10.1016/j.freeradbiomed.2012.10.536.

151. Dreher, I.; Schütze, N.; Baur, A.; Hesse, K.; Schneider, D.; Köhrle, J.; Jakob, F. Selenoproteins are expressed in fetal human osteoblast-like cells. *Biochem Biophys Res Commun* 1998, 245, 101–107. doi: 10.1006/bbrc.1998.8393.

152. Fuller, K.; Lean, J.M.; Bayley, K.E.; Wani, M.R.; Chambers, T.J. A role for TGFbeta(1) in osteoclast differentiation and survival. *J Cell Sci* 2000, 113(Pt 13), 2445–2453.

153. Sheweita, S.A.; Khoshhal, K.I. Calcium metabolism and oxidative stress in bone fractures: Role of antioxidants. *Curr Drug Metab* 2007, 8, 519–525. doi: 10.2174/138920007780866852.

154. Altindag, O.; Erel, O.; Soran, N.; Celik, H.; Selek, S. Total oxidative/anti-oxidative status and relation to bone mineral density in osteoporosis. *Rheumatol Int* 2008, 28, 317–321. doi: 10.1007/s00296-007-0452-0.

155. Kim, J.H.; Singhal, V.; Biswal, S.; Thimmulappa, R.K.; DiGirolamo, D.J. Nrf2 is required for normal postnatal bone acquisition in mice. *Bone Res* 2014, 2, 14033. doi: 10.1038/boneres.2014.33.

156. Almeida, M.; Han, L.; Martin-Millan, M.; O'Brien, C.A.; Manolagas, S.C. Oxidative stress antagonizes Wnt signaling in osteoblast precursors by diverting beta-catenin from T cell factor- to forkhead box O-mediated transcription. *J Biol Chem* 2007, 282, 27298–27305. doi: 10.1074/jbc.M702811200.

157. Ducy, P.; Starbuck, M.; Priemel, M.; Shen, J.; Pinero, G.; Geoffroy, V.; Amling, M.; Karsenty, G. A Cbfa1-dependent genetic pathway controls bone formation beyond embryonic development. *Genes Dev* 1999, 13, 1025–1036. doi: 10.1101/gad.13.8.1025.

158. Hinoi, E.; Fujimori, S.; Wang, L.; Hojo, H.; Uno, K.; Yoneda, Y. Nrf2 negatively regulates osteoblast differentiation via interfering with Runx2-dependent transcriptional activation. *J Biol Chem* 2006, 281, 18015–18024. doi: 10.1074/jbc.M600603200.

159. Kanzaki, H.; Shinohara, F.; Kajiya, M.; Kodama, T. The Keap1/Nrf2 protein axis plays a role in osteoclast differentiation by regulating intracellular reactive oxygen species signaling. *J Biol Chem* 2013, 288, 23009–23020. doi: 10.1074/jbc.M113.478545.

160. Baek, K.H.; Oh, K.W.; Lee, W.Y.; Lee, S.S.; Kim, M.K.; Kwon, H.S.; Rhee, E.J.; Han, J.H.; Song, K.H.; Cha, B.Y., et al. Association of oxidative stress with postmenopausal osteoporosis and the effects of hydrogen peroxide on osteoclast formation in human bone marrow cell cultures. *Calcif Tissue Int* 2010, 87, 226–235. doi: 10.1007/s00223-010-9393-9.

161. Asagiri, M.; Sato, K.; Usami, T.; Ochi, S.; Nishina, H.; Yoshida, H.; Morita, I.; Wagner, E.F.; Mak, T.W.; Serfling, E., et al. Autoamplification of NFATc1 expression determines its essential role in bone homeostasis. *J Exp Med* 2005, 202, 1261–1269. doi: 10.1084/jem.20051150.

162. Lippross, S.; Beckmann, R.; Streubesand, N.; Ayub, F.; Tohidnezhad, M.; Campbell, G.; Kan, Y.W.; Horst, F.; Sönmez, T.T.; Varoga, D., et al. Nrf2 deficiency impairs fracture healing in mice. *Calcif Tissue Int* 2014, 95, 349–361. doi: 10.1007/s00223-014-9900-5.

163. Al-Sawaf, O.; Clarner, T.; Fragoulis, A.; Kan, Y.W.; Pufe, T.; Streetz, K.; Wruck, C.J. Nrf2 in health and disease: Current and future clinical implications. *Clin Sci (Lond)* 2015, 129, 989–999. doi: 10.1042/cs20150436.

164. Ilyas, A.; Odatsu, T.; Shah, A.; Monte, F.; Kim, H.K.; Kramer, P.; Aswath, P.B.; Varanasi, V.G. Amorphous silica: A new antioxidant role for rapid critical-sized bone defect healing. *Adv Healthc Mater* 2016, 5, 2199–2213. doi: 10.1002/adhm.201600203.

165. Kelpke, S.S.; Reiff, D.; Prince, C.W.; Thompson, J.A. Acidic fibroblast growth factor signaling inhibits peroxynitrite-induced death of osteoblasts and osteoblast precursors. *J Bone Miner Res* 2001, 16, 1917–1925. doi: 10.1359/jbmr.2001.16.10.1917.

166. Turgut, A.; Göktürk, E.; Köse, N.; Kaçmaz, M.; Oztürk, H.S.; Seber, S.; Acar, S. Oxidant status increased during fracture healing in rats. *Acta Orthop Scand* 1999, 70, 487–490. doi: 10.3109/17453679909000986.

167. Mody, N.; Parhami, F.; Sarafian, T.A.; Demer, L.L. Oxidative stress modulates osteoblastic differentiation of vascular and bone cells. *Free Radic Biol Med* 2001, 31, 509–519. doi: 10.1016/s0891-5849(01)00610-4.

168. Morita, K.; Miyamoto, T.; Fujita, N.; Kubota, Y.; Ito, K.; Takubo, K.; Miyamoto, K.; Ninomiya, K.; Suzuki, T.; Iwasaki, R., et al. Reactive oxygen species induce chondrocyte hypertrophy in endochondral ossification. *J Exp Med* 2007, 204, 1613–1623. doi: 10.1084/jem.20062525.

169. Manolagas, S.C.; Parfitt, A.M. What old means to bone. *Trends Endocrinol Metab* 2010, 21, 369–374. doi: 10.1016/j.tem.2010.01.010.

170. Phillips, A.M. Overview of the fracture healing cascade. *Injury* 2005, 36(Suppl. 3), S5–S7. doi: 10.1016/j.injury.2005.07.027.

171. Wauquier, F.; Leotoing, L.; Coxam, V.; Guicheux, J.; Wittrant, Y. Oxidative stress in bone remodelling and disease. *Trends Mol Med* 2009, 15, 468–477. doi: 10.1016/j.molmed.2009.08.004.

172. Yeler, H.; Tahtabas, F.; Candan, F. Investigation of oxidative stress during fracture healing in the rats. *Cell Biochem Funct* 2005, 23, 137–139. doi: 10.1002/cbf.1199.

173. Hernlund, E.; Svedbom, A.; Ivergård, M.; Compston, J.; Cooper, C.; Stenmark, J.; McCloskey, E.V.; Jönsson, B.; Kanis, J.A. Osteoporosis in the European Union: Medical management, epidemiology and economic burden. A report prepared in collaboration with the International Osteoporosis Foundation (IOF) and the European Federation of Pharmaceutical Industry Associations (EFPIA). *Arch Osteoporos* 2013, 8, 136. doi: 10.1007/s11657-013-0136-1.

174. Klotzbuecher, C.M.; Ross, P.D.; Landsman, P.B.; Abbott, T.A., 3rd; Berger, M. Patients with prior fractures have an increased risk of future fractures: A summary of the literature and statistical synthesis. *J Bone Miner Res* 2000, 15, 721–739. doi: 10.1359/jbmr.2000.15.4.721.

175. Johnell, O.; Oden, A.; Caulin, F.; Kanis, J.A. Acute and a long-term increase in fracture risk after hospitalization for vertebral fracture. *Osteoporos Int* 2001, 12, 207–214. doi: 10.1007/s001980170131.

176. Johnell, O.; Kanis, J.A.; Odén, A.; Sernbo, I.; Redlund-Johnell, I.; Petterson, C.; De Laet, C.; Jönsson, B. Fracture risk following an osteoporotic fracture. *Osteoporos Int* 2004, 15, 175–179. doi: 10.1007/s00198-003-1514-0.

177. Lindsay, R.; Silverman, S.L.; Cooper, C.; Hanley, D.A.; Barton, I.; Broy, S.B.; Licata, A.; Benhamou, L.; Geusens, P.; Flowers, K., et al. Risk of new vertebral fracture in the year following a fracture. *JAMA* 2001, 285, 320–323. doi: 10.1001/jama.285.3.320.

178. Díez-Pérez, A.; Hooven, F.H.; Adachi, J.D.; Adami, S.; Anderson, F.A.; Boonen, S.; Chapurlat, R.; Compston, J.E.; Cooper, C.; Delmas, P., et al. Regional differences in treatment for osteoporosis: The global longitudinal study of osteoporosis in women (GLOW). *Bone* 2011, 49, 493–498. doi: 10.1016/j.bone.2011.05.007.

179. Guggina, P.; Flahive, J.; Hooven, F.H.; Watts, N.B.; Siris, E.S.; Silverman, S.; Roux, C.; Pfeilschifter, J.; Greenspan, S.L.; Díez-Pérez, A., et al. Characteristics associated with anti-osteoporosis medication use: Data from the global longitudinal study of osteoporosis in women (GLOW) USA cohort. *Bone* 2012, 51, 975–980. doi: 10.1016/j.bone.2012.08.130.

180. Jennings, L.A.; Auerbach, A.D.; Maselli, J.; Pekow, P.S.; Lindenauer, P.K.; Lee, S.J. Missed opportunities for osteoporosis treatment in patients hospitalized for hip fracture. *J Am Geriatr Soc* 2010, 58, 650–657. doi: 10.1111/j.1532-5415.2010.02769.x.

181. Freedman, K.B.; Kaplan, F.S.; Bilker, W.B.; Strom, B.L.; Lowe, R.A. Treatment of osteoporosis: Are physicians missing an opportunity? *J Bone Joint Surg Am* 2000, 82, 1063–1070. doi: 10.2106/00004623-200008000-00001.
182. Giangregorio, L.; Papaioannou, A.; Cranney, A.; Zytaruk, N.; Adachi, J.D. Fragility fractures and the osteoporosis care gap: An international phenomenon. *Semin Arthritis Rheum* 2006, 35, 293–305. doi: 10.1016/j.semarthrit.2005.11.001.
183. Nayak, S.; Roberts, M.S.; Greenspan, S.L. Factors associated with diagnosis and treatment of osteoporosis in older adults. *Osteoporos Int* 2009, 20, 1963–1967. doi: 10.1007/s00198-008-0831-8.
184. Vaile, J.; Sullivan, L.; Bennett, C.; Bleasel, J. First fracture project: Addressing the osteoporosis care gap. *Intern Med J* 2007, 37, 717–720. doi: 10.1111/j.1445-5994.2007.01496.x.
185. Chen, L.R.; Ko, N.Y.; Chen, K.H. Medical treatment for osteoporosis: From molecular to clinical opinions. *Int J Mol Sci* 2019, 20, 2213. doi: 10.3390/ijms20092213.
186. Faienza, M.F.; Chiarito, M.; D'Amato, G.; Colaianni, G.; Colucci, S.; Grano, M.; Brunetti, G. Monoclonal antibodies for treating osteoporosis. *Expert Opin Biol Ther* 2018, 18, 149–157. doi: 10.1080/14712598.2018.1401607.
187. Kling, J.M.; Clarke, B.L.; Sandhu, N.P. Osteoporosis prevention, screening, and treatment: A review. *J Womens Health (Larchmt)* 2014, 23, 563–572. doi: 10.1089/jwh.2013.4611.
188. Wong, S.K.; Chin, K.Y.; Ima-Nirwana, S. Quercetin as an agent for protecting the bone: A review of the current evidence. *Int J Mol Sci* 2020, 21, 6448. doi: 10.3390/ijms21176448.
189. Singh, B.; Singh, J.P.; Kaur, A.; Singh, N. Phenolic compounds as beneficial phytochemicals in pomegranate (Punica granatum L.) peel: A review. *Food Chem* 2018, 261, 75–86. doi: 10.1016/j.foodchem.2018.04.039.
190. Braun, K.F.; Ehnert, S.; Freude, T.; Egaña, J.T.; Schenck, T.L.; Buchholz, A.; Schmitt, A.; Siebenlist, S.; Schyschka, L.; Neumaier, M., et al. Quercetin protects primary human osteoblasts exposed to cigarette smoke through activation of the antioxidative enzymes HO-1 and SOD-1. *ScientificWorldJournal* 2011, 11, 2348–2357. doi: 10.1100/2011/471426.
191. Hassan, A.R.; Amer, K.F.; El-Toumy, S.A.; Nielsen, J.; Christensen, S.B. A new flavonol glycoside and other flavonoids from the aerial parts of Taverniera aegyptiaca. *Nat Prod Res* 2019, 33, 1135–1139. doi: 10.1080/14786419.2018.1460834.
192. Woo, H.D.; Kim, J. Dietary flavonoid intake and risk of stomach and colorectal cancer. *World J Gastroenterol* 2013, 19, 1011–1019. doi: 10.3748/wjg.v19.i7.1011.
193. Welch, A.A.; Hardcastle, A.C. The effects of flavonoids on bone. *Curr Osteoporos Rep* 2014, 12, 205–210. doi: 10.1007/s11914-014-0212-5.
194. Panche, A.N.; Diwan, A.D.; Chandra, S.R. Flavonoids: An overview. *J Nutr Sci* 2016, 5, e47. doi: 10.1017/jns.2016.41.
195. Chen, H.; Lin, H.; Xie, S.; Huang, B.; Qian, Y.; Chen, K.; Niu, Y.; Shen, H.M.; Cai, J.; Li, P., et al. Myricetin inhibits NLRP3 inflammasome activation via reduction of ROS-dependent ubiquitination of ASC and promotion of ROS-independent NLRP3 ubiquitination. *Toxicol Appl Pharmacol* 2019, 365, 19–29. doi: 10.1016/j.taap.2018.12.019.
196. Al-Anazi, A.F.; Qureshi, V.F.; Javaid, K.; Qureshi, S. Preventive effects of phytoestrogens against postmenopausal osteoporosis as compared to the available therapeutic choices: An overview. *J Nat Sci Biol Med* 2011, 2, 154–163. doi: 10.4103/0976-9668.92322.
197. Wang, Z.; Wang, D.; Yang, D.; Zhen, W.; Zhang, J.; Peng, S. The effect of icariin on bone metabolism and its potential clinical application. *Osteoporos Int* 2018, 29, 535–544. doi: 10.1007/s00198-017-4255-1.
198. Zhao, B.J.; Wang, J.; Song, J.; Wang, C.F.; Gu, J.F.; Yuan, J.R.; Zhang, L.; Jiang, J.; Feng, L.; Jia, X.B. Beneficial effects of a flavonoid fraction of herba epimedii on bone metabolism in ovariectomized rats. *Planta Med* 2016, 82, 322–329. doi: 10.1055/s-0035-1558294.
199. Jiang, J.; Xiao, S.; Xu, X.; Ma, H.; Feng, C.; Jia, X. Isomeric flavonoid aglycones derived from Epimedii Folium exerted different intensities in anti-osteoporosis through OPG/RANKL protein targets. *Int Immunopharmacol* 2018, 62, 277–286. doi: 10.1016/j.intimp.2018.07.017.

200. Weaver, C.M.; Alekel, D.L.; Ward, W.E.; Ronis, M.J. Flavonoid intake and bone health. *J Nutr Gerontol Geriatr* 2012, 31, 239–253. doi: 10.1080/21551197.2012.698220.
201. Niture, S.K.; Kaspar, J.W.; Shen, J.; Jaiswal, A.K. Nrf2 signaling and cell survival. *Toxicol Appl Pharmacol* 2010, 244, 37–42. doi: 10.1016/j.taap.2009.06.009.
202. Li, Y.; Yao, J.; Han, C.; Yang, J.; Chaudhry, M.T.; Wang, S.; Liu, H.; Yin, Y. Quercetin, inflammation and immunity. *Nutrients* 2016, 8, 167. doi: 10.3390/nu8030167.
203. Khan, A.; Ali, T.; Rehman, S.U.; Khan, M.S.; Alam, S.I.; Ikram, M.; Muhammad, T.; Saeed, K.; Badshah, H.; Kim, M.O. Neuroprotective effect of quercetin against the detrimental effects of LPS in the adult mouse brain. *Front Pharmacol* 2018, 9, 1383. doi: 10.3389/fphar.2018.01383.
204. Tang, S.M.; Deng, X.T.; Zhou, J.; Li, Q.P.; Ge, X.X.; Miao, L. Pharmacological basis and new insights of quercetin action in respect to its anti-cancer effects. *Biomed Pharmacother* 2020, 121, 109604. doi: 10.1016/j.biopha.2019.109604.
205. Aziz, T.A. Cardioprotective effect of quercetin and sitagliptin in doxorubicin-induced cardiac toxicity in rats. *Cancer Manag Res* 2021, 13, 2349–2357. doi: 10.2147/cmar.S300495.
206. Wei, Y.; Fu, J.; Wu, W.; Ma, P.; Ren, L.; Yi, Z.; Wu, J. Quercetin prevents oxidative stress-induced injury of periodontal ligament cells and alveolar bone loss in periodontitis. *Drug Des Devel Ther* 2021, 15, 3509–3522. doi: 10.2147/dddt.S315249.
207. Wattel, A.; Kamel, S.; Mentaverri, R.; Lorget, F.; Prouillet, C.; Petit, J.P.; Fardelonne, P.; Brazier, M. Potent inhibitory effect of naturally occurring flavonoids quercetin and kaemp-ferol on in vitro osteoclastic bone resorption. *Biochem Pharmacol* 2003, 65, 35–42. doi: 10.1016/s0006-2952(02)01445-4.
208. Guo, C.; Hou, G.Q.; Li, X.D.; Xia, X.; Liu, D.X.; Huang, D.Y.; Du, S.X. Quercetin triggers apoptosis of lipopolysaccharide (LPS)-induced osteoclasts and inhibits bone resorption in RAW264.7 cells. *Cell Physiol Biochem* 2012, 30, 123–136. doi: 10.1159/000339052.
209. Qi, Z.; Ci, X.; Huang, J.; Liu, Q.; Yu, Q.; Zhou, J.; Deng, X. Asiatic acid enhances Nrf2 signaling to protect HepG2 cells from oxidative damage through Akt and ERK activation. *Biomed Pharmacother* 2017, 88, 252–259. doi: 10.1016/j.biopha.2017.01.067.
210. Ganesh Yerra, V.; Negi, G.; Sharma, S.S.; Kumar, A. Potential therapeutic effects of the simultaneous targeting of the Nrf2 and NF-κB pathways in diabetic neuropathy. *Redox Biol* 2013, 1, 394–397. doi: 10.1016/j.redox.2013.07.005.
211. Messer, J.G.; Hopkins, R.G.; Kipp, D.E. Quercetin metabolites up-regulate the antioxidant response in osteoblasts isolated from fetal rat calvaria. *J Cell Biochem* 2015, 116, 1857–1866. doi: 10.1002/jcb.25141.
212. Vimalraj, S.; Rajalakshmi, S.; Raj Preeth, D.; Vinoth Kumar, S.; Deepak, T.; Gopinath, V.; Murugan, K.; Chatterjee, S. Mixed-ligand copper(II) complex of quercetin regulate osteogenesis and angiogenesis. *Mater Sci Eng C Mater Biol Appl* 2018, 83, 187–194. doi: 10.1016/j.msec.2017.09.005.
213. Dixon, R.A.; Ferreira, D. Genistein. *Phytochemistry* 2002, 60, 205–211. doi: 10.1016/s0031-9422(02)00116-4.
214. Albertazzi, P.; Steel, S.A.; Bottazzi, M. Effect of pure genistein on bone markers and hot flushes. *Climacteric* 2005, 8, 371–379. doi: 10.1080/13697130500345257.
215. Anderson, J.J.; Ambrose, W.W.; Garner, S.C. Biphasic effects of genistein on bone tissue in the ovariectomized, lactating rat model. *Proc Soc Exp Biol Med* 1998, 217, 345–350. doi: 10.3181/00379727-217-44243.
216. Fanti, P.; Monier-Faugere, M.C.; Geng, Z.; Schmidt, J.; Morris, P.E.; Cohen, D.; Malluche, H.H. The phytoestrogen genistein reduces bone loss in short-term ovariectomized rats. *Osteoporos Int* 1998, 8, 274–281. doi: 10.1007/s001980050065.
217. Ha, H.; Lee, H.Y.; Lee, J.H.; Jung, D.; Choi, J.; Song, K.Y.; Jung, H.J.; Choi, J.S.; Chang, S.I.; Kim, C. Formononetin prevents ovariectomy-induced bone loss in rats. *Arch Pharm Res* 2010, 33, 625–632. doi: 10.1007/s12272-010-0418-8.

218. Liao, Q.C.; Xiao, Z.S.; Qin, Y.F.; Zhou, H.H. Genistein stimulates osteoblastic differentiation via p38 MAPK-Cbfa1 pathway in bone marrow culture. *Acta Pharmacol Sin* 2007, 28, 1597–1602. doi: 10.1111/j.1745-7254.2007.00632.x.

219. Zhang, H.P.; Zheng, F.L.; Zhao, J.H.; Guo, D.X.; Chen, X.L. Genistein inhibits ox-LDL-induced VCAM-1, ICAM-1 and MCP-1 expression of HUVECs through heme oxygenase-1. *Arch Med Res* 2013, 44, 13–20. doi: 10.1016/j.arcmed.2012.12.001.

220. Lee, S.H.; Kim, J.K.; Jang, H.D. Genistein inhibits osteoclastic differentiation of RAW 264.7 cells via regulation of ROS production and scavenging. *Int J Mol Sci* 2014, 15, 10605–10621. doi: 10.3390/ijms150610605.

221. Zhai, X.; Lin, M.; Zhang, F.; Hu, Y.; Xu, X.; Li, Y.; Liu, K.; Ma, X.; Tian, X.; Yao, J. Dietary flavonoid genistein induces Nrf2 and phase II detoxification gene expression via ERKs and PKC pathways and protects against oxidative stress in Caco-2 cells. *Mol Nutr Food Res* 2013, 57, 249–259. doi: 10.1002/mnfr.201200536.

222. Li, Y.Q.; Xing, X.H.; Wang, H.; Weng, X.L.; Yu, S.B.; Dong, G.Y. Dose-dependent effects of genistein on bone homeostasis in rats' mandibular subchondral bone. *Acta Pharmacol Sin* 2012, 33, 66–74. doi: 10.1038/aps.2011.136.

223. Kim, M.; Lim, J.; Lee, J.H.; Lee, K.M.; Kim, S.; Park, K.W.; Nho, C.W.; Cho, Y.S. Understanding the functional role of genistein in bone differentiation in mouse osteoblastic cell line MC3T3-E1 by RNA-seq analysis. *Sci Rep* 2018, 8, 3257. doi: 10.1038/s41598-018-21601-9.

224. Ming, L.G.; Chen, K.M.; Xian, C.J. Functions and action mechanisms of flavonoids genistein and icariin in regulating bone remodeling. *J Cell Physiol* 2013, 228, 513–521. doi: 10.1002/jcp.24158.

225. Wong, S.K.; Chin, K.Y.; Ima-Nirwana, S. The osteoprotective effects of Kaempferol: The evidence from in vivo and in vitro studies. *Drug Des Devel Ther* 2019, 13, 3497–3514. doi: 10.2147/dddt.S227738.

226. Trivedi, R.; Kumar, S.; Kumar, A.; Siddiqui, J.A.; Swarnkar, G.; Gupta, V.; Kendurker, A.; Dwivedi, A.K.; Romero, J.R.; Chattopadhyay, N. Kaempferol has osteogenic effect in ovariectomized adult Sprague-Dawley rats. *Mol Cell Endocrinol* 2008, 289, 85–93. doi: 10.1016/j.mce.2008.02.027.

227. Zhu, J.; Tang, H.; Zhang, Z.; Zhang, Y.; Qiu, C.; Zhang, L.; Huang, P.; Li, F. Kaempferol slows intervertebral disc degeneration by modifying LPS-induced osteogenesis/adipogenesis imbalance and inflammation response in BMSCs. *Int Immunopharmacol* 2017, 43, 236–242. doi: 10.1016/j.intimp.2016.12.020.

228. Zhao, J.; Wu, J.; Xu, B.; Yuan, Z.; Leng, Y.; Min, J.; Lan, X.; Luo, J. Kaempferol promotes bone formation in part via the mTOR signaling pathway. *Mol Med Rep* 2019, 20, 5197–5207. doi: 10.3892/mmr.2019.10747.

229. Zhou, J.; Liao, Y.; Xie, H.; Liao, Y.; Zeng, Y.; Li, N.; Sun, G.; Wu, Q.; Zhou, G. Effects of combined treatment with ibandronate and pulsed electromagnetic field on ovariectomy-induced osteoporosis in rats. *Bioelectromagnetics* 2017, 38, 31–40. doi: 10.1002/bem.22012.

230. Zhou, X.; Li, Z.; Zhou, J. Tumor necrosis factor α in the onset and progression of leukemia. *Exp Hematol* 2017, 45, 17–26. doi: 10.1016/j.exphem.2016.10.005.

231. Pang, J.L.; Ricupero, D.A.; Huang, S.; Fatma, N.; Singh, D.P.; Romero, J.R.; Chattopadhyay, N. Differential activity of kaempferol and quercetin in attenuating tumor necrosis factor receptor family signaling in bone cells. *Biochem Pharmacol* 2006, 71, 818–826. doi: 10.1016/j.bcp.2005.12.023.

232. Alshehri, A.S. Kaempferol attenuates diabetic nephropathy in streptozotocin-induced diabetic rats by a hypoglycaemic effect and concomitant activation of the Nrf-2/Ho-1/antioxidants axis. *Arch Physiol Biochem* 2021, 1–14. doi: 10.1080/13813455.2021.1890129.

233. Alshehri, A.S.; El-Kott, A.F.; El-Gerbed, M.S.A.; El-Kenawy, A.E.; Albadrani, G.M.; Khalifa, H.S. Kaempferol prevents cadmium chloride-induced liver damage by upregulating Nrf2 and suppressing NF-κB and keap1. *Environ Sci Pollut Res Int* 2021. doi: 10.1007/s11356-021-16711-3.

234. Gao, S.S.; Choi, B.M.; Chen, X.Y.; Zhu, R.Z.; Kim, Y.; So, H.; Park, R.; Sung, M.; Kim, B.R. Kaempferol suppresses cisplatin-induced apoptosis via inductions of heme oxygenase-1 and glutamate-cysteine ligase catalytic subunit in HEI-OC1 cell. *Pharm Res* 2010, 27, 235–245. doi: 10.1007/s11095-009-0003-3.

235. Rajendran, P.; Ammar, R.B.; Al-Saeedi, F.J.; Mohamed, M.E.; ElNaggar, M.A.; Al-Ramadan, S.Y.; Bekhet, G.M.; Soliman, A.M. Kaempferol inhibits zearalenone-induced oxidative stress and apoptosis via the PI3K/Akt-mediated Nrf2 signaling pathway: In vitro and in vivo studies. *Int J Mol Sci* 2020, 22, 217. doi: 10.3390/ijms22010217.

236. Wang, J.; Wu, Q.; Ding, L.; Song, S.; Li, Y.; Shi, L.; Wang, T.; Zhao, D.; Wang, Z.; Li, X. Therapeutic effects and molecular mechanisms of bioactive compounds against respiratory diseases: Traditional Chinese medicine theory and high-frequency use. *Front Pharmacol* 2021, 12, 734450. doi: 10.3389/fphar.2021.734450.

237. Yao, H.; Sun, J.; Wei, J.; Zhang, X.; Chen, B.; Lin, Y. Kaempferol protects blood vessels from damage induced by oxidative stress and inflammation in association with the Nrf2/HO-1 signaling pathway. *Front Pharmacol* 2020, 11, 1118. doi: 10.3389/fphar.2020.01118.

238. Chiou, W.F.; Lee, C.H.; Liao, J.F.; Chen, C.C. 8-Prenylkaempferol accelerates osteoblast maturation through bone morphogenetic protein-2/p38 pathway to activate Runx2 transcription. *Life Sci* 2011, 88, 335–342. doi: 10.1016/j.lfs.2010.12.009.

239. Guo, A.J.; Choi, R.C.; Zheng, K.Y.; Chen, V.P.; Dong, T.T.; Wang, Z.T.; Vollmer, G.; Lau, D.T.; Tsim, K.W. Kaempferol as a flavonoid induces osteoblastic differentiation via estrogen receptor signaling. *Chin Med* 2012, 7, 10. doi: 10.1186/1749-8546-7-10.

240. Huang, J.; Wu, C.; Tian, B.; Zhou, X.; Ma, N.; Qian, Y. Myricetin prevents alveolar bone loss in an experimental ovariectomized mouse model of periodontitis. *Int J Mol Sci* 2016, 17, 422. doi: 10.3390/ijms17030422.

241. Gupta, G.; Siddiqui, M.A.; Khan, M.M.; Ajmal, M.; Ahsan, R.; Rahaman, M.A.; Ahmad, M.A.; Arshad, M.; Khushtar, M. Current pharmacological trends on myricetin. *Drug Res (Stuttg)* 2020, 70, 448–454. doi: 10.1055/a-1224-3625.

242. Fu, Y.X.; Wang, Y.H.; Tong, X.S.; Gong, Z.; Sun, X.M.; Yuan, J.C.; Zheng, T.T.; Li, C.; Niu, D.Q.; Dai, H.G., et al. EDACO, a derivative of myricetin, inhibits the differentiation of Gaoyou duck embryonic osteoclasts in vitro. *Br Poult Sci* 2019, 60, 169–175. doi: 10.1080/00071668.2018.1564239.

243. Wu, C.; Wang, W.; Tian, B.; Liu, X.; Qu, X.; Zhai, Z.; Li, H.; Liu, F.; Fan, Q.; Tang, T., et al. Myricetin prevents titanium particle-induced osteolysis in vivo and inhibits RANKL-induced osteoclastogenesis in vitro. *Biochem Pharmacol* 2015, 93, 59–71. doi: 10.1016/j.bcp.2014.10.019.

244. Pan, X.; Chen, T.; Zhang, Z.; Chen, X.; Chen, C.; Chen, L.; Wang, X.; Ying, X. Activation of Nrf2/HO-1 signal with myricetin for attenuating ECM degradation in human chondrocytes and ameliorating the murine osteoarthritis. *Int Immunopharmacol* 2019, 75, 105742. doi: 10.1016/j.intimp.2019.105742.

245. Lee, K.H.; Choi, E.M. Myricetin, a naturally occurring flavonoid, prevents 2-deoxy-D-ribose induced dysfunction and oxidative damage in osteoblastic MC3T3-E1 cells. *Eur J Pharmacol* 2008, 591, 1–6. doi: 10.1016/j.ejphar.2008.06.004.

246. Hwang, E.; Lin, P.; Ngo, H.T.T.; Gao, W.; Wang, Y.S.; Yu, H.S.; Yi, T.H. Icariin and icaritin recover UVB-induced photoaging by stimulating Nrf2/ARE and reducing AP-1 and NF-κB signaling pathways: A comparative study on UVB-irradiated human keratinocytes. *Photochem Photobiol Sci* 2018, 17, 1396–1408. doi: 10.1039/c8pp00174j.

247. Sze, S.C.; Tong, Y.; Ng, T.B.; Cheng, C.L.; Cheung, H.P. Herba Epimedii: Anti-oxidative properties and medical implications. *Molecules* 2010, 15, 7861–7870. doi: 10.3390/molecules15117861.
248. Chen, S.H.; Wang, X.L.; Zheng, L.Z.; Dai, Y.; Zhang, J.Y.; Guo, B.L.; Yang, Z.J.; Yao, X.S.;
Qin, L. Comparative study of two types of herbal capsules with different Epimedium species for the prevention of ovariectomised-induced osteoporosis in rats. *J Orthop Translat*
2016, 4, 14–27. doi: 10.1016/j.jot.2015.07.001.
249. Xu, Q.; Chen, G.; Liu, X.; Dai, M.; Zhang, B. Icariin inhibits RANKL-induced osteoclastogenesis via modulation of the NF-κB and MAPK signaling pathways. *Biochem Biophys
Res Commun* 2019, 508, 902–906. doi: 10.1016/j.bbrc.2018.11.201.
250. Zhao, J.; Ohba, S.; Shinkai, M.; Chung, U.I.; Nagamune, T. Icariin induces osteogenic
differentiation in vitro in a BMP- and Runx2-dependent manner. *Biochem Biophys Res
Commun* 2008, 369, 444–448. doi: 10.1016/j.bbrc.2008.02.054.
251. Fu, S.; Yang, L.; Hong, H.; Zhang, R. Wnt/β-catenin signaling is involved in the icariin
induced proliferation of bone marrow mesenchymal stem cells. *J Tradit Chin Med* 2016,
36, 360–368. doi: 10.1016/s0254-6272(16)30050-4.
252. Hsieh, T.P.; Sheu, S.Y.; Sun, J.S.; Chen, M.H.; Liu, M.H. Icariin isolated from Epimedium
pubescens regulates osteoblasts anabolism through BMP-2, SMAD4, and Cbfa1 expression. *Phytomedicine* 2010, 17, 414–423. doi: 10.1016/j.phymed.2009.08.007.
253. Song, Y.H.; Cai, H.; Zhao, Z.M.; Chang, W.J.; Gu, N.; Cao, S.P.; Wu, M.L. Icariin attenuated oxidative stress induced-cardiac apoptosis by mitochondria protection and ERK activation. *Biomed Pharmacother* 2016, 83, 1089–1094. doi: 10.1016/j.biopha.2016.08.016.
254. Hsieh, T.P.; Sheu, S.Y.; Sun, J.S.; Chen, M.H. Icariin inhibits osteoclast differentiation and
bone resorption by suppression of MAPKs/NF-κB regulated HIF-1α and PGE(2) synthesis.
Phytomedicine 2011, 18, 176–185. doi: 10.1016/j.phymed.2010.04.003.
255. Kim, T.H.; Jung, J.W.; Ha, B.G.; Hong, J.M.; Park, E.K.; Kim, H.J.; Kim, S.Y. The effects of
luteolin on osteoclast differentiation, function in vitro and ovariectomy-induced bone loss.
J Nutr Biochem 2011, 22, 8–15. doi: 10.1016/j.jnutbio.2009.11.002.
256. Choi, E.M. Modulatory effects of luteolin on osteoblastic function and inflammatory
mediators in osteoblastic MC3T3-E1 cells. *Cell Biol Int* 2007, 31, 870–877. doi: 10.1016/j.
cellbi.2007.01.038.
257. Nash, L.A.; Sullivan, P.J.; Peters, S.J.; Ward, W.E. Rooibos flavonoids, orientin and luteolin, stimulate mineralization in human osteoblasts through the Wnt pathway. *Mol Nutr
Food Res* 2015, 59, 443–453. doi: 10.1002/mnfr.201400592.
258. Chen, C.Y.; Peng, W.H.; Tsai, K.D.; Hsu, S.L. Luteolin suppresses inflammation-associated
gene expression by blocking NF-kappaB and AP-1 activation pathway in mouse alveolar
macrophages. *Life Sci* 2007, 81, 1602–1614. doi: 10.1016/j.lfs.2007.09.028.
259. Trzeciakiewicz, A.; Habauzit, V.; Mercier, S.; Barron, D.; Urpi-Sarda, M.; Manach, C.;
Offord, E.; Horcajada, M.N. Molecular mechanism of hesperetin-7-O-glucuronide, the
main circulating metabolite of hesperidin, involved in osteoblast differentiation. *J Agric
Food Chem* 2010, 58, 668–675. doi: 10.1021/jf902680n.
260. Trzeciakiewicz, A.; Habauzit, V.; Mercier, S.; Lebecque, P.; Davicco, M.J.; Coxam, V.;
Demigne, C.; Horcajada, M.N. Hesperetin stimulates differentiation of primary rat osteoblasts involving the BMP signalling pathway. *J Nutr Biochem* 2010, 21, 424–431. doi:
10.1016/j.jnutbio.2009.01.017.
261. Kim, S.Y.; Lee, J.Y.; Park, Y.D.; Kang, K.L.; Lee, J.C.; Heo, J.S. Hesperetin alleviates the
inhibitory effects of high glucose on the osteoblastic differentiation of periodontal ligament stem cells. *PLoS One* 2013, 8, e67504. doi: 10.1371/journal.pone.0067504.
262. Horcajada, M.N.; Habauzit, V.; Trzeciakiewicz, A.; Morand, C.; Gil-Izquierdo, A.; Mardon,
J.; Lebecque, P.; Davicco, M.J.; Chee, W.S.; Coxam, V., et al. Hesperidin inhibits ovari-
ectomized-induced osteopenia and shows differential effects on bone mass and strength
in young and adult intact rats. *J Appl Physiol* (1985) 2008, 104, 648–654. doi: 10.1152/
japplphysiol.00441.2007.

263. Zhang, X.; Zhou, C.; Zha, X.; Xu, Z.; Li, L.; Liu, Y.; Xu, L.; Cui, L.; Xu, D.; Zhu, B. Apigenin promotes osteogenic differentiation of human mesenchymal stem cells through JNK and p38 MAPK pathways. *Mol Cell Biochem* 2015, 407, 41–50. doi: 10.1007/s11010-015-2452-9.

264. Lee, J.H.; Zhou, H.Y.; Cho, S.Y.; Kim, Y.S.; Lee, Y.S.; Jeong, C.S. Anti-inflammatory mechanisms of apigenin: Inhibition of cyclooxygenase-2 expression, adhesion of mono-cytes to human umbilical vein endothelial cells, and expression of cellular adhesion mol-ecules. *Arch Pharm Res* 2007, 30, 1318–1327. doi: 10.1007/bf02980273.

265. Zhang, X.; Wang, G.; Gurley, E.C.; Zhou, H. Flavonoid apigenin inhibits lipopolysaccha-ride-induced inflammatory response through multiple mechanisms in macrophages. *PLoS One* 2014, 9, e107072. doi: 10.1371/journal.pone.0107072.

266. Choi, E.M. Apigenin increases osteoblastic differentiation and inhibits tumor necrosis fac-tor-alpha-induced production of interleukin-6 and nitric oxide in osteoblastic MC3T3-E1 cells. *Pharmazie* 2007, 62, 216–220.

267. Dang, Z.; Löwik, C.W. The balance between concurrent activation of ERs and PPARs determines daidzein-induced osteogenesis and adipogenesis. *J Bone Miner Res* 2004, 19, 853–861. doi: 10.1359/jbmr.040120.

268. Jia, T.L.; Wang, H.Z.; Xie, L.P.; Wang, X.Y.; Zhang, R.Q. Daidzein enhances osteoblast growth that may be mediated by increased bone morphogenetic protein (BMP) production. *Biochem Pharmacol* 2003, 65, 709–715. doi: 10.1016/s0006-2952(02)01585-x.

269. Yu, B.; Tang, D.Z.; Li, S.Y.; Wu, Y.; Chen, M. Daidzein promotes proliferation and differen-tiation in osteoblastic OCT1 cells via activation of the BMP-2/Smads pathway. *Pharmazie* 2017, 72, 35–40. doi: 10.1691/ph.2017.6502.

270. De Wilde, A.; Lieberherr, M.; Colin, C.; Pointillart, A. A low dose of daidzein acts as an ERbeta-selective agonist in trabecular osteoblasts of young female piglets. *J Cell Physiol* 2004, 200, 253–262. doi: 10.1002/jcp.20008.

271. Tyagi, A.M.; Srivastava, K.; Sharan, K.; Yadav, D.; Maurya, R.; Singh, D. Daidzein pre-vents the increase in CD4+CD28null T cells and B lymphopoesis in ovariectomized mice: A key mechanism for anti-osteoclastogenic effect. *PLoS One* 2011, 6, e21216. doi: 10.1371/journal.pone.0021216.

272. Karieb, S.; Fox, S.W. Phytoestrogens directly inhibit TNF-α-induced bone resorption in RAW264.7 cells by suppressing c-fos-induced NFATc1 expression. *J Cell Biochem* 2011, 112, 476–487. doi: 10.1002/jcb.22935.

273. Jin, X.; Sun, J.; Yu, B.; Wang, Y.; Sun, W.J.; Yang, J.; Huang, S.H.; Xie, W.L. Daidzein stimulates osteogenesis facilitating proliferation, differentiation, and antiapoptosis in human osteoblast-like MG-63 cells via estrogen receptor-dependent MEK/ERK and PI3K/Akt activation. *Nutr Res* 2017, 42, 20–30. doi: 10.1016/j.nutres.2017.04.009.

274. Sakai, E.; Shimada-Sugawara, M.; Yamaguchi, Y.; Sakamoto, H.; Fumimoto, R.; Fukuma, Y.; Nishishita, K.; Okamoto, K.; Tsukuba, T. Fisetin inhibits osteoclastogenesis through prevention of RANKL-induced ROS production by Nrf2-mediated up-regulation of phase II antioxidant enzymes. *J Pharmacol Sci* 2013, 121, 288–298. doi: 10.1254/jphs.12243fp.

275. Wang, Y.; Liu, J.; Pang, Q.; Tao, D. Alpinumisoflavone protects against glucocorticoid-induced osteoporosis through suppressing the apoptosis of osteoblastic and osteocytic cells. *Biomed Pharmacother* 2017, 96, 993–999. doi: 10.1016/j.biopha.2017.11.136.

276. Xu, X.K.; Chen, Z.Y.; Li, Z.Q.; Zhang, Y.M.; Liao, L.P.; Zhou, Q.; Zhang, Z.J. Absorption mechanism of neobavaisoflavone in Caco-2 cell monolayer model *Zhongguo Zhong Yao Za Zhi* 2016, 41, 2922–2926. doi: 10.4268/cjcmm20161528.

277. Chen, H.; Fang, C.; Zhi, X.; Song, S.; Gu, Y.; Chen, X.; Cui, J.; Hu, Y.; Weng, W.; Zhou, Q., et al. Neobavaisoflavone inhibits osteoclastogenesis through blocking RANKL signalling-mediated TRAF6 and c-Src recruitment and NF-κB, MAPK and Akt pathways. *J Cell Mol Med* 2020, 24, 9067–9084. doi: 10.1111/jcmm.15543.

278. Zhu, Z.; Wang, X.; Wang, Z.; Zhao, Z.; Zhou, P.; Gao, X. Neobavaisoflavone protects osteoblasts from dexamethasone-induced oxidative stress by upregulating the CRNDE-mediated Nrf2/HO-1 signaling pathway. *Drug Dev Res* 2021, 82, 1044–1054. doi: 10.1002/ddr.21811.

279. Fang, J. Bioavailability of anthocyanins. *Drug Metab Rev* 2014, 46, 508–520. doi: 10.3109/03602532.2014.978080.

280. Zhang, Q.; Liu, J.; Duan, H.; Li, R.; Peng, W.; Wu, C. Activation of Nrf2/HO-1 signaling: An important molecular mechanism of herbal medicine in the treatment of atherosclerosis via the protection of vascular endothelial cells from oxidative stress. *J Adv Res* 2021, 34, 43–63. doi: 10.1016/j.jare.2021.06.023.

Role of Nrf2 in Cardiovascular Diseases and Flavonoid Action

9

Seth Kwabena Amponsah
University of Ghana Medical School

Emmanuel Boadi Amoafo
North Dakota State University

Contents

THE CELLULAR ANTIOXIDANT DEFENSE SYSTEM

The human body is equipped with a defense system that mops up reactive oxygen species (ROS). The body does this mop-up by producing enzymes that include super-oxide dismutase (SOD), catalase (CAT), peroxiredoxin (Prx), and glutathione peroxidase (GSH-Px). In addition, the body defends itself against ROS via non-enzymatic compounds such as tocopherol, beta-carotene, ascorbic acid, and glutathione (GSH) [1]. These compounds mop up and neutralize free radicals, thus mitigating the harmful effects of ROS. Also of mention is the transcription factor nuclear factor erythroid 2–related factor (Nrf2) that regulates the expression of genes involved in protection against oxidative injury. Nrf2 is known to regulate antioxidant systems that are related to GSH and thioredoxin.

Reduced activity of the antioxidant defense system can lead to an increased risk for cardiovascular diseases (CVDs). Reports suggest that low levels of plasma SOD are associated with myocardial infarction (MI) in patients [2]. Singh and colleagues were able to establish that plasma levels of vitamin C and E were inversely related to congestive heart disease [3,4]. Data also suggest that agents that modulate oxidative stress may be promising therapeutic agents against CVDs [5].

TRANSCRIPTION FACTOR NUCLEAR FACTOR ERYTHROID 2–RELATED FACTOR (Nrf2)

Transcription factor nuclear factor erythroid 2–related factor (Nrf2) belongs to the cap "n" collar (CNC) family of transcription factors. Nrf2 binds to the antioxidant response element (ARE) and regulates expression of genes involved in protection against oxidative injury [6]. The activity of Nrf2 is inhibited by Kelch-like ECH-associated protein (Keap) 1 by preventing its binding to the ARE. Nrf2 is unremittingly degraded in Keap1 via a proteasome pathway [7,8]. However, under stressful conditions, such as increased ROS or electrophiles, there is disruption of Keap1-mediated repression. This then leads to the stabilization of Nrf2. Thus, Nrf2 accumulates in the nucleus, where it activates target genes that are responsible for cytoprotection. Nrf2 also regulates antioxidant systems that are related to GSH and thioredoxin [9,10].

Nrf2 AND CARDIOVASCULAR DISEASES

CVDs are a major cause of morbidity and mortality worldwide. In 2016, about 17.6 million deaths were attributed to CVD, representing a 14.5% increase compared to 2006 [11]. Common CVDs include stroke, heart failure, ischemic heart disease, and peripheral arterial disease [12–14].

One of the major players in the pathophysiology of CVDs is oxidative stress. Damage caused by oxidative stress can be at the cellular or tissue level. The human body is equipped with an antioxidant defense system that helps to regulate ROS production. Reports suggest that Nrf2 plays an important role in mitigating oxidative injury; hence, it may be beneficial in CVDs management [15].

Activation of Nrf2, either via endogenous or exogenous (pharmacological) processes, can lead to the regulation of more than 200 cytoprotective genes such SOD, CAT, Prx, and GSH-Px [16].

It has been established that activation of the renin-angiotensin system (RAS) is heavily involved in cardiovascular disorders (hypertension, heart failure, and MI). Activation of RAS and increased production of angiotensin II disturb the delicate balance of redox homeostasis. This has the tendency to cause excess production of nicotinamide adenine dinucleotide phosphate (NADPH) oxidases, as seen in models of hypertension and metabolic syndrome [17]. Nrf2 can counteract the redox imbalance caused by the overproduction of angiotensin II and its associated NADPH oxidases. Hence, Nrf2 is likely to slow down the progression of CVDs. Reports also suggest that pharmacological activators of Nrf2 may be beneficial in the management of many metabolic disorders and drug-induced organ injuries [18].

ROLE OF Nrf2 IN ENDOTHELIAL DYSFUNCTION

There is enough evidence pointing to the fact that endothelial dysfunction is the first step in the pathophysiology of several CVDs. The vascular endothelium produces and releases a number of active biomolecules that regulate the structure and function of blood vessels [19]. When the integrity of the endothelium is compromised, there is a likelihood that CVDs would occur. Reports suggest that low levels of nitric oxide (NO) coupled with excessive production of ROS can lead to cellular damage and endothelial dysfunction [20]. Nrf2 is activated in endothelial cells by shear stress through elevated levels of ROS and the P13K-Akt signaling pathway [20].

FLAVONOIDS

Generally, the body has the propensity to deal with changes in the levels of free radicals. However, sometimes these free radicals may overwhelm the body. This can occur as a result of an ineffective endogenous cellular defense system and risk factors such as smoking, drugs, and radiation. Therefore, dietary or pharmacological antioxidants help to augment the endogenous cellular defense system [21,22]. Over the years, growing research has found that certain phytochemicals found in plants are good antioxidants. These compounds are prevalent in all plant foods, usually at high levels, and include phenols, phenolic acids, flavonoids, lignin, and tannins.

Flavonoids are secondary plant metabolites that are known as the characteristic red, blue, and purple anthocyanin pigments of plant tissues [23]. They are produced in plants from aromatic amino acids such as phenylalanine, tyrosine, and malonate [24].

Flavonoids can be subdivided into different subgroups, namely, flavones, flavonols, flavanones, flavanonols, flavanols (catechins), anthocyanins, and chalcones [25,26]. Structures of the flavonoid subgroups are shown in Figure 9.1. Some flavonoids and their dietary sources are also listed in Table 9.1.

Flavonoids have been widely investigated, and data suggests that they are potent antioxidants. Some reports indicate that the antioxidant strength of flavonoids may be higher than vitamins C and E [32]. Most, if not all, of the subgroups of flavonoids, can act as antioxidants, with flavones and catechins being the most potent in counteracting ROS [31].

Some mechanisms by which flavonoids counteract ROS in the body include direct scavenging of ROS, activating antioxidant enzymes, inhibition of oxidases, alleviating oxidative stress caused by NO, and increasing antioxidant properties of low molecular antioxidants [33–35]. When we consider the role oxidative stress plays in the pathophysiology of most CVDs, the antioxidant prospect of flavonoids may be key in the management or remission of these chronic conditions [36,37]. In fact, there is data that shows that people who consumed large amounts of flavonoids had 18% lower mortality risk of CVDs [38,39]. An algorithm showing the role of flavonoids in reducing CVDs is summarized in Figure 9.2.

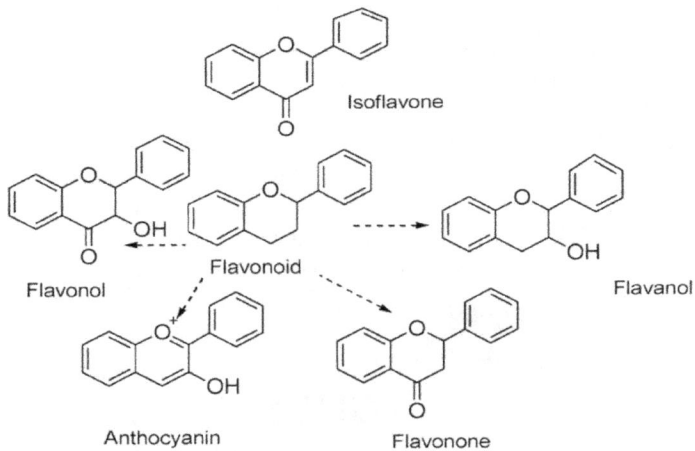

FIGURE 9.1 Basic structure of flavonoid and its subgroups.

TABLE 9.1 Flavonoids and their dietary sources

FLAVONOID	SUBGROUP	DIETARY SOURCES	REFERENCES
Quercetin	Flavonols	Vegetables, fruits, spices	[27]
Genistein	Isoflavone	Tofu, soybean	[28]
Taxifolin	Flavanonol	Vinegar	[29]
Theaflavin	Catechins	Tea leaves, black tea	[30]
Peonidin	Anthocyanidin	Cranberries, blueberries, grapes	[31]

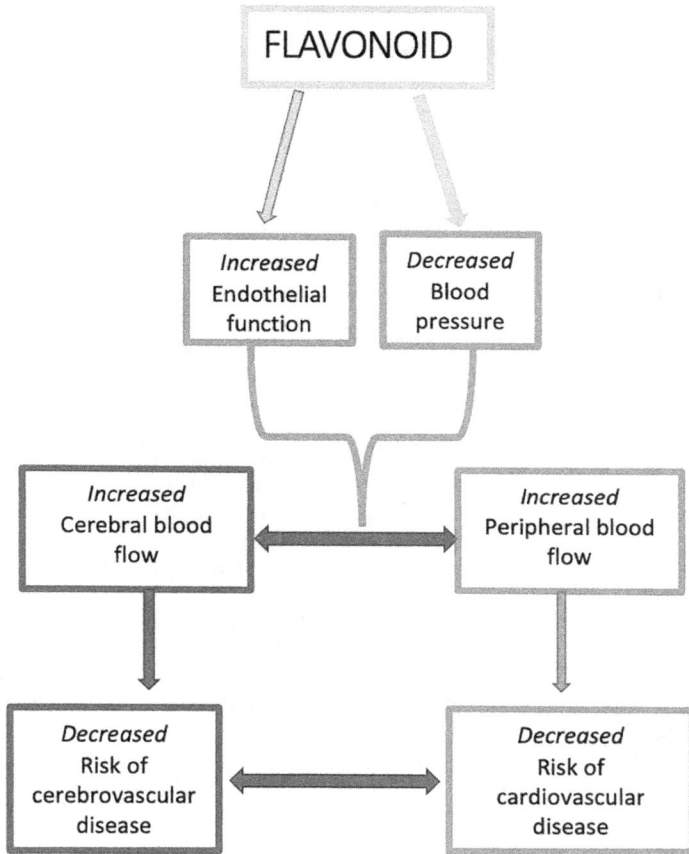

FIGURE 9.2 The role of flavonoids on vascular and cerebrovascular function.

EFFECT OF FLAVONOIDS ON Nrf2

Flavonoids are known to cause upregulation of Nrf2 under both normal physiological and induced conditions [40]. The subgroup flavones are the more potent in upregulating Nrf2 expression during in vitro and pre-clinical studies [41]. Cheng et al. [42] showed that resveratrol modulated inflammation and oxidative damage by stimulating Nrf2. Eriodictyol, a flavonoid found in citrus fruits, was found to induce the nuclear translocation of Nrf2 and increase the levels of intracellular glutathione [43]. Inflammation and oxidative stress are key players in the pathophysiology of CVDs. By targeting the Nrf2 pathway, damage to the cardiovascular system can be prevented or slowed. Agents that target this pathway either endogenously or exogenously may play a vital role in maintaining redox homeostasis in the body. Since flavonoids are potent antioxidants (from plant sources) and are known to induce Nrf2, they can be helpful in controlling oxidative stress and managing CVDs.

REFERENCES

1. Senoner, T. and W. Dichtl, Oxidative stress in cardiovascular diseases: Still a therapeutic target? *Nutrients*, 2019. 11(9): p. 2090.
2. Wang, X., et al., Plasma extracellular superoxide dismutase levels in an Australian population with coronary artery disease. *Arterioscler Thromb Vasc Biol*, 1998. 18(12): pp. 1915–1921.
3. Gey, K., et al., Inverse correlation between plasma vitamin E and mortality from ischemic heart disease in cross-cultural epidemiology. *Am J Clin Nutr*, 1991. 53(1): pp. 326S–334S.
4. Singh, R.B., et al., Dietary intake, plasma levels of antioxidant vitamins, and oxidative stress in relation to coronary artery disease in elderly subjects. *Am J Cardiol*, 1995. 76(17): pp. 1233–1238.
5. Poprac, P., et al., Targeting free radicals in oxidative stress-related human diseases. *Trends Pharmacol Sci*, 2017. 38(7): pp. 592–607.
6. Kaspar, J.W., S.K. Niture, and A.K. Jaiswal, Nrf2:INrf2 (Keap1) signaling in oxidative stress. *Free Radic Biol Med*, 2009. 47(9): pp. 1304–9.
7. Itoh, K., et al., Keap1 represses nuclear activation of antioxidant responsive elements by Nrf2 through binding to the amino-terminal Neh2 domain. *Genes Dev*, 1999. 13(1): pp. 76–86.
8. McMahon, M., et al., Keap1-dependent proteasomal degradation of transcription factor Nrf2 contributes to the negative regulation of antioxidant response element-driven gene expression. *J Biol Chem*, 2003. 278(24): pp. 21592–21600.
9. Itoh, K., et al., An Nrf2/small Maf heterodimer mediates the induction of phase II detoxifying enzyme genes through antioxidant response elements. *Biochem Biophys Res Commun*, 1997. 236(2): pp. 313–322.
10. Itoh, K., K.I. Tong, and M. Yamamoto, Molecular mechanism activating Nrf2–Keap1 pathway in the regulation of adaptive response to electrophiles. *Free Rad Biol Med*, 2004. 36(10): pp. 1208–1213.
11. Naghavi. Global, regional, and national age-sex specific mortality for 264 causes of death, 1980–2016: A systematic analysis for the Global Burden of Disease Study 2016. *The Lancet*. 2017, 390(10100). https://doi.org/10.1016/S0140-6736(17)32152-9.
12. Tattersall, I. and J.H. Schwartz, Hominids and hybrids: The place of Neanderthals in human evolution. *Proc Nat Acad Sci*, 1999. 96(13): pp. 7117–7119.
13. Nitsa, A., et al., Vitamin D in cardiovascular disease. *In Vivo*, 2018. 32(5): pp. 977–981.
14. Sun, S., et al., Differential circular RNA expression analysis for screening the potential biomarkers in atrial fibrillation patients. 2021.
15. Cuadrado, A., et al., Transcription factor NRF2 as a therapeutic target for chronic diseases: A systems medicine approach. *Pharmacol Rev*, 2018. 70(2): pp. 348–383.
16. Pall, M.L. and S. Levine, Nrf2, a master regulator of detoxification and also antioxidant, anti-inflammatory, and other cytoprotective mechanisms, is raised by health-promoting factors. *Sheng Li Xue Bao*, 2015. 67(1): pp. 1–18.
17. Dovinová, I., et al., Effects of PPARγ agonist pioglitazone on redox-sensitive cellular signaling in young spontaneously hypertensive rats. *Paper Res*, 2013. 2013.

18. Lee, C., Collaborative power of Nrf2 and PPARγ activators against metabolic and drug-induced oxidative injury. *Oxid Med Cell Longev*, 2017. 2017.
19. Chen, B., et al., The role of Nrf2 in oxidative stress-induced endothelial injuries. *J Endocrinol*, 2015. 225(3): pp. R83–99.
20. Chen, B., et al., The role of Nrf2 in oxidative stress-induced endothelial injuries. *J Endocrinol*, 2015. 225(3): pp. R83–99.
21. Wayner, D., et al., The relative contributions of vitamin E, urate, ascorbate, and proteins to the total peroxyl radical-trapping antioxidant activity of human blood plasma. *Biochimica Et Biophysica Acta (BBA) – Gen Subjects*, 1987. 924(3): pp. 408–419.
22. Halliwell, B., Free radicals, antioxidants, and human disease: Curiosity, cause, or Consequence? *The Lancet*, 1994. 344(8924): pp. 721–724.
23. Winkel-Shirley, B., Flavonoid biosynthesis. A colorful model for genetics, biochemistry, cell biology, and biotechnology. *Plant Physiology*, 2001. 126(2): pp. 485–493.
24. Cody, V., Plant flavonoids in biology and medicine. *Prog Clin Biol Res*, 1988. 280.
25. Mulvihill, E.E. and M.W. Huff, Antiatherogenic properties of flavonoids: Implications for cardiovascular health. *Can J Cardiol*, 2010. 26(Suppl A): pp. 17a–21a.
26. Ullah, A., et al., Important Flavonoids and Their Role as a Therapeutic Agent. *Molecules (Basel, Switzerland)*, 2020. 25(22): p. 5243.
27. Hertog, M.G., P.C. Hollman, and B. Van de Putte, Content of potentially anticarcinogenic flavonoids of tea infusions, wines, and fruit juices. *J Agric Food Chem*, 1993. 41(8): pp. 1242–1246.
28. Thompson, L.U., et al., Phytoestrogen content of foods consumed in Canada, including isoflavones, lignans, and coumestan. *Nutr Cancer*, 2006. 54(2): pp. 184–201.
29. Cerezo, A.B., et al., Effect of wood on the phenolic profile and sensory properties of wine vinegars during ageing. *J Food Comp Analys*, 2010. 23(2): pp. 175–184.
30. Leung, L.K., et al., Theaflavins in black tea and catechins in green tea are equally effective antioxidants. *J Nutr*, 2001. 131(9): pp. 2248–51.
31. Truong, V.D., et al., Characterization of anthocyanins and anthocyanidins in purple-fleshed sweetpotatoes by HPLC-DAD/ESI-MS/MS. *J Agric Food Chem*, 2010. 58(1): pp. 404–10.
32. Prior, R.L. and G. Cao, Antioxidant phytochemicals in fruits and vegetables: Diet and health implications. *Hortscience*, 2000. 35(4): pp. 588–592.
33. Nijveldt, R.J., et al., Flavonoids: A review of probable mechanisms of action and potential applications. *Am J Clin Nutr*, 2001. 74(4): pp. 418–425.
34. Heim, K.E., A.R. Tagliaferro, and D.J. Bobilya, Flavonoid antioxidants: Chemistry, metabolism and structure-activity relationships. *J Nutr Biochem*, 2002. 13(10): pp. 572–584.
35. Bast, A., Flavonoids as scavengers of nitric oxide radical. *Biochemical And*, 1995.
36. Satta, S., et al., The role of Nrf2 in cardiovascular function and disease. *Oxid Med Cell Longev*, 2017. 2017: p. 9237263.
37. Abd El-Twab, S.M., H.M. Mohamed, and A.M. Mahmoud, Taurine and pioglitazone attenuate diabetes-induced testicular damage by abrogation of oxidative stress and up-regulation of the pituitary-gonadal axis. *Can J Physiol Pharmacol*, 2016. 94(6): pp. 651–61.
38. Faggio, C., et al., Flavonoids and platelet aggregation: A brief review. *Eur J Pharmacol*, 2017. 807: pp. 91–101.
39. Rees, A., G.F. Dodd, and J.P.E. Spencer, The effects of flavonoids on cardiovascular health: A review of human intervention trials and implications for cerebrovascular function. *Nutrients*, 2018. 10(12): p. 1852.
40. Li, L., et al., Luteolin protects against diabetic cardiomyopathy by inhibiting NF-κB-mediated inflammation and activating the Nrf2-mediated antioxidant responses. *Phytomedicine*, 2019. 59: p. 152774.
41. Zhang, H.B., et al., Baicalin reduces early brain injury after subarachnoid hemorrhage in rats. *Chin J Integr Med*, 2020. 26(7): pp. 510–518.

42. Cheng, L., et al., Resveratrol attenuates inflammation and oxidative stress induced by myocardial ischemia-reperfusion injury: Role of Nrf2/ARE pathway. *Int J Clin Exp Med*, 2015. 8(7): pp. 10420–10428.
43. Johnson, J., et al., The flavonoid, eriodictyol, induces long-term protection in ARPE-19 cells through its effects on Nrf2 activation and phase 2 gene expression. *Invest Ophthalmol Vis Sci*, 2009. 50(5): pp. 2398–2406.

Nrf2 and the Aging Liver

10

Aparoop Das and Kalyani Pathak
Dibrugarh University

Manash Pratim Pathak
Assam Downtown University

Urvashee Gogoi and Riya Saikia
Dibrugarh University

Contents

DOI: 10.1201/9781003225225-10

INTRODUCTION

Aging is the gradual accumulation of changes over time that are linked to or cause the ever-increasing predisposition to disease and mortality that comes with getting older. Aging causes a steady loss of homeostasis at the genetic, cellular, tissue, and whole-organism levels, reducing survival and fertility while raising illness and mortality risks. At the molecular level, aging is determined by a multitude of processes known as the "Hallmarks of Aging": epigenetic changes, genomic instability, telomere attrition, loss of proteostasis, dysregulation of nutrient sensing, altered intracellular communication, mitochondrial dysfunction, stem cell exhaustion, cellular senescence, inflammation, and impaired stress adaptation [1,2]. The nature of the aging process has sparked much debate. The accumulation of data presently shows that the aggregate of the harmful free radical reactions occurring continually throughout the cells and tissues constitutes or is a key component of the aging process [3]. Because the liver is a complex metabolic organ that regulates energy metabolism, xenobiotic, endobiotic clearance, and molecular biosynthesis to maintain whole-body homeostasis, age-related alterations in liver function contribute to systemic vulnerability to age-related illnesses [4].

Hallmarks of the Aging Liver: Morphological, Physiological, and Functional

Aging has various effects on different organs, tissues, and cell types in the same organism; the amount of age-related structural and functional changes is site-specific [5]. Impaired proliferative and metabolic activities are linked to liver aging. All kinds of liver cells, including hepatocytes, liver sinusoidal endothelial cells, hepatic stellate cells, and Küpffer cells, are affected by the hallmarks of aging (KCs).

Morphological Changes

The liver undergoes various morphological changes as people age, but the processes behind these changes are unknown. The liver suffers "brown atrophy" with old age on a macroscopic level [6]. Initially, it was discovered that aging was linked to a 20% decline in male liver weight and an 11% loss in female liver weight [7]. According to research by Woodhouse et al. the liver shrinks with age, with a significant decrease in volume after the sixth decade of life, as measured by ultrasonography [8]. According to Wynne et al. [9], in research of 65 volunteers aged 24–91, there was a 35% drop in hepatic blood flow in persons over 65 years compared with those under 40 years in a study of 65 volunteers aged 24–91. Reduced liver volume and hepatic blood flow in the elderly have unknown consequences, although they might significantly influence the pharmacokinetic profiles of medicines that must pass hepatic oxidation. There is evidence that age-related hepatic morphological changes, such as a loss of hepatic volume and a decrease in hepatic perfusion, can impair key liver functions, such as first-pass pharmacokinetics [10]. Hepatocytes show signs of genetic instability as they age [11]. During aging, the human liver develops macrohepatocytes and polyploidy and an increase in nuclei and nucleoli, notably near the terminal hepatic veins [5]. Senescent hepatocytes release cytokines such as interleukin 6 (IL-6), tumor necrosis factor 1 (TNF), and interleukin 8 (IL-8) that contribute to age-related inflammation (referred to as the senescence-associated secretory phenotype) and have reduced mitochondrial enzymes (mitochondrial nitric oxide synthase, manganese superoxide dismutase [SOD], complexes I and IV [12–14]. In hepatocytes, there are several age-related alterations in mitochondria. Reduced mitochondrial biogenesis and autophagic destruction of mitochondria (mitophagy) and dissociation of ATP synthase, and increased ROS buildup contribute to mitochondrial DNA damage and respiratory chain complex dysfunction [15–17]. Autophagy is a eukaryotic cell recycling mechanism that degrades defective intracellular components and recycles the basic chemicals. It is important for maintaining cell homeostasis and coping with environmental stress. With age, the rate of autophagy-mediated proteolysis slows, and insufficient clearance of damaged proteins leads to the development of protein aggregates such as lipofuscins, which are frequent in old hepatocytes [18,19]. In aged rats, the rough endoplasmic reticulum (RER) appears to be diminished, along with decreased glucose-6-phosphatase production and increased A-glutamyltransferase production in periportal hepatocytes. The decrease in RER with age could be due to a change in the hepatocytes' ability to synthesize proteins [5]. A decline in hepatic blood flow of roughly 35%–40% is also unmistakably linked to old age. This has been conclusively demonstrated using various technological methods, such as dye dilution and indicator clearance, indicator distribution, and Doppler ultrasound [10,20,21].

Physiological and Functional Changes

Although aging has been linked to various alterations in hepatic function, clinically critical biochemical markers of liver function in the elderly are typically normal.

Metabolic Activities

The liver plays a critical role in the regulation of carbohydrate, protein, and lipid metabolism. Protein, lipid, and glucose synthesis decreases with age [22,23]. Although aging has been linked to a variety of changes in hepatic physiology, clinically relevant biochemical parameters of liver function in the elderly are generally normal [24].

Protein and Albumin Metabolism

The senescence of liver cells is characterized by a decline in hepatic protein synthesis and the accumulation of some aberrant proteins in aged liver cells [25]. Current findings on age-related variations in protein synthesis in isolated rat hepatocytes have indicated that such effects are strain and sex-dependent [26,27]. Albumin synthesis is a significant component of protein synthesis in the liver. Animal experiments have shown mixed results when it comes to age-related alterations in albumin production. Some have found an age-related reduction in hepatic albumin production and reduced albumin plasma concentrations [28], whereas others have not [29]. Fibrinogen is another critical liver protein with specific roles; research shows that fibrinogen's fractional synthesis rate declines with age [30]. Protein synthesis and transcriptional and translational processes both slow down. Changes in cellular protein breakdown may have significant implications for the cell life cycle and may be a key element of the aging process. In older rats, albumin levels in the serum might drop by 10%–20%. This may be related to lower albumin gene expression [13]. A DNAse I hypersensitive site exists in the gene, but it is noticeably less sensitive in aged rats. Its 5'-CCGG-3' sequences get more methylated with age, and its transcription rate is likewise reduced [24].

Lipid Metabolism
Lipid metabolism is largely controlled by the liver. Depending on the species, it is the center of fatty acid synthesis and lipid circulation via lipoprotein synthesis. Dysregulation of glucose and lipid metabolism is linked to aging. The number of hepatic triglycerides and cholesterol increases with age, whereas the quantity of phospholipids stays the same [31]. Hepatic lipid accumulation can cause serious hepatic and systemic problems, such as steatohepatitis, cirrhosis, impaired systemic glucose metabolism, and metabolic syndrome, all of which contribute to age-related diseases. Insulin, leptin, and adiponectin are key regulators of hepatic lipid metabolism's various physiologic processes [32]. The lipid composition of liver microsomal membranes is also thought to affect the activity of the hepatic microsomal monooxygenase system. Furthermore, the fatty acid content of phospholipids alters membrane fluidity [33].

Carbohydrate Metabolism
Spence recognized the decline in glucose tolerance with age in subjects over 60 in 1920 [34]. Plasma glucose levels are kept stable in the post-prandial state by a synchronized balance in both hepatic glucose production and glucose uptake by peripheral tissues. Increased peripheral glucose uptake and decreased hepatic glucose output (HGO), improved splanchnic glucose utilization, and the rate of ingested glucose entry into the systemic circulation all influence the glucose tolerance curve [35]. Changes in carbohydrate metabolism with age can influence the capacity of the liver to metabolize drugs. The elderly population has had prolonged exposure to a sedentary lifestyle and has easy access to a high-caloric diet. They, therefore, tend to have a higher percentage of body weight as fat and a more detrimental fat distribution. Available evidence suggests that the effect of age on the ability of insulin to suppress HGO is not affected by age per se but rather by differences in body composition [36].

Excretory Functions
Exogenous chemicals such as eosin, bromsulfophthalein (BSP), and indocyanine green, which are taken from the blood and excreted in the bile, are also expelled by the liver. During the first year of life, rats' biliary excretion of eosin was shown to be lower [37]. Rats showed a rise in BSP retention with age, notably within the first 12 months [38]. The greater retention of BSP in the serum of aged rats was attributed to a reduction in the maximum excretion capacity (Tm), whereas the liver's relative storage capacity (S)

for BSP remained unchanged [39]. The conclusion drawn from a comparison of in vivo and in vitro data is that the deterioration in the liver's ability to eliminate foreign compounds is at least partially attributable to an age-related decrease in the retention power of individual hepatocytes for those substances [38].

Drug Metabolism
In general, drugs are digested by the liver in two stages. The processes in which lipophilic drugs are converted via oxidation, hydrolysis, and reduction are referred to as phase I metabolism. Phase II metabolism refers to the processes in which drugs or their phase I metabolites are conjugated with tiny endogenous molecules like glucuronic acid to produce less lipophilic metabolites. Phase I responses have received the greatest attention. The cytochrome P450 system in hepatocytes' smooth endoplasmic reticulum (SER) frequently catalyzes them [40]. It was discovered that there is a negative association between chronological age and in vitro hepatic microsomal drug-metabolizing enzymes using inbred male rats. A drop in SER and total phospholipid content, together with a rise in the cholesterol/phospholipid ratio, is thought to be the cause [5]. Sotaniemi et al. (1997) found a 30% drop in hepatic drug metabolism beyond 70 years of age in 226 human participants, showing a gradual deterioration in drug metabolism with aging [41]. Studies on phase II enzyme activity are few, contradictory, and confined to a few chosen drugs. Some studies show no change in conjugation rates with age, while others show a little reduction [8].

Liver Regeneration
The ability of the liver to recover its bulk after partial hepatectomy is a unique trait. According to reports, aging reduces the liver's regeneration potential, both in terms of the rate and extent to which the organ's original volume is recovered [42]. There is little conclusive evidence that the cellular and molecular systems that regulate liver regeneration are impacted by aging. In aged animals, changes in hepatic responsiveness to growth hormones, such as epidermal growth factor (EGF), appear to impact regeneration. Following EGF stimulation, studies have shown (a) a 60% decrease in EGF binding to hepatocyte plasma membranes, (b) decreased expression of the hepatic high-affinity EGF receptor, and (c) a block between the G1 and S phases of the cell cycle in aged rats [43]. Recent research suggests that decreased phosphorylation and dimerization of the EGF receptor, both of which are required for the activation of the extracellular signal-regulated kinase pathway and consequent cell proliferation, are to blame [44]. In another research, aging has been shown to impact the overexpression of FoxM1B, a Forkhead Box transcription factor that is required for growth hormone-stimulated liver regeneration in hepatectomy mice [45]. Aging appears to impair liver regeneration by interfering with various pathways, resulting in a slower rate of regeneration but not the ability to restore the organ to its previous volume.

Mechanisms of the Free Radical Generation in the Aging Liver

Aging in the liver is accompanied by several alterations in the functional, physiological, and morphological set [46]. Changes in volume, apoptosis, lipofuscin accumulation, impaired hepatic clearance function, decreased SER area, and decreased mitochondrial number and functions are some of the hallmarks of the aging liver [47,48]. As per available studies, oxidative stress is one of the main causes responsible for the above-mentioned pathological conditions. Aging is a natural phenomenon, and the generation of reactive oxygen species (ROS) throughout the lifespan is one of the many reasons for aging. The theory of aging proposed by Harman was widely accepted in the 1950s. However, there has been a shift in the acceptability of the theory, and now the generation of ROS is only regarded as one of the many reasons of aging [49,50]. ROS, a type of molecule that comprises a number of free radicals like superoxide, is mainly generated in the mitochondria [51]. The main reason behind the generation of ROS in mitochondria is the electron transport chain (ETC) that consumes 90% of the oxygen and yields superoxide (O_2^-), hydrogen peroxide (H_2O_2), and hydroxyl radical (OH) [52] under aerobic condition, and oxygen is reduced directly to water by cytochrome oxidase [53]. Any chemical species (atom, ion, or molecule) with an unpaired or odd number of electrons is known as a free radical, and oxygen is by far the most prevalent generator of free radicals in biological systems [54]. As a result of both enzymatic and nonenzymatic reactions, free radicals are generated continuously in cells. The respiratory chain, phagocytosis, prostaglandin synthesis, and the cytochrome P-450 system are all examples of enzymatic processes, and free radicals generated by the interactions of oxygen with organic molecules and those initiated by ionizing processes fall under the nonenzymatic reactions [55]. A free electron is present in both the superoxide and hydroxyl radicals in their outer orbit, and they are oxidants of an extremely reactive nature. Hydrogen peroxide is damaging to cells, especially the cell membrane, and becomes more active, especially when it reacts with reduced transition metals to produce hydroxyl radicals. Although biological metabolism and energy generation require molecular oxygen (O_2), however, the breakdown of oxygen releases highly reactive chemicals that have the ability to harm biological tissues significantly [56]. When an imbalance between ROS synthesis and detoxification or repair leads to an increase in ROS-dependent damage, cells and organisms are said to be under oxidative stress [52]. ROS oxidizes and destroys macromolecules such as proteins, lipids, and nucleic acids. However, there is an endogenous repairing system that repairs the harm produced by the ROS. SOD is the first defensive antioxidant enzyme (AOE) against free radicals, followed by many other protective factors termed antioxidants [57]. An antioxidant is a stable molecule which donates an electron to a free radical, neutralizing it and decreasing the free radical's ability to cause damage to the cells. Because of their ability to scavenge free radicals, these antioxidants can prevent or eliminate cellular damage [58]. AOEs are the body's initial line of defense against oxygen free radicals, working together and in unison to decrease the superoxide radical, the first product of monoelectric oxygen reduction, in water. SOD transforms the superoxide radical to hydrogen peroxide (H_2O_2), catalase (CAT) quenches the produced radical by converting H_2O_2 to water, and glutathione peroxidase (GPx) detoxifies H_2O_2 but mostly scavenges phospholipid and other organic hydroperoxides [59]. Initially, it was speculated that although the livers of older adults have decreased responsiveness to adaptive and reserve capacity, clinical testing shows that an aging liver still functions well [60]. However, later many studies have found that the senescent liver has a variety of traits consistent with oxidative injury, and ROS tissue levels impact liver functioning and are closely linked to the majority of age-related disorders [61]. Cellular senescence, a type of irreversible replicative suspension, is linked to aging, and hepatocytes also undergo senescence during aging. Several mechanisms reported where mechanisms of free radical generation in the aging liver are reported. One such mechanism is the formation of the spontaneous point mutation in genomic DNA. In ETC, about 2% of the total oxygen employed is reduced to monoelectronic produces superoxide anion and hydrogen peroxide, and finally, the formation of a more harmful species of hydroxyl radicals. These harmful species of free radicals have the ability to assault and change genomic DNA, and during old age, the DNA lesion 8-oxo-deoxyguanine is a common kind that accumulates with age. If this adduct in genomic DNA is not fixed, it may cause a point mutation during DNA replication. 8-oxo-deoxyguanines on either strand of DNA can mix and pair with adenosines during DNA replication, resulting in G: C T: A transversion mutations. The same mutational pattern can be caused by misincorporating an 8-oxodeoxyguanine as a substrate nucleotide [61,62]. This spontaneous point mutation owing to the generation of ROS in the aging liver was studied in the big blue transgenic mouse, and it was found that such type of mutation is larger in the liver compared with other tissues like neurons and male germ cells [63]. Apart from the spontaneous point mutation, ROS-backed DNA lesions are one of such mechanisms that occurs due to free radical generation and results in the aging of the liver. Exogenous sources of ROS and environmental agents or pollutants might damage DNA, resulting in DNA lesions. 8-oxo-2'-deoxyguanosine (8-oxo-dG) is the major promutagenic DNA lesion that results from the generation of ROS and leads to the transversion of G: C $\rightarrow$ T: A [64,65]. Increased levels of oxidized proteins and lipid peroxidation, protein misfolding and aggregation, and in vivo elevation of alanine transaminase are all linked to age-related declines in macroautophagy and chaperone-mediated autophagy [66].

Role of Nrf2 in the Regulation of Free Radicals in the Aging Liver

NF-E2-related factor 2 (Nrf2) is a major transcription factor in the liver that controls the production of detoxifying and antioxidant defense genes and is regarded as a "master regulator" of the antioxidant defenses at the cellular level. It stimulates the expression of its target genes by activating the response to oxidative stress and binding to the antioxidant response element [67]. Chemical and radiation-induced oxidative/electrophilic stressors are detected by Nrf2 [68]. Increased ROS activates Nrf2, the transcription of various antioxidant and detoxification enzymes, including several glutathione-S-transferase classes (GST) [69]. Nrf2 is negatively controlled by cytoplasmic Kelch-like ECH-associated protein 1 (Keap1). Through NADPH oxidase, the Keap1-Nrf2 pathway regulates both the generation of mitochondrial and cytosolic ROS [70]. In the absence of oxidative stress, Nrf2 is sequestered by cytoplasmic Keap1 and targeted for proteasomal destruction. However, when oxidative stress occurs, Nrf2 detaches from Keap1 and translocates to the nucleus, where it heterodimers with one of the small Maf (musculoaponeurotic fibrosarcoma oncogene homolog) proteins [71]. As a response to oxidative stress, Nrf2, after being released from the oxidized Keap1, gets translocated to the nucleus and binds to the target genes like HO-1 (haem oxygenase-1), and NQO1 (NAD(P)H: quinone oxidoreductase-1) as well as CAT which is in the promoter region.

After entering the nucleus, dissociated Nrf2 binds to the antioxidative response element (ARE) and increases the production of HO-1. HO-1, the pathway's final and most important component, is an inducible isoform of heme oxygenase that catalyzes heme breakdown to produce biliverdin and bilirubin, ferrous iron, and carbon monoxide, as well as being potent free radical scavengers in the body [72]. Nrf2 is associated with many liver anomalies that include acute hepatotoxicity, non-alcoholic fatty liver disease (NAFLD), hepatitis, liver fibrosis, and primary hepatic malignancies [73]. Many studies reported that Nrf2 is closely associated with the aged liver. Despite the inflammatory milieu present in the livers of older rats, the level of Nrf2 protein levels drops in the liver. It was found that an increase in microRNA suppression of Nrf2 translation with aging may contribute to the decrease of Nrf2 protein production [74]. In both aged humans and animals, there is downregulation of Nrf2, and decreased Nrf2 target gene expression is associated with increased muscle ROS generation, glutathione (GSH) depletion, and oxidative damage to proteins, DNA, and lipids [75,76].

The depletion of the Nrf2 level in the aged liver is reported to be upregulated by the intervention of various antioxidants. In a recent study, chitosan oligosaccharide (COS) administration elevated the expression of Nrf2 and its downstream target genes HO-1, NQO1, and CAT in a significant manner in D-galactose-treated mice [77]. In another study, *Lactobacillus plantarum* AR501, isolated from traditional Chinese fermented food, is reported to elevate the Nrf2-mediated AOE expression in a D-galactose-induced model of aging mice [78]. A study reported that activation of the Nrf2-ARE signaling pathway ameliorates the levels of Nrf2, HO-1, and NQO1 in substantia nigra and ventral tegmental area as well as in the liver with the administration of testosterone propionate [79,80]. From the above discussion, it is pertinent that the activity of Nrf2 declines in the aging liver with the simultaneous increment of ROS generation, due to which functions of a number of organs and tissues in the body subside. Also, it is shown above that the activity of Nrf2 may be alleviated by external supplementation of antioxidants and functional foods.

MECHANISMS OF Nrf2 REGULATION IN AGING LIVER SUFFERING FROM

Nrf2 is normally found in the cytoplasm coupled to its inhibitor protein Keap1 and is destroyed rapidly via the ubiquitin-proteasome pathway [81]. Under oxidative conditions, however, the Keap1-Nrf2 association is disrupted, resulting in Nrf2 stability and accumulation in the nucleus, where it heterodimers with one of the small musculoaponeurotic fibrosarcoma oncogene homolog (small Maf, sMAF) proteins [82]. These Nrf2-sMaf heterodimers detect ARE sequences, resulting in the transcription of ARE-responsive genes such as HO-1, NQO1, GST, GSH-Px, glutamate-cysteine ligase catalytic subunit (GCLC), and extracellular SOD, which are all necessary for oxidative damage repair. Additionally, Nrf2-sMaf complexes contribute significantly to the regulation of anti-inflammatory responses, autophagy, and proteasome activity [83]. Nrf2 inactivation is primarily mediated by Keap1, which facilitates poly-ubiquitination of Nrf2 by the Cullin 3-Ring box protein (Cul3-Rbx) complex and subsequent degradation of Nrf2 by the 26S proteasome [83]. Cys151, Cys273, and Cys288 are the primary cysteine residues in human Keap1 that are implicated in stress sensing. ROS can change Keap1 cysteines via an electrophile process, resulting in the generation of adducts that inhibit Nrf2 ubiquitination and promote its nuclear translocation and transcriptional activation of Nrf2 target genes [84]. Additionally, a serine/threonine-protein kinase glycogen synthase kinase 3 (GSK-3) and the E3 ligase adaptor β-TrCP can regulate Nrf2 activity [85]. β-TrCP acts as a substrate receptor for the S-phase kinase-associated protein 1 (Skp1)-Cul1-Rbx1/Regulator of cullins-1 (Roc1) ubiquitin ligase complex, which ubiquitinates and degrades Nrf2, whereas GSK-3 is a critical protein involved in Nrf2 stabilization and regulation in the absence of Keap1. GSK-3 activity can phosphorylate Nrf2 in the Neh6 domain, boosting Nrf2 recognition by TrCP and thus Nrf2 protein degradation [86].

Finally, a degradation mechanism involving the E3 ubiquitin ligase Hrd1, a component of the unfolded protein response's (UPR) inositol-required protein 1 pathway, can modulate Nrf2 activation.

Non-Alcoholic Fatty Liver Disease

NAFLD is a degenerative condition caused by lipid accumulation in hepatocytes, which is increasing in prevalence worldwide [87]. Around one-third of people with NAFLD develop severe non-alcoholic steatohepatitis (NASH), a condition associated with inflammation and cirrhosis [88]. Recent research indicates that ROS and electrophiles are involved in the etiology of NASH; consequently, inducing Nrf2 appears to be a feasible strategy for preventing and treating NAFLD; investigated the therapeutic potential of Nrf2 activation using osteocalcin and discovered that it could ameliorate NAFLD by reducing oxidative stress and blocking the JNK pathway, a key mechanism involved in the pathogenesis of NAFLD [88,89]. Scutellarin, a flavonoid glycoside with antioxidative stress activity, significantly decreased blood lipid levels and increased antioxidative capacity by activating PPAR and its coactivator-1, Nrf2, HO-1, GST, and NQO1 and suppressing nuclear factor B and Keap1 at the mRNA and protein levels, thereby ameliorating NAFLD [90]. Additionally, apigenin, a PPAR modulator, was shown to ameliorate NAFLD via Nrf2-associated modulation of oxidative stress and hepatocyte lipid metabolism [90]. Additionally, scutellarin, a natural compound derived from breviscapine, was demonstrated to be helpful in preventing NAFLD by boosting the Nrf2-mediated antioxidant system in rats fed a high-fat diet (HFD) and exposed to chronic stress [91]. A major regulator of NASH prevention has been discovered as nuclear erythroid 2-related factor 2.

In comparison, it has been proven that the absence of Nrf2 or its deletion results in the progression of benign steatosis to NASH and leads to disease aggravation [92,93]. Ramadori et al. [95] revealed that overexpression of Nrf2 inhibited the detrimental effect of hepatocyte-specific c-met deletion on the course of NASH and that Nrf2 repaired liver damage in hepatocyte-specific c-met-deficient mice by preserving cellular redox homeostasis balance [94]. Green tea extract and ezetimibe (a Niemann-Pick-C1-Like 1 inhibitor) have been shown to augment Nrf2's protective action against lipid accumulation and the inflammatory response in NASH [95,96]. However, Nrf2-associated therapy strategies for NASH are unlikely to be used in a real-world clinical area in the coming years.

Non-Alcoholic Steatohepatitis

Oxidative stress is the primary cause of hepatocellular injury, and it may aggravate inflammation and fibrosis in persons with NASH [96]. Additionally, increased CYP2E1 activity is a significant source of free radicals in NASH. Hepatocytes with NASH had decreased SOD and catalase activity and enhanced lipid peroxidation [61].

Apoptosis, inflammation, and fibrosis are all caused by lipid peroxidation [97]. Due to lipid peroxidation, nucleotide and protein synthesis are compromised, resulting in apoptosis, inflammation, and liver fibrosis [98]. The UPR in NASH is critical for cellular stress and inflammation. Nrf2 plays a critical function in NASH, and activation of this gene has been shown to protect against the disease [97]. When fed an MCD or an HFD, Nrf2-KO mice develop NASH. Nrf2 activation suppresses the activity of the liver X receptor-alpha (LXR_) and LXR-dependent steatosis in the liver [99]. It has been observed that genetic activation of Nrf2 in Keap1-KD mice inhibits steatohepatitis. However, after 24 weeks on an HFD, Keap1-KD animals developed hepatic steatosis and inflammation [100]. Upregulation of genes such as Gpx2, thioredoxin 1 (Trx1), and NQO1 was detected in hepatocyte-specific Nrf2-overexpressing animals regardless of whether they were fed regular chow or an MCD diet [99,100]. This conclusion is consistent with a prior study demonstrating that hepatic Nrf2 overexpression protects mice from oxidative stress generated by long-term MCD diet exposure [101]. The Nrf2 protein was abundant in the nucleus in NASH patients, while Gpx2, Txn1, and HO-1 expression were increased [99].

A 28-day MCD diet elevated the expression of genes involved in triglyceride export and oxidation, but not oxidative stress or inflammation [102]. MCD-fed mice showed higher liver mass but decreased fat accumulation following a combined liver-specific KO ofc-met and Keap1 (where Nrf2 is overactivated). Green tea extract and ezetimibe have been demonstrated to improve Nrf2's protective effect in NASH patients with lipid buildup and inflammation [99]. Protandim boosted the activities of SOD and catalase in human erythrocytes [100]. TBE-31, a tricyclic acetylenic bis(cyanoenone), decreased insulin resistance, steatosis, fibrosis, and oxidative stress in C57BL/6 mice but not in Nrf2-KO mice [102].

Alcoholic Liver Disease

Over decades, it has been established that alcohol intake is highly connected with the development and progression of liver illnesses [103]. In the liver, ethanol is oxidized by alcohol dehydrogenase in hepatocytes, and microsomal oxidation is facilitated by

CYP2E1 [104]. Alcohol dehydrogenase-mediated ethanol metabolism produces acetaldehyde, which has a number of downstream consequences, including GSH depletion, lipid peroxidation, and the formation of ROS. Additionally, it was discovered that the dysregulation of antioxidant GSH caused ALD development by creating pathological circumstances, whereas the Nrf2-mediated antioxidant response provided protection against alcohol-induced oxidative stress by regulating GSH metabolism [105]. It is believed that oxidative stress–induced Nrf2 overexpression favorably modulates the expression of VLDLR, which leads to ALD. The role of Nrf2-induced antioxidant factors was initially investigated in ethanol-exposed mice using the Nrf2 inducer D3T. D3T therapy dramatically lowered the formation of ethanol-induced ROS and apoptosis, indicating that activating Nrf2 may mitigate ethanol-induced apoptosis and improve disease status [104]. Additionally, Zhou et al. [107] demonstrated that Nrf2-mediated cytoprotective enzymes could ameliorate alcohol-induced liver steatosis in both in vivo and in vitro models [106]. They also administered sulforaphane, an Nrf2 activator that is abundant in brassica vegetables such as broccoli, cabbage, and kale, and discovered that it was beneficial in reversing alcohol-induced liver steatosis. Additionally, current research reveals that activating the Nrf2 pathway protects against alcohol-induced liver fibrosis and hepatotoxicity, whereas Nrf2 deficiency results in enhanced hepatocyte necroptosis triggered by alcohol [107]. By contrast, a recent study demonstrated that ethyl pyruvate, which possesses antibacterial, anti-inflammatory, antiviral, vasodilatory, antioxidant, and anti-apoptotic properties, decreases ALT, AST, hepatic morphological changes, triglycerides, free fatty acids, and proinflammatory factor expression while increasing anti-inflammatory factor and peroxisome proliferator expression. Taken together, the data suggest that Nrf2 activation is required for the formation of ALD and that concurrent Nrf2 downregulation with ROS and VLDLR may potentially be beneficial in reversing ALD. Additional research is needed to investigate the extent to which Nrf2 overexpression and downregulation alleviate when ROS and VLDLR expression levels are decreased in ALD [108].

Viral Hepatitis B and C

Oxidative stress has been implicated with viral hepatitis-associated liver diseases, including HBV and HCV infections [109]. Previously, it was demonstrated that HCV could phosphorylate and activate Nrf2, which was regulated by mitogen-activated protein kinases. Furthermore, the researchers concluded that increasing Nrf2-derived survival in HCV-infected cells could induce carcinogenesis [110]. Another study shows that HCV-infected cells' core proteins regulate Nrf2 and antioxidant response elements by causing the delocalization of small Maf proteins associated with NS proteins NS3, consequently lowering the expression of cytoprotective genes [110]. According to the authors, inhibiting Nrf2 and antioxidant response element-regulated genes may contribute to the pathogenesis of HCV by impairing the induction of reactive oxygen intermediates by cytoprotective genes, resulting in host cell DNA damage, and increasing the viral genome's genetic variability. Additionally, Ivanov et al. (2011) demonstrated that HCV proteins, including the core, E1, E2, NS5A, and NS4B, activate the antioxidant-protective

Nrf2/antioxidant response element pathway in both ROS-dependent and -independent ways. Additionally, an early-stage elevation of the antioxidant-protective system was seen, indicating that Nrf2 is activated to protect against oxidative stress generated by HCV [109]. It has been observed that Nrf2-mediated heme oxygenase-1 (HO-1) inducible factor (lucidone), a phytocompound isolated from Lindera erythrocarpa Makino fruits, and celastrol, a quinone methide triterpene derived from *Tripterygium wilfordii* root extract, inhibit HCV replication [76]. Similarly, a Japanese study revealed that suppressing Nrf2 significantly reduced HCV infection and steatosis in in vitro cell lines [111]. Recent studies have demonstrated the in vitro anti-HCV activity of brusatol, an Nrf2 inhibitor.

Infection with hepatitis B virus, which causes acute or chronic liver inflammation and eventually results in the development of hepatocellular carcinoma (HCC), activates Nrf2 and antioxidative response elements in vivo and in vitro via c-Raf and mitogen-activated protein kinase [112]. Additionally, we were able to induce the overexpression of glucose-6-phosphate dehydrogenase by activating Nrf2 via HBx proteins, reprogramming glucose metabolism, and perhaps contributing to the formation of HCC [111,112].

Thus, Nrf2 is a critical protein that is activated in response to oxidative stress caused by viral hepatitis and a protective factor implicated in viral hepatitis-infected cell survival and hepatocarcinogenesis.

Hepatocellular Carcinoma

HCC is one of the most frequently occurring tumor forms worldwide, accounting for more than 80% of all hepatic malignancies. HCC is more prevalent in people with chronic liver disease caused by HCV than in patients with NASH [113]. Male and female Nrf2-KO mice treated with 2-amino-3-methylimidazo [4,5-f] quinoline developed liver tumors at a similar rate. Additionally, indazolo [3,2-b] quinazolinones cause cell death in HCC cells by impairing Nrf2 signaling [114]. Pomegranate inhibited hepatocarcinogenesis in a rat model via Nrf2 overexpression. In the early stages of carcinogenesis, HCC exhibits molecular changes, including activation of the Nrf2 pathway, which leads to the advancement of preneoplastic lesions down the route of malignant transformation. Additionally, elevated Nrf2 expression has been seen in HCC patient samples. In general, liver cancer frequently develops in a chronic inflammatory state of the liver [115]. Disruption of Nrf2 may contribute to inflammatory progression and, ultimately, to the formation and progression of cancer [113]. Multiple HCC cohorts have been discovered with KEAP1 loss-of-function mutations. NFE2L2 mutations, which encode Nrf2, are more prevalent in HCC than Keap1 mutations; these mutations occur late in HCC, as they were discovered in advanced stages of human liver carcinogenesis [116]. Mallory–Denk bodies (MDBs) and intracellular hyaline bodies (IHBs) are cytoplasmic inclusions found in a subtype of HCC. MDBs are made up of the intermediate filament proteins keratin 8 (K8) and K18, as well as p62 and ubiquitin, whereas IHBs are made up of p62 and/or ubiquitin. Hibs were reported to be strongly linked with worse overall survival in patients with HCC [114,115]. Numerous studies have demonstrated that autophagy inhibits liver carcinogenesis; for example, autophagy has been found to prevent tumor growth in the early stages of HCC by suppressing inflammation, maintaining genomic stability, and regulating p62 accumulation [116]. There has been evidence of a link between defective autophagy and Nrf2 activation in HCC. Persistent Nrf2 activation was related to p62 accumulation, promoting HCC progression, and causing robust GSH synthesis, which confers chemoresistance and improves the proliferative capacity of hepatoma cells [117]. Increased expression of the anti-apoptotic factor Bcl-xL results in decreased expression of the pro-apoptotic factor Bax and caspase 3/7 activity; consequently, Nrf2 promotes cancer cell survival. In HCC cells, mutations in NFE2L2 or KEAP1 activate the Keap1/Nrf2 pathway, boosting Nrf2 nuclear abundance and subsequent activation of its target genes, resulting in tumor cell survival and carcinogenesis promotion. Nrf2 is also thought to be involved in the proliferation, motility, and invasiveness of HCC cells [118].

Through the production of matrix metalloproteinase-9 (MMP-9) and BCL-xL, Nrf2 promotes the proliferation and invasion of HCC. Nrf2 overexpression activates metabolic enzymes such as glucose-6-phosphate dehydrogenase (G6PD) and 6-phosphogluconate dehydrogenase, promoting glutamine and glucose metabolism further and ultimately enhancing purine synthesis and cell proliferation [112,113]. Finally, activation of Nrf2 has been linked to HCC development and metastasis [118]. Numerous investigations have demonstrated that miR-340, miR-144, camptothecin, and valproic acid inhibit Nrf2 signaling, sensitizing HCC cells to anti-cancer therapies [117,118]. Additionally, inhibiting the p62/Keap1/Nrf2 pathway enhanced the suppression of HCC caused by elastin and sorafenib. HCC cells with defective KEAP1 were less responsive to sorafenib therapy in the short and long term than wild-type cells. Inactivation of KEAP1 resulted in resistance to sorafenib, lenvatinib, and regorafenib in HCC cells via upregulation of Nrf2 target genes and reduction of ROS levels [119]. Other substances, including the flavonoids apigenin and luteolin, as well as the powerful Nrf2 inhibitor chrysin, have been demonstrated to block Nrf2 and its target genes, implying that these compounds may be evaluated as possible anti-cancer treatments [120]. As a result, Nrf2 is a promising molecular target for preventing and treating liver cancer.

Acute Liver Failure

The activation of Nrf2 has been found to protect against acute liver damage [121]. Wu et al. [123] investigated serum ALT, LDH, hepatic hemorrhage, and necrosis levels in Nrf2-null and Nrf2-enhanced mice in a cadmium-induced acute liver injury model; they discovered that Nrf2-enhanced mice had lower serum ALT and LDH levels and less morphological changes [122]. Cytoprotective genes, such as sulfiredoxin-1, glutamate-cysteine ligase, and GSH peroxidase-2, were expressed exclusively in Nrf2-enhanced mice, implying that Nrf2 activation protects against oxidative stress and acute liver injury via the regulation of antioxidant defense-associated genes. Following that, the protective effects of Nrf2 were evaluated in LPS and D-GalN-induced liver injury animal models using mangiferin, a compound that can dose-dependently increase Nrf2 gene expression [88]. Mangiferin therapy decreased serum ALT, AST, IL-1, TNF-, and ROS levels, further demonstrating that activating the Nrf2 pathway protects against acute liver injury.

Biochanin A, morin, curcumin, andrographolide, oxymatrine, and madecassoside were also reported to protect mice against acute liver injury caused by LPS and D-GalN via Nrf2 activation [123]. Additionally, the antioxidant pathway of Nrf2 was examined and found to be efficient in mice acute liver injury models caused by carbon tetrachloride and acetaminophen [124]. Numerous investigations have also established the role of Nrf2 in hepatic IRI [125]. Ke et al. [128] demonstrated that the Keap1–Nrf2 complex might protect mice receiving orthotopic liver transplants from oxidative damage via Keap1 signaling. The protective effects were identified by decreasing hepatic inflammatory reactions and hepatocellular necrosis [126]. Research studies recently identified that the cytoprotective CDDO is a potent Nrf2 activator in hepatic IRI. Inducing Nrf2 target gene HO-1 expression results in increased autophagy in hepatocytes, resulting in increased clearance of damaged mitochondria, decreased mtDNA release, and ROS production, resulting in decreased DAMP release-induced inflammatory responses and subsequent secondary hepatocyte injury [127]. Despite mounting evidence, Nrf2-based treatment for acute liver failure has yet to enter clinical trials worldwide.

Ischemia-Reperfusion Damage to the Liver

Hepatic ischemia-reperfusion (IR) injury is often regarded as the primary cause of liver damage and functioning. Nrf2 is a transcription factor that is required for cells to be protected against oxidative damage. As a result, it is hypothesized that activating Nrf2 protects the liver from I/R harm [128]. Compared with wild-type livers, Nrf2-deficient livers demonstrated increased tissue damage, impaired GSTm1, NQO1, and GCLc inductions disrupted redox status, and increased tumor necrosis factor mRNA expression following hepatic I/R.15d-PGJ2 therapy protected wild-type mice's livers against I/R injury by increasing GSTm1, NQO1, and GCLc expression; maintaining redox status; and decreasing tumor necrosis factor induction. These effects were not observed in the livers of Nrf2 (–/–) mice and were not abolished by a peroxisome proliferator-activated receptor antagonist in Nrf2 (+/+) mice, indicating that the protective effect of 15d-PGJ2 is mediated by an Nrf2-dependent antioxidant response [129,130].

CURRENT THERAPEUTIC ADVANCES TARGETING Nrf2 PATHWAYS IN AGING LIVER

A wide number of compounds have been identified that are found to be effective in treating liver diseases. Different drugs, both of the herbal origin and synthetic origin, have been found to prevent liver damage and associated disorders via positive modification of Nrf2 signaling pathways [131].

Drugs from the Natural Source

Resveratrol

Resveratrol (RSV) is a polyphenol obtained from berries, red wine, peanuts, and fresh grapes' skin and exhibits antioxidant properties. Experimental studies on HCC model have indicated that RSV can prevent the induction of iNOS (inducible nitric oxide synthase), lipid peroxidation, and accumulation of carbonylated protein and increase the expression level of Nrf2. Hence, these properties of RSV make the compound attractive for the prevention of oxidative damages produced during the pathogenesis of HCC. In the case of experiments performed in a murine model, RSV has been found to diminish the methylation of Nrf2 induced by HFD. Hence, it diminishes the activity of genes SREBP-1c and FAS associated to hepatic lipogenesis. Even though a demonstration on the safety and efficacy profile of RSV has been presented, its therapeutic use is limited in both clinical and clinical studies because of its poor bioavailability and rapid metabolism [132–134].

Curcumin

Curcumin derived from the rhizomes of *Curcuma longa* is categorized under the polyphenol class of compounds [135]. Experimental studies on curcumin indicated that it could stimulate the expression of Nrf2 in furazolidone and quinocetone-induced liver damage and can also active Nrf2 in case of liver damage accelerated by CCl_4 (carbon tetrachloride) [136,137]. Furthermore, the administration of curcumin in an experimental model induced with alcoholic liver damage was found to be effective in the reduction of lipid deposition through the stimulated expression of Nrf2 and FXR (farnesoid X receptor) [138,139]. Newer discoveries on curcumin have also indicated its ability to elevate the demethylation of DNA and inhibit the activity of enzyme histone deacetylases, thereby repressing the development of HCC [140]. In a clinical trial study, administration of curcumin at the dose of 1,000 mg/day for a time period of 8 weeks was found to be safe and effective in the reduction of fatty liver content. Thus, curcumin was found to be efficacious in treating different liver-associated disorders through the activation of the Nrf2 signaling pathway [141,142].

Quercetin

Quercetin is derived in higher concentrations from apples and onions and is categorized under the flavonoid class of secondary metabolites. Even though it exhibits widespread properties, it also has a vital role to play in liver damage. The antioxidant property of quercetin in liver damage is exerted by increasing the gene expression CAT (catalase) and SOD and upregulating HO-1 (Hemeoxygenase-1). However, quercetin also exhibits the capacity to modulate the expression of Nrf2 and promote its translocation to the nucleus, followed by its binding to ARE to increase the level of GSH and expression GPx. Two different metabolites of quercetin, namely quercetin 3-O-glucuronide (Q3GA) and 30-O-methyl quercetin (30MQ), were found to be active in producing cytoprotective effects against liver damage caused due to the consumption of alcohol [143,144].

Drugs from a Non-Natural Source

Oltipraz, chemically named 4-methyl-5(pyrazinyl-2)-1–2-dithiole-3-thione, is a synthetic compound categorized as dithiolethione that effectively stimulates Nrf2 and promotes the transcription of different antioxidant genes. The drug has the capacity to express the enzyme-like NQO1b (NAD(P)H quinone oxidoreductase 1) related to phase II biotransformation and can also promote the biosynthesis of GSH [145]. Experimental in vivo studies have indicated that Oltipraz can prevent damage to the liver induced by acetaminophen and CCl_4 [146].Ursodeoxycholic acid, another compound, acted as an antioxidant moiety and was effective in several liver disorders like biliary cirrhosis and hepatitis [147]. Also, this compound produces the antioxidant effect by enhancing the expression of the enzyme glutamine-cysteine ligase plays a vital role in the synthesis of GSH, and stimulates the expression of Nrf2 by promoting its translocation at the nuclear level in an experimental model with cholestatic liver damage [148,149]. Currently, the acetylated precursor of both GSH and L-cysteine called N-acetyl cysteine (NAC) is considered to be the prime antidote against the overdose of acetaminophen [150]. Further studies have illustrated the antioxidant capacity of NAC and its potential for the treatment of liver diseases [151]. However, studies have also indicated other alternative antioxidant mechanisms of NAC whereby it can modulate the signaling pathway of Nrf2 and increase the mRNA levels of HO-1 and Nrf2 to prevent injuries related to the hepatic system [152,153].

CONCLUSIONS

Oxidative stress can promote inflammation and fibrosis, which can progress to more severe liver damage, such as cirrhosis or cancer, regardless of the etiology of the disease. As a potential therapeutic target for liver illness, recent studies have focused on the Nrf2 transcription factor as well as epigenetic alterations that enhance Nrf2's ability to function. A number of different antioxidant compounds, including curcumin, quercetin, and pirfenidone, have been shown to exert their effects via altering the Nrf2 pathway; however, few investigations have explained in detail the molecular alterations exerted by these medications, specifically in the liver. When it comes to liver disease, there is currently no effective medication to counteract the damage. It is hoped that studying the antioxidant properties of various compounds will make them good candidates for the treatment of these diseases, especially by focusing beyond their roles as ROS scavengers and specifically on their effects as modulators of Nrf2 signaling and/or as modulators of epigenetic mechanisms. Nrf2 plays a critical role in the mechanism of hepatic I/R injury and would be a new therapeutic target for preventing hepatic I/R injury during liver surgery.

ACKNOWLEDGMENTS

The authors would like to thank Dibrugarh University for providing the necessary infrastructure and technical support in proceeding with this work. The authors are also grateful to the All India Council for Technical Education (AICTE), Department of Biotechnology (DBT), Indian Council of Medical Research (ICMR), University Grants Commission (UGC), New Delhi, Govt. of India, for providing financial support.

CONFLICT OF INTEREST

There are no conflicts of interest among the authors to report with respect to this chapter.

REFERENCES

1. López-Otín C, Blasco MA, Partridge L, Serrano M, Kroemer G. The hallmarks of aging. *Cell* 2013;153(6):1194–1217.
2. Hunt NJ, Kang SW (Sophie), Lockwood GP, Le Couteur DG, Cogger VC. Hallmarks of aging in the liver. *Comput Struct Biotechnol J.* 2019;17:1151–1161.
3. Harman D. The aging process. *Proc Natl Acad Sci.* 1981;78(11):7124–7128.
4. Rui L. Energy metabolism in the liver. *Compr Physiol.* 2014;4(1):177.
5. Schmucker DL. Aging and the liver: An update. *Journals Gerontol Ser A* 1998;53A (5):B315–B321.
6. Wynne HA, James OFW. The ageing liver. *Age Ageing* 1990;19(1):1–3.
7. Wiener E, Rabinovici N. Liver haemodynamics and age. *Proc Soc Exp Biol Med.* 2016;108(3):752–754.
8. Woodhouse KW, James FW. Hepatic drug metabolism and ageing. 1990;46(1):22–35.
9. Wynne HA, Cope LH, Mutch E, Rawlins MD, Woodhouse KW, James OFW. The effect of age upon liver volume and apparent liver blood flow in healthy man. *Hepatology* 1989;9(2):297–301.
10. Wynne HA, Cope LH, Mutch E, Rawlins MD, Woodhouse KW, James OFW. The effect of age upon liver volume and apparent liver blood flow in healthy man. *Hepatology* 1989;9(2):297–301.
11. Basso A, Piantanelli L, Rossolini G, Roth GS. Reduced DNA synthesis in primary cultures of hepatocytes from old mice is restored by thymus grafts. *J Gerontol A Biol Sci Med Sci.* 1998;53(2).
12. Navarro A, Boveris A. Rat brain and liver mitochondria develop oxidative stress and lose enzymatic activities on aging. *Am J Physiol – Regul Integer Comp Physiol.* 2004;287(5) 56–55.

13. Campisi J. Aging, Cellular senescence, and cancer. *Annu Rev Physiol.* 2013;75:685–705.
14. A. Lasry YB-N. Senescence-associated inflammatory responses: Aging and cancer perspectives. *Trends Immunol.* 2015;36(4):217–228.
15. Daum B, Walter A, Horst A, Osiewacz HD, Kühlbrandt W. Age-dependent dissociation of atp synthase dimers and loss of inner-membrane cristae in mitochondria. *Natl Acad Sci.* 2013;110(38):15301–15306.
16. Kim H, Kisseleva T, In DB-C opinion, 2015 U. Aging and liver disease. *Curr Opin Gastroenterol.* 2015;31(3):184.
17. Hagen TM, Yowe DL, Bartholomew JC, Wehr CM, Do KL, Park J-Y, Ames BN. Mitochondrial decay in hepatocytes from old rats: Membrane potential declines, heterogeneity and oxidants increase. *Natl Acad Sci.* 1997;94:3064–3069.
18. Swanlund J, Kregel K, Autophagy TO. Autophagy following heat stress: The role of aging and protein nitration. *Taylor Fr.* 2008;4(7):936–939.
19. X. Xu L, Hueckstaedt JR. Deficiency of insulin-like growth factor 1 attenuates aging-induced changes in hepatic function: Role of autophagy. *J Hepatol.* 2013;59(2):308–317.
20. Woodhouse K, Wynne HA. Age-related changes in hepatic function: Implications for drug therapy. *Drugs Aging* 1992;2(3):243–255.
21. Zoli M, Magalotti D, Bianchi G, Gueli C, Orlandini C, Grimaldi M, Marchesini G. Total and functional hepatic blood flow decrease in parallel with ageing. *Age Ageing.* 1999;28(1):29–33.
22. Bezooijen CFAVA. Influence of age-related changes in rodent liver morphology and physiology on drug metabolism—A review. *Mechanisms of Ageing and Development.* 1984;25(1–2):1–22.
23. Sastre J, Pallardó F V, Plá R, Pellín A, Juan G, O'Connor JE, Estrela JM, Miquel J, Viña J. Aging of the liver: Age-associated mitochondrial damage in intact hepatocytes. *Hepatology.* 1996;24(5):1199–1205.
24. Anantharaju A, Feller A, Chedid A. Aging liver: A review. *Gerontology.* 2002;48(6):343–353.
25. de Castro TG, Manickavasagan H, Muñoz SJ. Liver disease in the elderly. *Handb Liver Dis.* 2018:351–361.
26. Ricca GA, Liu DSH, Coniglio JJ, Richardson A. Rates of protein synthesis by hepatocytes isolated from rats of various ages. *J Cell Physiol.* 1978;97(2):137–146.
27. Bezooijen C Van, Grell T, and DK-M of Ageing, 1977 U. The effect of age on protein synthesis by isolated liver parenchymal cells. *Mech Ageing Dev.* 1977;6:293–304.
28. Durnas C, Loi CM, Cusack BJ. Hepatic drug metabolism and aging. *Clin Pharmacokinet.* 1990;19(5):359–389.
29. Shah GN, Mooradian AD. Age-related shortening of poly(a) tail of albumin mRNA. *Arch Biochem Biophys.* 1995;324(1):105–110.
30. Fu A, Nair KS. Age effect on fibrinogen and albumin synthesis in humans. *Am J Physiol – Endocrinol Metab.* 1998;275:638–6.
31. Schneeman BO, Richter D. Changes in plasma and hepatic lipids, small intestinal histology and pancreatic enzyme activity due to aging and dietary fiber in rats. *J Nutr.* 1993;123(7):1328–1337.
32. Gong Z, Tas E, Yakar S, Muzumdar R. Hepatic lipid metabolism and non-alcoholic fatty liver disease in aging. *Mol Cell Endocrinol.* 2017;455:115–130.
33. van Bezooijen CFA. Influence of age-related changes in rodent liver morphology and physiology on drug metabolism – A review. *Mech Ageing Dev.* 1984;25(1–2):1–22.
34. Spence J. Some observations on sugar tolerance, with special reference to variations found at different ages. *QJM An Int J Med.* 1921;56:314–326.
35. Jackson RA, Hawa MI, Roshania RD, Sim BM, DiSilvio L, Jaspan JB. Influence of aging on hepatic and peripheral glucose metabolism in humans. *Diabetes* 1988;37(1):119–129.

36. Chia CW, Egan JM, Ferrucci L. Age-related changes in glucose metabolism, hyperglycemia, and cardiovascular risk. *Circ Res.* 2018;123(7):886–904.
37. Varga F, Fischer E. Age dependent changes in blood supply of the liver and in the biliary excretion of eosine in rats. *Liver and aging.* 1978:327–342.
38. C.F.A. Van Bezooijen DLK. A comparison of age-related changes in bromsulfophthalein metabolism of the liver and isolated hepatocytes. In: Liver and Aging; North-Holland/Amsterdam: Elsevier/Biomedical Press. 1978;131–141.
39. Kitani K, Zurcher C, van Bezooijen K. The effect of aging on the hepatic metabolism of sulfobromophthalein in BN/Bi female and Wag/Rij male and female rats. *Mechanisms of Ageing and Development.* 1981;17(4):381–393.
40. Durnas C, Loi CM, Cusack BJ. Hepatic drug metabolism and aging. *Clin Pharmacokinet.* 1990;19(5):359–389.
41. Rovaniemi EA, Arranto AJ, Pelkonen O, Pasanen M. Age and cytochrome p450-linked drug metabolism in humans: An analysis of 226 subjects with equal histopathologic conditions. *Clin Pharmacol Ther.* 1997;61(3):331–339.
42. Schmucker DL, Sanchez H. Liver regeneration and aging: A current perspective. *Curr Gerontol Geriatr Res.* 2011;2011.
43. Sawada N. Hepatocytes from old rats retain responsiveness of C-myc expression to EGF in primary culture but do not enter S phase. *Exp Cell Res.* 1989;181(2):584–588.
44. Palmer H, Tuzon C, Chemistry KP-J of B, 1999 U. Age-dependent decline in mitogenic stimulation of hepatocytes: Reduced association between shc and the epidermal growth factor receptor is coupled to decreased. *J Biol Chem.* 1999;274(16):11424–11430.
45. Wang X, Quail E, Hung N-J, Tan Y, Ye H, Costa RH. Increased levels of forkhead box M1B transcription factor in transgenic mouse hepatocytes prevent age-related proliferation defects in regenerating liver. *Natl Acad Sci.* 2001;98(20):11468–11473.
46. Bloomer SA, Han O, Kregel KC, et al. Altered expression of iron regulatory proteins with aging is associated with transient hepatic iron accumulation after environmental heat stress. *Blood Cells Mol Dis.* 2014. 52(1):19–26.
47. Schmucker DL. Age-related changes in liver structure and function: Implications for disease? *Exp Gerontol.* 2005. 40(8–9):650–659.
48. Zhong HH, Hu SJ, Yu Bo, et al. Apoptosis in the aging liver. *Oncotarget.* 2017. 8(60):102640.
49. Harman D. Aging: A theory based on free radical and radiation chemistry. *J Gerontol.* 1957. 2:298–300.
50. Gladyshev VN. The free radical theory of aging is dead. Long live the damage theory! *Antioxid Redox Signal.* 2014. 20(4):727–731.
51. Chance B, Sies H, and Boveris A. Hydroperoxide metabolism in mammalian organs. *Physiol Rev.* 1979. 59(3):527–605.
52. Hekimi S, Lapointe J, Wen Y. Taking a "good" look at free radicals in the aging process. *Trends Cell Biol.* 2011. 21(10):569–576.
53. Ott M, Gogvadze V, Orrenius S, et al. Mitochondria, oxidative stress, and cell death. *Apoptosis.* 2007. 12(5):913–922.
54. Halliwell B, Gutteridge JM. Free Radicals in Biology and Medicine, 2nd ed. Oxford: Oxford University Press. 1989.
55. Lobo V, Patil A, Phatak A, et al. Free radicals, antioxidants, and functional foods: Impact on human health. *Pharmacogn Rev.* 2010. 4(8):118.
56. Wickens AP. Ageing and the free radical theory. *Respir Physiol.* 2001. 128(3):379–391.
57. McCord JM, Fridovich I. Superoxide dismutase: An enzymic function for erythrocuprein (hemocuprein). *J Biol Chem.* 1969. 244(22):6049–6055.
58. Halliwell B. How to characterize an antioxidant: An update. *Biochemical Society Symposium.* 1995. 61:73–101.

59. Hauck SJ, Bartke A. Free radical defenses in the liver and kidney of human growth hormone transgenic mice: Possible mechanisms of early mortality. *J Gerontol A Biol Sci Med Sci.* 2001. 56(4): B153–B162.
60. Schmucker DL. Aging and the liver: An update. *J Gerontol A Biol Sci Med Sci.* 1998. 53(5): B315–B321.
61. Lebel M, de Souza-Pinto NC, Bohr VA. Metabolism, genomics, and DNA repair in the mouse aging liver. *Curr Gerontol Geriatr Res.* 2011.
62. Dizdaroglu M. Characterization of free radical-induced damage to DNA by the combined use of enzymatic hydrolysis and gas chromatography-mass spectrometry. *J Chromatogr A.* 1986. 367:57–366.
63. Cheng KC, Cahill DS, Kasai H, et al. 8-Hydroxyguanine, an abundant form of oxidative DNA damage, causes GT and AC substitutions. *J Biol Chem.* 1992. 267(1):166–172.
64. Hill KA, Halangoda A, Heinmoeller PW, et al. Tissue-specific time courses of spontaneous mutation frequency and deviations in mutation pattern are observed in middle to late adulthood in Big Blue mice. *Environ Mol Mutagen.* 2005. 45(5):442–454.
65. Jüngst C, Cheng B, Gehrke R, et al. Oxidative damage is increased in human liver tissue adjacent to hepatocellular carcinoma. *Hepatology.* 2004;39(6):1663–1672.
66. Mikkelsen L, Bialkowski K, Risom L, et al. Aging and defense against generation of 8-oxo-7, 8-dihydro-2'-deoxyguanosine in DNA. *Free Radic Biol Med.* 2009. 47(5):608–615.
67. Hunt NJ, Kang SWS, Lockwood GP, et al. Hallmarks of aging in the liver. *Comput Struct Biotechnol J.* 2019. 17:1151–1161.
68. Kim KM, and Ki SH, et al. Nrf2: A key regulator of redox signaling in liver diseases. In: Liver Pathophysiology. Academic Press. 2017:355–374.
69. Nature SK, Jaiswal AK. 2.26-antioxidant induction of gene expression. In: McQueen, C.A. (Ed.), Comprehensive Toxicology, 2nd ed. Oxford: Elsevier. 2010:523–528.
70. Frohlich DA, McCabe MT, Arnold RS, et al. The role of Nrf2 in increased reactive oxygen species and DNA damage in prostate tumorigenesis. *Oncogene.* 2008. 27(31):4353–4362.
71. Kovac S, Angelova PR, Holmström KM, Nrf2 regulates ROS production by mitochondria and NADPH oxidase. *Biochim Biophys Acta Gen Subj.* 2015. 1850(4):794–801.
72. Bellezza I, Giambanco I, Minelli A, et al. Nrf2-Keap1 signaling in oxidative and reductive stress. *Biochim Biophys Acta – Mol C.* 2018. 1865(5):721–733.
73. Xu D, Xu M, Jeong S, et al. The role of Nrf2 in liver disease: Novel molecular mechanisms and therapeutic approaches. *Front Pharmacol.* 2019. 9:1428.
74. Smith EJ. Shay KP, Thomas NO, et al. Age-related loss of hepatic Nrf2 protein homeostasis: Potential role for heightened expression of miR-146a. *Free Radic Biol Med.* 2015. 89:1184–1191.
75. Kalt W, Cassidy A, Howard LR, Krikorian R, Stull AJ, Tremblay F, Zamora-Ros R. Recent research on the health benefits of blueberries and their anthocyanins. *Advances in Nutrition.* 2020 Mar 1;11(2):224–36.
76. Suh JH, Shenvi SV, Dixon BM, et al. Decline in transcriptional activity of Nrf2 causes age-related loss of glutathione synthesis, which is reversible with lipoic acid. *PNAS.* 2004. 101(10):3381–3386.
77. Safdar A, deBeer J, Tarnopolsky MA. Dysfunctional Nrf2–Keap1 redox signaling in skeletal muscle of the sedentary old. *Free Radic Biol Med.* 2010. 49(10):487–1493.
78. Wang Y, Xiong Y, Zhang A. Oligosaccharide attenuates aging-related liver dysfunction by activating Nrf2 antioxidant signaling. *Food Sci Nutr.* 2020 8(7):3872–3881.
79. Lin X, Xia Y, Wang G., et al. Lactobacillus plantarum AR501 alleviates the oxidative stress of D-galactose-induced aging mice liver by upregulation of Nrf2-mediated antioxidant enzyme expression. *J Food Sci.* 2018. 83(7):1990–1998.
80. Gao J, Yu Z, Jin S, et al. Protective effect of Anwulignan against D-galactose-induced hepatic injury through activating p38 MAPK–Nrf2–HO-1 pathway in mice. *Clin Interv Aging.* 2018. 13:1859.

81. Zhang G, Cui R, Kang Y, et al. Testosterone propionate activated the Nrf2-ARE pathway in ageing rats and ameliorated the age-related changes in liver. *Sci Rep.* 2019. 9(1):1–9.
82. Bryan HK, Olayanju CE, Parks BK. The Nrf2 cell defense pathway: Keap1-dependent and-independent mechanisms of regulation. *Biochem Pharmacol.* 2013;85:705–717.
83. Jadeda RN, Upadhyay KK, Devkar RV, Khurana S. Naturally occurring Nrf2 activators: Potential in treatment of liver injury. *Oxid Med Cell Longev.* 2016;2016:1–13.
84. Petri S, Körner S, Kiaei M. Nrf2/ARE signaling pathway: Key mediator in oxidative stress and potential therapeutic target in ALS. *Neurol Res Int.* 2012;2012:878030.
85. Hayes JD, Dinkova-Kostova AT. The Nrf2 regulatory network provides an interface between redox and intermediary metabolism. *Trends Biochem Sci.* 2014;39(4):199–218.
86. Saito R, Suzuki T, Hiramoto K, et al. Characterizations of three major cysteine sensors of Keap1 in stress response. *Mol Cell Biol.* 2016;36(2):271–284.
87. Robledinos-Antón N, Fernández-Ginés R, Manda G, Cuadrado A. Activators, and inhibitors of Nrf2: A review of their potential for clinical development. *Oxid Med Cell Longev.* 2019;2019:9372182.
88. Bender D, Hildt E. Effect of hepatitis viruses on the Nrf2/Keap1-signaling pathway and its impact on viral replication and pathogenesis. *Int J Mol Sci.* 2019;20(18):4659.
89. Satapathy SK, Sanyal AJ. Epidemiology and natural history of non-alcoholic fatty liver disease. *Semin Liver Dis.* 2015;35(3):221–235. doi: 10.1055/s-0035-1562943.
90. Tarantino G, Finelli C. Pathogenesis of hepatic steatosis: The link between hypercortisolism and non-alcoholic fatty liver disease. *World J Gastroenterol.* 2013;19(40):6735–6743.
91. Dietrich P, Hellerbrand C. Non-alcoholic fatty liver disease, obesity, and the metabolic syndrome. *Best Pract Res Clin Gastroenterol.* 2014;28(4):637–653.
92. Gupte AA, Lyon CJ, Hsueh WA. Nuclear factor (erythroid-derived 2)-like-2 factor (Nrf2), a key regulator of the antioxidant response to protect against atherosclerosis and non-alcoholic steatohepatitis. *Curr Diabetes Rep.* 2013;13(3):362–371.
93. Zhang X, Ji R, Sun H, et al. Scutellarin ameliorates non-alcoholic fatty liver disease through the PPARgamma/PGC-1alpha-Nrf2 pathway. *Free Radic Res.* 2018;52(2):198–211.
94. Chowdhry S, Nazmy MH, Meakin PJ, et al. Loss of Nrf2 markedly exacerbates non-alcoholic steatohepatitis. *Free Radic Biol Med.* 2010;48(2):357–371.
95. Ramadori P, Drescher H, Erschfeld S, et al. Genetic Nrf2 overactivation inhibits the deleterious effects induced by hepatocyte-specific c-met deletion during the progression of NASH. *Oxid Med Cell Longev.* 2017;2017:3420286.
96. Zhang X, Ji R, Sun H, et al. Scutellarin ameliorates non-alcoholic fatty liver disease through the PPARgamma/PGC-1alpha-Nrf2 pathway. *Free Radic Res.* 2018;52(2):198–211.
97. Shin SM, Yang JH, Ki SH. Role of the Nrf2-ARE pathway in liver diseases. *Oxid Med Cell Longev.* 2013;2013:763257.
98. Slocum SL, Skoko JJ, Wakabayashi N, et al. Keap1/Nrf2 pathway activation leads to a repressed hepatic gluconeogenic and lipogenic program in mice on a high-fat diet. *Arch Biochem Biophys.* 2016;591:57–65.
99. Bazick J, Donithan M, Neuschwander-Tetri BA, et al. Clinical model for NASH and advanced fibrosis in adult patients with diabetes and NAFLD: Guidelines for referral in NAFLD. *Diabetes Care.* 2015;38(7):1347–1355.
100. Abdelmegeed MA, Banerjee A, Yoo SH, Jang S, Gonzalez FJ, Song BJ. Critical role of cytochrome P450 2E1 (CYP2E1) in the development of high fat-induced non-alcoholic steatohepatitis. *J Hepatol.* 2012;57(4):860–866.
101. Bataille AM, Manautou JE. Nrf2: A potential target for new therapeutics in liver disease. *Clin Pharmacol Ther.* 2012;92(3):340–348.
102. Takahashi Y, Kobayashi Y, Kawata K, et al. Does hepatic oxidative stress enhance activation of nuclear factor-E2-related factor in patients with non-alcoholic steatohepatitis? *Antioxid Redox Signal.* 2014;20(3):538–543.

103. Bae SH, Sung SH, Cho EJ, et al. Concerted action of sulfiredoxin and peroxiredoxin I protect against alcohol-induced oxidative injury in mouse liver. *Hepatology.* 2011;53(3):945–953.
104. Shepard BD, Tuma DJ, Tuma PL. Chronic ethanol consumption induces global hepatic protein hyperacetylation. *Alcohol Clin Exp Res.* 2010;34(2):280–291.
105. Rejitha S, Prathibha P, Indira M. Nrf2-mediated antioxidant response by ethanolic extract of Sida cordifolia provides protection against alcohol-induced oxidative stress in liver by upregulation of glutathione metabolism. *Redox Rep.* 2015;20(2):75–80.
106. Harvey CJ, Thimmulappa RK, Singh A, et al. Nrf2-regulated glutathione recycling independent of biosynthesis is critical for cell survival during oxidative stress. *Free Radic Biol Med.* 2009;46(4):443–453.
107. Zhou R, Lin J, Wu D. Sulforaphane induces Nrf2 and protects against CYP2E1-dependent binge alcohol-induced liver steatosis. *Biochim Biophys Acta.* 2014;1840(1):209–218.
108. Lu C, Xu W, Zhang F, Shao J, Zheng S. Nrf2 knockdown disrupts the protective effect of curcumin on alcohol-induced hepatocyte necroptosis. *Mol Pharm.* 2016;13(12):4043–4053. doi: 10.1021/acs.molpharmaceut.6b00562.
109. Ni YH, Huo LJ, Li TT. Antioxidant axis Nrf2-keap1-ARE in inhibition of alcoholic liver fibrosis by IL-22. *World J Gastroenterol.* 2017;23(11):2002–2011.
110. Ivanov AV, Bartosch B, Smirnova OA, Isaguliants MG, Kochetkov SN. HCV and oxidative stress in the liver. *Viruses.* 2013;5(2):439–469.
111. Bataille AM, Manautou JE. Nrf2: A potential target for new therapeutics in liver disease. *Clin Pharmacol Ther.* 2012;92(3):340–348.
112. Tseng CK, Hsu SP, Lin CK, Wu YH, Lee JC, Young KC. Celastrol inhibits hepatitis C virus replication by upregulating heme oxygenase-1 via the JNK MAPK/Nrf2 pathway in human hepatoma cells. *Antiviral Res.* 2017;146:191–200.
113. Satapathy SK, Sanyal AJ. Epidemiology and natural history of non-alcoholic fatty liver disease. *Semin Liver Dis.* 2015;35(3):221–235.
114. Schaedler S, Krause J, Himmelsbach K, et al. Hepatitis B virus induces expression of antioxidant response element-regulated genes by activation of Nrf2. *J Biol Chem.* 2010;285(52):41074–41086.
115. Ascha MS, Hanouneh IA, Lopez R, Tamimi TA, Feldstein AF, Zein NN. The incidence and risk factors of hepatocellular carcinoma in patients with non-alcoholic steatohepatitis. *Hepatology.* 2010;51(6):1972–1978.
116. Cazanave SC, Sanyal AJ. KEAP the balance between life and death. *Mol Cell Oncol.* 2015;2(2): E968065.
117. Zhou J, Zhang X, Tang H, et al. Nuclear factor erythroid 2 (NF-E2)-related factor 2 (Nrf2) in autophagy-induced hepatocellular carcinoma. *Clin Chim Acta.* 2020;506:1–8.
118. Deshmukh P, Unni S, Krishnappa G, Padmanabhan B. The Keap1-Nrf2 pathway, promising therapeutic target to counteract ROS-mediated damage in cancers and neurodegenerative diseases. *Biophys Rev.* 2017;9(1):41–56.
119. Aigelsreiter A, Neumann J, Pichler M, et al. Hepatocellular carcinomas with intracellular hyaline bodies have a poor prognosis. *Liver Int.* 2017;37(4):600–610.
120. Sun X, Ou Z, Chen R, et al. Activation of the p62-Keap1-NRF2 pathway protects against ferroptosis in hepatocellular carcinoma cells. *Hepatology.* 2016;63(1):173–184.
121. Zheng A, Chevalier N, Calderoni M, et al. CRISPR/Cas9 genome-wide screening identifies KEAP1 as a sorafenib, lenvatinib, and regorafenib sensitivity gene in hepatocellular carcinoma. *Oncotarget.* 2019;10(66):7058–7070.
122. Xu D, Xu M, Jeong S, et al. The role of Nrf2 in liver disease: Novel molecular mechanisms and therapeutic approaches. *Front Pharmacol.* 2018;9:1428.
123. Wu KC, Liu JJ, Klaassen CD. Nrf2 activation prevents cadmium induced acute liver injury. *Toxicol Appl Pharmacol.* 2012;263(1):14–20.

124. Pan CW, Pan ZZ, Hu JJ, et al. Mangiferin alleviates lipopolysaccharide and D-galactosamine-induced acute liver injury by activating the Nrf2 pathway and inhibiting NLRP3inflammasome activation. *Eur J Pharmacol.* 2016;770:85–91.

125. Pan CW, Yang SX, Pan ZZ, et al. Andrographolide ameliorates d-galactosamine/lipopoly-saccharide-induced acute liver injury by activating Nrf2 signaling pathway. *Oncotarget.* 2017;8(25):41202–41210.

126. Peng X, Dai C, Liu Q, Li J, Qiu J. Curcumin attenuates on carbon tetrachloride-induced acute liver injury in mice via modulation of the Nrf2/HO-1 and TGF-beta1/Smad3 pathway. *Molecules.* 2018;23(1): E215.

127. Ge M, Yao W, Yuan D, et al. Brg1-mediated Nrf2/HO-1 pathway activation alleviates hepatic ischemia-reperfusion injury. *Cell Death Dis.* 2017;8(6): E2841.

128. Ke B, Shen XD, Zhang Y, et al. KEAP1-NRF2 complex in ischemia-induced hepatocellular damage of mouse liver transplants. *J Hepatol.* 2013;59(6):1200–1207.

129. Xu D, Chen L, Chen X, et al. The triterpenoid CDDO-imidazolide ameliorates mouse liver ischemia-reperfusion injury through activating the Nrf2/HO-1 pathway enhanced autophagy. *Cell Death Dis.* 2017;8(8): E2983.

130. Cichoż-Lach H, Michalak A. Oxidative stress as a crucial factor in liver diseases. *World J Gastroenterol.* 2014;20(25):8082–8091.

131. Ahmed SM, Luo L, Namani A, Wang XJ, Tang X. Nrf2 signaling pathway: Pivotal roles in inflammation. *Biochim Biophys Acta Mol Basis Dis.* 2017;1863(2):585–597.

132. Robledinos-Anton N, Fernandez-Gines R, Manda G, Cuadrado A. Activators, and inhibitors of Nrf2: A review of their potential for clinical development. *Oxid Med Cell Longev.* 2019;14:9–72.

133. Singh AP, Singh R, Verma SS, Rai V, Kaschula CH, Maiti P, Gupta SC. Health benefit of resveratrol: Evidence from clinical studies. *Med Res Rev.* 2019;39(5):1851–1891.

134. Bishayee A, Barnes KF, Bhatia D, Darvesh AS, Carroll RT. Resveratrol suppressed oxidative stress and inflammatory response in diethylnitrosamine-initiated rat hepatocarcinogenesis. *Cancer Prev Res.* 2010;3(6):753–763.

135. Hosseini H, Teimouri M, Shabani M, Koushki M, Babaei Khorzoughi R, Namvarjah F, Izadi P, Meshkani R. Resveratrol alleviates non-alcoholic fatty liver disease through epigenetic modification of the Nrf2 signaling pathway. *Int J Biochem Cell Biol.* 2020;119: 105667.

136. Punithavathi D, Venkatesan N, Babu M. Protective effects of curcumin against amiodarone-induced pulmonary fibrosis in rats. *Br J Pharmacol.* 2003;139(7):1342–1350.

137. Charoensuk L, Pinlaor P, Prakobwong S, Hiraku Y, Laothong U, Ruangjirachuporn W, Yongvanit P, Pinlaor S. Curcumin induces a nuclear factor-erythroid 2-related factor 2-driven response against oxidative and nitrative stress after praziquantel treatment in liver fluke-infected hamsters. *Int J Parasitol.* 2011;41(6):615–626.

138. Dai C, Lei L, Li B, Lin Y, Xiao X, Tang S. Involvement of the activation of Nrf2/HO-1, p38 MAPK signaling pathways and endoplasmic reticulum stress in furazolidone induced cytotoxicity and S phase arrest in human hepatocyte L02 cells: Modulation of curcumin. *Toxicol Mech Methods.* 2017;27(3):165–172.

139. Korean PR, Veerapur VP, Kunwar A, Mishra B, Barik A, Priyadarsini IK, Mazhuvancherry UK. Effect of curcumin and curcumin copper complex (1:1) on radiation-induced changes of antioxidant enzymes levels in the livers of Swiss albino mice. *J Radiat Res.* 2007;48(3):241–245.

140. Lu C, Zhang F, Xu W, Wu X, Lian N, Jin H, Chen Q, Chen L, Shao J, Wu L, Lu Y, Zheng S. Curcumin attenuates ethanol-induced hepatic steatosis through modulating Nrf2/FXR signaling in hepatocytes. *IUBMB Life.* 2015;67(8):645–658.

141. Moreno FS, Heidor R, Pogribny IP. Nutritional epigenetics and the prevention of hepatocellular carcinoma with bioactive food constituents. *Nutr Cancer.* 2016;68(5):719–733.

142. Panahi Y, Kianpour P, Mohtashami R, Jafari R, Simental-Mendía LE, Sahebkar A. Efficacy, and safety of phytosomal curcumin in non-alcoholic fatty liver disease: A randomized controlled trial. *Drug Res.* 2017;67(4):244–251.
143. Farzaei MH, Zobeiri M, Parvizi F, El-Senduny FF, Marmouzi I, Coy-Barrera EC, Naseri R, Nabavi SM, Rahimi R, Abdollahi M. Curcumin in liver diseases: A systematic review of the cellular mechanisms of oxidative stress and clinical perspective. *Nutrients.* 2018;10(7):855.
144. Lee YJ, Beak SY, Choi I, Sung JS. Quercetin and its metabolites protect hepatocytes against ethanol-induced oxidative stress by activation of Nrf2 and AP-1. *Food Sci Biotechnol.* 2018;27(3):809–817.
145. Granado-Serrano AB, Martín MA, Bravo L, Goya L, Ramos S. Quercetin modulates Nrf2 and glutathione-related defenses in Hep G2 cells: Involvement of p38. *Chem Biol Interact.* 2012;195(2):154–164.
146. Kensler TW, Qian GS, Chen JG, Groopman JD. Translational strategies for cancer prevention in liver. *Nat Rev Cancer.* 2003;3(5):321–329.
147. Answer SS, Dolan P, Budding E. Chemoprotective effects of two dithiolthiones and of butyl hydroxy anisole against carbon tetrachloride and acetaminophen toxicity. *Hepatology.* 1983;3(6):932–935.
148. Compact I, Micu L, Iliescu L, Voiculescu M. New therapeutical indications of ursodeoxycholic acid. *Rom J Gastroenterol.* 2005;14(3):259–266. PMID 16200237.
149. Okada K, Shoda J, Taguchi K, Maher JM, Ishizaki K, Inoue Y, Ohtsuki M, Goto N, Takeda K, Utsunomiya H, Oda K, Warabi E, Ishii T, Osaka K, Hyodo I, Yamamoto M. Ursodeoxycholic acid stimulates Nrf2-mediated hepatocellular transport, detoxification, and antioxidative stress systems in mice. *Am J Physiol Gastrointest Liver Physiol.* 2008;295(4): G735–G747.
150. Arisawa S, Ishida K, Kameyama N, Ueyama J, Hattori A, Tatsumi Y, Hayashi H, Yano M, Hayashi K, Kanato Y, et al. Ursodeoxycholic acid induces glutathione synthesis through activation of PI3K/Akt pathway in HepG2 cells. *Biochem Pharmacol.* 2008;77:858–866.
151. Bunchorntavakul C, Reddy KR. Acetaminophen (APAP or N-acetyl-p-aminophenol) and acute liver failure. *Clin Liver Dis.* 2018;22(2):325–346.
152. Galicia-Moreno M, Rodríguez-Rivera A, Reyes-Gordillo K, Segovia J, Shibayama M, Tsutsumi V, Vergara P, Moreno MG, Muriel P. N-acetylcysteine prevents carbon tetrachloride-induced liver cirrhosis: Role of liver transforming growth factor-beta and oxidative stress. *Eur J Gastroenterol Hepatol.* 2009;21(8):908–914.
153. Cai Z, Lou Q, Wang F, Li E, Sun J, Fang H, Xi J, Ju L. N-acetylcysteine protects against liver injury induced by carbon tetrachloride via activation of the Nrf2/HO-1 pathway. *Int J Clin Exp Pathol.* 2015;8(7):8655–8662.

Nrf2 Flavonoid-Based Functional Foods

11

Archita Jha and Yashwant V. Pathak
University of South Florida

Contents

DOI: 10.1201/9781003225225-11

INTRODUCTION

What Are Flavonoids?

Flavonoids are defined as a class of secondary metabolites having a polyphenolic structure. They are natural constituents most commonly found in various plants, specifically fruits and vegetables [1]. More than 9,000 individual flavonoids have been isolated from plants, with numerous more constantly being identified [2]. Their 15-carbon structure consists of two phenyl rings joined to a heterocyclic ring [3]. Currently, six subclasses of flavonoids have been recognized, which are flavonols, isoflavones, flavanones, flavones, anthocyanidins, and flavan-3-ol [3]. Each subclass varies specifically by the structure of the heterocyclic ring. The significance of discovering flavonoids is profound due to their biological importance in almost all forms of life. For plants, flavonoids are responsible for the aroma, as well as their pigment. Additionally, flavonoids offer plants protection from various biotic and abiotic stresses, further displaying the beneficial nature of these products in plant success. For vegetables, flavonoids are essential for growth and defense against plaque. Fruits utilize flavonoids to attract pollinators, which in turn aid in the dispersion of seeds and spores [1]. Humans also benefit from flavonoids due to their applications in disease therapy. Anticancer, anti-inflammatory, and antiviral capabilities are just a few of their many attributes. Thus, further research is being conducted to fully understand and apply the usage of flavonoids to treat human diseases, such as Alzheimer's disease (AD).

The antioxidant activity of flavonoids is especially pertinent to humans due to their ability to neutralize free radicals, which could otherwise increase oxidative stress in the cell and impair numerous cellular structures. Antioxidants operate by donating a hydroxyl group to any free radical in the cell to support the free radical [4]. Antioxidants are natural products found in various plants, specifically vegetables and fruits, whose consumption could protect the human body from diseases such as cancer, AD, and Parkinson's disease [5]. The development of such human diseases can be attributed to reactive oxygen species (ROS), which include peroxynitrite, hydroxyl radicals, and superoxide. Hence, flavonoids exhibiting powerful antioxidant capabilities could provide a simple method of disease therapy [3]. Rather than undergoing tedious operations and consuming drugs with damaging side effects, we could simply resort to natural therapeutic measures and incorporate more fruits and vegetables into our diet.

Role of Nrf2?

Transcription factors are proteins that facilitate the process of transcription, in which DNA is converted into RNA [6]. Nuclear factor E2–related factor 2 (Nrf2) is a specific transcription factor primarily involved in the regulation of antioxidant and detoxification expression. The leucine zipper-structured modular protein is part of the Cap n' collar subfamily and is encoded by the gene NFE2L2. The Nrf2-antioxidant response is activated upon the occurrence of oxidative or electrophilic stress and serves as a cellular defense mechanism against them. Upon activation, genes that control detoxification of the reactive oxidants are expressed and offer a defense mechanism against potential cellular damage. Additionally, by activating Nrf2, our body can produce more antioxidants which reduce inflammation, repair the body after viral infections, and more. The consumption of antioxidant-rich natural foods could be a mechanism for activating the Nrf2 pathway. The consumption of these allows for the release of antioxidants contained in food while also activating antioxidant proteins within our bodies. Examples of antioxidant activators include red wine, legumes, and dark chocolate. Additionally, it has been tested through various studies that exercise could activate Nrf2, which could assist the body in responding to oxidative stress. Drugs have also been developed to carry out the same purpose. However, the drawback of utilizing drugs is their negative side effects which could wind up doing more harm than good. [7]. An inhibitor protein to turn off Nrf2 is Keap1, responsible for the polyubiquitination of Nrf2. Keap1 is utilized to regulate the Nrf2 pathway and prevent protein overexpression [8].

What Are Functional Foods?

There are many ways to define what functional foods are, varying based on how global researchers and health institutions approach them. Overall, it can be considered as foods that are consumed regularly by humans, however, contain physiological benefits, expand beyond the basic nutritional value, and reduce the risk of chronic diseases. Functional foods have been internationally recognized as being crucial to maintaining well-being, and a specific application of this is best seen in Japan, where functional foods are considered their own category. Additionally, the functional food market in Japan produces FOSHU, which are foods with specific health purposes ranging from blood pressure to heart conditions. Functional foods are not limited to being natural and could consist of synthesized or modified food sources. Conventional food sources contain substances that are naturally occurring. An example is β-gulan, which is commonly found in oat bran and consumed for cholesterol purposes. Modified food sources, on the other hand, could have bioactive substances that have been enriched, as seen with margarine which has been modified to contain phytosterol being utilized for serum cholesterol levels. Alternatively, certain food ingredients could be synthesized, such as specialized carbohydrates [9].

To create a functional food, it is recommended that components that could result in negative effects be removed, components that have beneficial effects be included, or replacement of a specific component with one that has displayed positive effects in the human body [10]. Examples of functional foods are green tea, fatty fish, cranberry sauce, spinach, kale, tomatoes, lamb, vegetables, soy, and more. Each contains bioactive components that could induce positive health benefits. As earlier mentioned, green tea is a functional food that consists of the bioactive component catechins. The effect of this is that the risk of certain cancers is reduced. Functional foods can also consist of antioxidants, which could then be utilized to activate the Nrf2 signaling pathway and further provide health benefits [11].

DARK CHOCOLATE

Flavonoid Properties

Theobroma cacao is the plant from which dark chocolate is derived. This flavonoid-rich food source provides health benefits to the consumer, specifically the reduction of cardiovascular diseases (CVDs). The flavonoid subclass to which dark chocolate belongs is flavanols, specifically epicatechin, known to produce a bitter flavor in their food products. The manufacturing of chocolate is broken down into three steps which are as follows: fermentation, roasting, and milling of the collected cacao. During the process of fermentation, the initial concentration of flavanol drops and, thus, lowers the concentration of antioxidants present, which is why regular, highly processed chocolate does not provide as much nutritional value as dark chocolate. Highly processed chocolates do not retain their bitter flavor and consist of lower flavanol content. Dark chocolate is recognized as containing higher percentages of cocoa content, undergoing fewer processes, and retaining more antioxidants, making them potent therapeutic substances against conditions such as CVD [12].

Additionally, it was studied that incorporating milk into chocolate could potentially interfere with the body's ability to absorb the antioxidant content. By doing so, any potential health benefits chocolate provides get significantly reduced. Adding milk forms secondary bonds between the flavonoids and the milk proteins, which decreases how accessible the flavonoids are to target substances. The inability to bond with flavonoids would reduce any antioxidant effect chocolate would have in vivo [13].

The wide range of benefits provided by dark chocolate is further supported by numerous studies being conducted. For example, a study done by Buijsse et al. stated that consuming dark chocolate daily could lower the risk of CVD by 45%–50%, and it reduces systolic blood pressure by 5.1 mm Hg and diastolic blood pressure by 1.8 mm Hg [14]. Overall, these data suggest that dark chocolate flavanol content is beneficial for our longevity and health.

Nrf2 Activation

Cancer

Cancer has been one of the leading causes of death worldwide, with no definitive cure to treating it. Many therapeutic approaches have been implemented. However, the mortality rate due to the disease remains high as large numbers of people develop cancer. Cancer is the process of uncontrolled cellular growth with three primary stages of development, which are initiation, promotion, and progression. It is during the initiation stage that ROS have resulted in DNA damage and abnormal gene expression and produced negative effects on the signaling pathways involved. By deregulating the signaling pathways, enhanced cell proliferation occurs, which is the driving factor for cancer progression. For this reason, the inhibition of ROS could reduce cell proliferation and be effective in slowing down cancer development, making it easier to treat therapeutically.

The antioxidants of flavonoids have the potential to neutralize the reactive oxidative species, thus inhibiting or slowing down the initiation of cancer and downregulating cell proliferation. Cocoa specifically has displayed antioxidant activity that could be anticarcinogenic and be utilized as natural therapeutic measures against cancer. One mechanism cocoa has neutralized the effects of oxidative stress is through its targeting Nrf2, which as mentioned earlier, is a transcription factor [15]. The regulation of the antioxidant response element (ARE), which are enhancer sequences found in genes producing detoxification enzymes. Upon oxidative stress, Nrf2 disassociates from Keap1 (Kelch-like ECH-associated protein 1) and translocates into the nucleus, where it then subsequently forms a heterodimer with Maf family transcriptional factors to bind to ARE and active antioxidant genes transcription [16]. Cocoa could enhance nuclear Nrf2 levels and further aid in the production of antioxidants to combat oxidative stress. In a 2016 study, it was observed through in vivo studies that a daily intake of chocolate or cocoa could provide a natural, easily accessible, and relatively cheap way to prevent colorectal cancer, which has been the leading cause of cancer-related mortality [15].

Neuroprotection

The flavan-2-ol compounds that have been found in cocoa beans are epicatechin and catechin, which can aid in composing the polymeric procyanidins type B-2. During the fermenting and processing stages of chocolate production, the concentration of these antioxidants varies. Consuming flavanol-rich chocolate, specifically dark chocolate, results in a large concentration of epicatechin observed in the plasma due to its high absorbance. Upon entering the brain, flavonoids bear the effects of protecting neurons, enhancing neuronal functions, and stimulating regeneration. In neurodegenerative diseases, neuronal loss is experienced due to neuroinflammation, endogenous antioxidants, and glutamatergic excitotoxicity. Diseases such as AD emerge due to neuroinflammation. Various studies done on rats have established that flavanol epicatechin has been effective in protecting neurons from oxidative damage and blocking oxidative-induced neuronal damage. In a study involving transgenic mice, the removal of Nrf2 was associated with abolishing any neuroprotection previously provided.

The transcription factor Nrf2 plays the role of inducing the transcription of genes that are responsible for producing antioxidant enzymes and, thus, neutralizing oxidative damage occurring in the brain [17]. This specifically occurs by Nrf2 targeting enzymes such as heme oxygenase (HO1) which regulate redux states within the cells. Nrf2 controls the HO1 enzyme and protects the cell by degrading heme (which is a pro-oxidant substrate) and producing antioxidants. Cerebral ischemic stroke is a particular neurodegenerative disease that is positively affected by Nrf2. This is done by epicatechin, found in dark chocolates, which can upregulate Nrf2 and HO1 and protect the brain. A 2018 study found that regarding transient middle cerebral artery occlusion, a brain disease, epicatechin offered protection to mice treated with 30 mg/kg of it. No mortality was observed posttreatment, as opposed to the control. Overall, it can be observed that epicatechin provided by consuming dark chocolate can activate the activity of Nrf2 and HO1, which ultimately produce the antioxidants, biliverdin, and bilirubin, capable of providing neuroprotection. Additionally, neural oxidative stress could be reduced by the degradation of heme [18].

GREEN TEA

Flavonoid Properties

Tea is extracted from the plant *Camellia sinensis*, which can be consumed in various forms internationally. Green tea is observed to be the most beneficial form of tea that is processed. The production of green tea occurs by harvesting tea leaves and steaming them to produce a dry form. The antioxidative, antibacterial, and anti-inflammatory properties present in green tea are increasingly being studied and encouraged as potential natural remedies for various diseases such as CVDs. The polyphenol content encompasses approximately 30% of the dry weight of the tea leaves. The polyphenols present in green tea are phenolic acids, flavonols, flavonoids, and flavandiols. The most abundant one is flavanols, specifically catechins, which are more commonly found in green tea as opposed to other forms of tea. The specific catechins found in green tea are epigallocatechin, epigallocatechin gallate (EGCG), epicatechin, and epicatechin-3-gallate. The catechin content in green tea decreases as the tea leaves are processed and prepared for consumption. For this reason, the ingested amount of catechins varies.

With minimal fermentation occurring in the process of green tea production, the levels of catechins are high and, thus, the most beneficial for human health. However, as you progressively ferment green tea, it becomes Oolong and ultimately black tea, which has less of an ability to preserve the polyphenol compounds and provides fewer advantages [19].

The catechins in green tea are able to increase the antioxidant activity present in vivo and provide cellular protection against ROS. This was primarily observed by studying the malondialdehyde levels, which are indicative of oxidative stress occurring in the cell. Additionally, further studies revealed that hepatotoxicity could be prevented due to the antiproliferative activity green tea displays on hepatoma cells. Green tea also displays effectiveness in neuroprotection by slowing down the progression of neurodegenerative diseases such as AD. The contribution of the Nrf2 system in our bodies upon consuming green tea is favorably seen in terms of anti-inflammatory and anticancer activity [19].

Nrf2 Activation

Liver Disease

The most common form of liver disorder in the United States is nonalcoholic fatty liver disease. Within this, numerous liver-associated diseases are included, such as nonalcoholic steatohepatitis (NASH), fibrosis, and hepatocellular carcinoma. The disorder is characterized as occurring in individuals who do not consume alcohol but still develop liver disease. Factors such as obesity and diabetes could contribute to the progression by accumulating hepatic lipids. This steatotic liver can then be affected by oxidative stress and inflammation to further aggravate the disease. For this reason, Nrf2 is increasingly drawing attention as a potential therapeutic approach to diseases such as NASH. Nrf2 can limit the oxidative stress that results in the development of liver diseases and reduce inflammation. Studying the effects of Nrf2 against NASH has presented insightful information regarding the hepatoprotective potential of the pathway. In the study, mice with no Nrf2 were fed a diet to aggravate NASH, inflammation, and biomarkers of liver peroxidation [20].

The risk of developing inflammation or liver injury decreases with a higher intake of green tea. The concentration of major catechin epigallocatechin gallate is high in green tea extract, thus resulting in the hypothesis that it would be effective as an antioxidant and anti-inflammatory measure. Specifically, the Nrf2-dependant pathways could detoxify ROS and provide the body protection against the development of conditions such as NASH. The results of the study indicated that mice lacking Nrf2 and fed a high-fat diet did develop NASH, observed by the increase in NF-κB-dependent proinflammatory response and greater hepatic lipid peroxidation. It was also found that by consuming green tea, there were fewer biomarker levels of inflammation and liver injury. By the presence of catechin epigallocatechin gallate, there is increased expression of Nrf2 resulting in the activation of the downstream target gene known as NADPH: quinone oxidoreductase 1 (Nqo1) whose antioxidant properties lower oxidative stress [19].

This further displays how the activation of the Nrf2 pathway by consuming green tea can reduce oxidative stress in the body as well as inflammation within the body, collectively contributing to hepatoprotection.

Cardiovascular Diseases

In CVDs, the Nrf2 pathway can prevent smoldering inflammation, which is essentially inflammation as a result of ROS. As mentioned, green tea consists of a high concentration of catechin flavanol and epigallocatechin gallate, which then activates the Nrf2 pathway and provide therapeutic potential for CVDs. Upon expression, Nrf2 binds to AREs, which are sequences in the DNA with the ability to respond to the dietary antioxidants consumed. This signaling pathway then can activate many antioxidants, such as NQO1 and GST, to combat the harmful effects of ROS within the body [21].

RED RASPBERRIES

Flavonoid Properties

Raspberries are members of the Rubus genera, which also consist of dewberries and blackberries. The dietary intake of raspberries provides many therapeutic benefits due to their nutritional value. The composition of raspberries includes but is not limited to vitamins A, B, C, and B1, folic acids, and ellagitannins. Consuming red raspberries, there can be noticeable effects on cancer, diabetes, obesity, infections, CVDs, and more [22]. Raspberries display antioxidant potential as well, primarily due to the phytochemicals in them. Other valuable aspects of phytochemicals are their contribution to providing pigmentation, IV radiation protection, antimicrobial, and antifungal defense. The function of antioxidants specifically could be to prevent further damage to cellular DNA and proteins that occur by ROS. The antioxidant activity is induced by the presence of flavonoids, predominantly anthocyanin. Forms of anthocyanin isolated from raspberries are cyanidin-3-glucoside, cyanidin-3-glucoside, cyanidin-3-rutinoside, cyanidin-3-sambubioside, and quercetin-3-glucoside [23]. Another predominant polyphenol present in raspberries is ellagitannin. By increasing our intake of raspberries, we would significantly enhance our consumption of ellagitannin, which can be utilized not only for antioxidants but for anticancer and anti-inflammation as well. The phenolic composition in red raspberries consists of 50% ellagitannins, 25% anthocyanins, and 20% vitamins [22]. In raspberries, the total content of anthocyanin is 92.1 mg/100 g, the majority of which is cyanidin glycosides. The common glycoside moieties included in red raspberries are rutinoside, glucoside, sophoroside, as well as glucorutinoside. The correlation between anthocyanins and antioxidant activity was strong, with a correlation coefficient of 0.85. This further reinforces that a positive relationship is present between anthocyanins concentration and level of antioxidant activity.

Nrf2 Activation

Anti-Aging

Caenorhabditis elegans are small nematodes whose lengths are approximately 1 mm [24]. These species are effective in their roles as model organisms due to their simplicity in being cultures, ability to undergo rapid reproduction and a short generation time, known genetic pathways, and low cost. For this reason, they have been used as effective ways to study aging. Aging is essentially the process in which an organism experiences a functional decline. Studies are currently being conducted to establish anti-aging methods. The main objective is to uncover the natural ways of slowing down again and to delay the occurrence of diseases that would normally be prevalent as we get older.

One significant factor contributing to aging is oxidative stress. To potentially combat this, fruits were considered to be effective natural products due to their presence of phytochemicals. Raspberries contain a high concentration of phytochemicals, specifically flavonoids, which could be utilized to reduce reactive oxidative stress and prevent the onset of chronic diseases. As potent model organisms, *C. elegans* regulated by the Skinhead-1 transcription factor (SKN-1) or the vertebrate homolog of it, Nrf2, could be utilized to test how specifically raspberries could be used in anti-aging processes. It was observed that upon oxidative stress, the SKN-1/Nrf2 proteins are activated via phosphorylation and found in the nucleus. The effect of activating SKN-1/Nrf2 is that the downstream target genes such as GST (glutathione S-transferase)-4 and GST-7 are switched on. The expression levels of these downstream targets were 3.37 ± 0.22 and 4.62 ± 0.27, respectively, which are significantly greater than the expression levels of *C. elegans* containing SKN-1/Nrf2 mutants. By consuming raspberries, the migration of SKN-1/Nrf2 to the nucleus occurs, which further facilitates the activation of the downstream target genes, which could relieve oxidative stress in *C. elegans*. This migration from the cytosol to the nucleus can be seen with the reduction in cytosolic SKN-1/Nrf2 concentration from 72.5% to 14.2% in the test subjects. Additionally, downregulation of ROS occurred by consuming raspberries and expressing antioxidant genes such as SKN-1/Nrf2. Overall, it was found that by consuming raspberries, the overall lifespan of *C. elegans* could increase between 13% and 29% depending on the concentration of fruit consumed [25]. The hope is that this can be translated into humans as well and have a similar influence in slowing down our rate of aging.

Cardiovascular Diseases

As established, the consumption of fruits and vegetables has displayed significant potential in reducing the likelihood of various diseases ranging from neurodegenerative (such as AD) to CVDs. Red raspberries have specifically displayed promise for therapeutic purposes due to their high concentration of nutrients and dietary fiber (approximately 6.5 g/100 g). Anthocyanins, the flavonoid compounds of red raspberries, are a contributor of 25% of their antioxidant activity, and the levels found in the fruit itself vary on when it is collected and the season.

CVDs are a high contributor to global annual deaths. While there are many contributors, inflammation and oxidative stress have been key factors in the occurrence of CVD. This is due to the endothelium in the tissues being highly vulnerable to any oxidative stress that occurs from ROS. An example of oxidants that are produced from ROS is hydroxyl radicals, which can then harm cellular components of the human body. A specific instance of the negative effects of ROS is when the radian oxidants produce modified products resulting in the oxidation of LDLs. This stimulated the formation of plaques and redox-sensitive pathways to upregulate proinflammatory gene expression and increase the risk of CVD. The anthocyanins found in raspberries mitigate the effects of this oxidative stress by enhancing the concentration of electrophilic compounds introduced to the body to alter the redox status of the cell and express endogenous antioxidant defense systems. The Nrf2 transcription factor functions by inducing the synthesis of glutathione and stimulating the transcription of ARE, which is effectively utilized as a method of antioxidant defense. Ultimately, by enhancing the antioxidant activity in the cell, any occurrences of inflammation that may occur due to ROS could be mitigated. Learning how to regulate this Nrf2 pathway can provide groundbreaking therapeutic relief to a disease that is largely widespread throughout the globe [26].

CABBAGE

Flavonoid Properties

Cabbage is a cruciferous vegetable belonging to the species *Brassica oleracea*. This species is comprised of numerous plant species such as broccoli, cauliflower, and brussels sprouts, suggesting that their properties are closely related. Various forms of cabbage, such as red cabbage or Chinese cabbage, have been cultivated throughout the world, as cabbage is one of the most important vegetables to be consumed. The primary health benefits provided are plentiful amounts of mineral elements such as iron, selenium, manganese, and zinc. Additionally, there is up to 3.3% of protein. The lack of fat in cabbage is one of the reasons why they are a good source of food to maintain cardio health. Nutritional value, primarily vitamin C, obtained from the daily consumption of this vegetable, offers growth and maintenance of body functions. Flavonoids contribute significantly to many of their key characteristics and benefits. For example, the active color compounds present in cabbage can be attributed to the presence of flavonoids. The formation of these flavonoids within these plants is dependent on light. Thus, they are found in the outer plant tissues [27].

Across many cruciferous vegetables, there are three essential flavanols: kaempferol, quercetin, and myricetin. Two flavones, specifically apigenin and luteolin, are commonly found as well. The concentration of each varies among the types of cabbage. In red cabbage, only quercetin is present, while in green cabbage, there is quercetin and kaempferol. Anthocyanin content is high as well, with up to 322 mg/100g in red cabbage [28]. A major discovery that further provides value to cabbages is that through the process of fermentation kaempferol value remains content. This is important because it suggests that no matter how fermented and processed the cabbage is, it can still provide the numerous benefits flavanols offer [27]. Overall, cabbage has displayed therapeutic potential against cancer, CVD, and diabetes.

Nrf2 Activation

Diabetes

Type 2 diabetes mellitus (T2DM) has developed into a global public health concern due to its increasing prevalence. In 2019, it was estimated that more than 463.8 million adults between the ages of 20 and 79 were affected by T2DM. The prediction is that by 2045, that number could increase to 700 million if left untreated [29]. T2DM is characterized by increased glucose levels due to the impaired secretion of insulin or insulin resistance. Oxidative stress results in the overproduction of ROS, which contributes to this inability to produce insulin. which could occur due to oxidative stress stimulated by ROS overproduction. It is more common than type 1 diabetes mellitus, and it is estimated that the rapid development of the disease worldwide is occurring due to physical inactivity, cigarette smoking, duration of sleep, and genetics [30]. Functional foods are increasingly becoming affordable and natural methods of controlling the rapid growth in T2DM cases. White, green, and red cabbage consumption can impact glucose homeostatic regulation and decrease damage done to the body by T2DM complications. The flavonoid sources in cabbage, such as quercetin, epicatechin, and epigallocatechin gallate, have antidiabetic effects, specifically in carbohydrate digestion regulation [29].

The activation of the Nrf2 pathway is a process involving ARE expression, upregulation of antioxidant enzymes, and subsequently, the decrease in ROS-induced oxidative stress. Additionally, transcriptional repression of G6P enzymes could reduce gluconeogenesis and hepatic glucose production. Quercetin induces the nuclear translocation of Nrf2, which increases the expression of ARE-dependent genes. This mechanism is effective in improving glucose metabolism by activating antioxidant endogen expression and reducing ROS expression. Another flavonoid, kaempferol, increased Nrf2 phosphorylation which triggered the antioxidant gene expression of HO-1 and NQO-1 in HpG2 cells. Rutin, however, results in G6P inhibition and provides erythrocytes defense mechanisms against any t-butyl hydroperoxide-induced oxidative stress by expression of antioxidant enzymes such as GST, GR, SOD, and CAT [29]. Overall, flavonoids in red cabbage are applicable to treating and preventing T2DM, and the extent to which cabbage could be utilized for other diseases is constantly being studied.

BLUEBERRY

Flavonoid Properties

Blueberries are commonly consumed fruits providing numerous health to the consumer. They belong to the genus *Vaccinium*, under which cranberries, huckleberries, and bilberries are as well. The commercially significant blueberries worldwide are low-bush (wild), highbush, rabbiteye blueberry, and European bilberry. In the United States, lowbush (wild) and highbush (cultivated) are the most common types of blueberries containing varying amounts of antioxidants and contributing differently to our bodies [31]. Blueberries are strongly recommended for consumption due to their high amounts of dietary fiber, 3%–3.5%. Additionally, the presence of manganese, iron, selenium, b-carotene, zeaxanthin, and lutein are other benefits of blueberry intake. Blueberries are vitamin-rich as well, with the most prevalent ones being vitamin A, B complex, C, and E [32].

The flavonoid content in this fruit is the majority of anthocyanins. Anthocyanins were observed to provide pigmentation in the blueberries as they ripen to specifically red, purple, or blue colors. The amount of anthocyanin increases during the ripening process to provide the distinction that the fruit has passed its early stages and is now ripe. Up to 60% of the polyphenolics in the now-ripened blueberries are anthocyanin flavonoids. Apart from anthocyanin, there are proanthocyanins and flavanols [31]. The abundant flavonoid amount found within blueberries contributes to many aspects of their ability to relieve many diseases. The antioxidant activity can suppress free radicals, slow cognitive decline, preserve the blood flow through LDL oxidation, and prolong epithelium function. A study analyzing the differences in phenolic content among blackberry, blueberry, and strawberry displayed that the total flavonoid content was 11.83, 36.08, and 7.04 mg rutin/g DW, respectively, further indicating that the consumption of blueberries specifically can display the most prominent effect in the therapeutic realm [4].

Nrf2 Activation

Anti-Inflammation

The accumulation of ROS can result in oxidative stress and inflammatory responses, which in turn could bring about their own subset of health-related problems. Obesity is one such effect of the building, which can then result in chronic diseases such as type 2 diabetes, cancer, and CVDs. The ROS accumulation can result in the activation of a transcription factor NF-κB that is responsible for the expression of this proinflammatory cytokine. Nrf2 is established to be an effective antioxidant defense mechanism to express genes such as glutamyl cysteine ligase catalytic subunit. The flavonoid anthocyanins have been observed to display anti-inflammatory properties that are attributed to the antioxidant capacity they contain.

Blueberries contain abundant amounts of anthocyanins, which led to the theory that they have the potential to combat inflammation. The major anthocyanins found in blueberries are malvidin-3-glucoside. A cell undergoing oxidative stress would release Nrf2 from the cytoplasm to the nucleus to enable the transcription of genes that can combat the stress [33]. By inhibiting the expression of genes such as IL-1ß AND TNFα, the suppression of proinflammatory factors could occur. The Nrf2 pathway in blueberries displayed increased effectiveness in lowering oxidative stress as well as the IL-1ß mRNA levels. This was done by inhibiting the nuclear translocation of NF-κB within macrophages, thus inhibiting the expression of proinflammatory genes. While the anti-inflammatory effect of anthocyanin in blueberries was not as high as its antioxidant potential, it is an important area of research due to the profound impact that can be made in the prevention of chronic diseases just by natural means of eating blueberries [33].

Diabetes Retinopathy

The elevation of blood glucose levels can lead to the development of diabetic retinopathy. The long-term spike in glucose levels can weaken the retinal small blood vessels causing neovascular glaucoma, diabetic macular edema, and retinal detachment. If untreated, diabetic retinopathy can ultimately result in blindness. Understanding the contributing factors to the disease can help in developing effective treatment methods to combat it. It was studied that chronic inflammation and oxidative stress were furthering the progression of the disease. This is furthered by the observation that increased levels of anti-inflammatory cytokines were present in diabetic retinopathy patients, as well as elevated levels of vascular endothelial growth factor (VEGF) [34]. The oxidative stress induces the production of mitochondrial superoxide and increases the peroxynitrite levels in the retinal capillary cells, which causes mitochondrial dysfunction. Additionally, high glucose levels are shown to increase NF-κB in the endothelial cells of the retina. The IL-1ß activity increases within the capillary cells, activate NF-κB and accelerates apoptosis of those capillary cells under hyperglycemic conditions. These factors further contribute to the development of diabetic retinopathy [35].

Consuming blueberries with high anthocyanin content can mitigate the risk of disease due to its effective inhibition of oxidative stress and proinflammatory molecule expression. Through numerous studies, it was displayed that the transcription of Nrf2 and nuclear translocation was increased upon consuming blueberries. The anthocyanin increases the expression of Nrf2, which then activates the synthesis of many antioxidants to reduce the effects of oxidative stress. As the anthocyanin concentration increased upon blueberry consumption, the levels of VEGF and IL-1ß decreased. Decreased amounts of these genes suppress proinflammatory factors to reduce the contributing effect of inflammation in the disease [34].

RED WINE

Flavonoid Properties

Red wine is a worldwide, commercially utilized alcoholic beverage made by the fermentation of grapes. The primary method of producing them is the fermentation process of collected grapes. Variations in the numerous types of wine occur based on the alcohol content, grape variety, sweetness, and carbon dioxide content. The process of producing red wine entails destemming and crushing grapes, which remain in contact with the skin and seeds. Sulfur dioxide is added as well as preventative measures against bacteria. Fermentation then occurs through the addition of yeast to make alcohol. The win will undergo many additional steps, such as aging and blending until it is ready for commercial use [36].

Major components of wine are glycerol, water, sugars, polysaccharides, and carbon dioxide. One key distinguishing factor between white and red wine is that red wine is fermented with the skin and seeds present while white wine is not. Fermentation of the solid parts in red wine then results in it containing 10-fold more phenolic compounds and the total content being 900–2,500 mg/L [37,38]. With over 200 various phenolic compounds being present, there are both flavonoids and nonflavonoids contributing to numerous biological functions. The grape skin for red wine production is rich in flavanol monomers epicatechin, gallocatechin, epigallocatechin, and catechin, while the seeds consist of flavanol polymers proanthocyanidins. The flavanol monomers are retained during the production of red wine. However, the flavanol polymer is poorly absorbed and is present at minimal levels [39]. The flavanols that contribute to red wine maceration are in control of the bitter taste in red wines. Additional other predominant flavonoids include quercetin and anthocyanins such as malvidin-3-glucoside, which are responsible for the dark red pigment of the beverage [40,41]. Red wine has displayed significant potential in being used for therapeutic purposes, as 20%–30% mortality rate has been observed for all diseases [40].

Nrf2 Activation

Neuroprotection

Neurodegenerative diseases can develop because of cellular damage experienced by ROS, and they are combated by the activation of Nrf2 transcription factors. The most severe neurodegenerative disease today is AD, which has affected more than 40 million people in 2016 alone. Increased levels of ß-amyloid peptide, mitochondrial dysfunction, and various other factors could increase ROS levels and oxidative stress, which have a role in the accumulation of AD. The expression of Nrf2 to combat oxidative stress activates HO-1, the effect being anti-neuroinflammatory responses to protect neurons, improve cognitive deficits, and reduce the rate of apoptosis from neurotoxins. The second most severe neurodegenerative disease is Parkinson's, affecting 10 million people globally. Oxidative stress harms lipids and DNA, reduces GSH levels while increasing oxidized GSH levels, decreases antioxidant activity, and induces apoptosis. Like AD, the Nrf2 pathway activated HO-1; however, it also improved GSH levels and lowered oxidative markers such as ROS. The epicatechin and catechin flavonoids in red wine provide defense mechanisms against the contributing factors of ROS in neurodegenerative diseases. By activating the Nrf2 pathway, GSH levels could be upregulated to lower oxidative stress. The mechanism of this, as mentioned above, is through the expression of HO-1. Ultimately, it could provide natural methods of delaying the progression of AD and Parkinson's disease [41].

Cerebral ischemia is another leading cause of death stemming from a decrease in cerebral flow. The peroxidation of lipids can be triggered by the release of ROS, DNA injury, and increasing Ca^{2+} are some of the observed mechanisms by which the release of transcription factors HIF-1, STAT3, and NF-κB produce inflammatory cytokines and recruit activated leukocytes. To combat the influx of ROS, antioxidant enzymes are produced by the assistance of Nrf2 transcription factors, and neurological deficits and infarct size associated with the disease are ameliorated. The procyanidin administered through the consumption of red wine can restore the Nrf2 levels to activate NQO1, GSTα, NQO1, and HO-1 in the ischemic brain area and decrease any neurological damage by reducing ROS [41]. Overall, the flavonoid content in red wine has displayed significant amounts of importance in treating or alleviating neurodegenerative diseases.

SOYBEANS

Flavonoid Properties

Soybeans of the species *Glycine max* have been used in various forms throughout the world. These legumes are produced through the process of germination, maturation, and flowering, after which the soybean flowers can be collected and prepared for commercial use [42]. A significant feature of soybeans is their nitrogen-fixating capabilities through the formation of a symbiotic relationship with rhizobium (*Bradyrhizobium japonicum*). The total uptake of nitrogen from the atmosphere can be as high as 98%, resulting in the efficient formation of large seed sizes to seed biomass [43]. Soybeans provide many health benefits due to their increased content of isoflavones and soy protein. The protein content in soy ranges from 36% to 46%, and isoflavones vary between 1,176 and 3,309 mg in the United States. Soybeans also contain vitamin B, zinc, fiber, iron, and calcium, which further contribute to their benefits as functional foods [44]. All these sources make soybean an of nutrients, and bioactive compounds make soybeans a sustaining source of nutrients and protein for vegetarians.

The flavonoids in soybeans have been known to provide numerous health benefits upon consumption. The most predominant subclass of flavonoids in soybeans are isoflavones, also known as phytoestrogens, with 5–30 mg/100 g found within the legumes [45]. The specific isoflavone conjugates that display the therapeutic effects are genistein, glycitein, and daidzein, which are prevalent as malonyl or acetyl glycosides which are genistein, glycitein, and daidzin. The abundance of derivatives in decreasing order are malonyl-genistin, malonyl-glucitin, genistin, daidzin, daidzein, genistein, and glycitein [46]. Overall, the isoflavone content in soybeans has contributed to discovering natural remedies against CVD and various cancers. With the many essential nutrients present in the legumes, their daily consumption is highly recommended.

Nrf2 Activation

Cardiovascular Diseases

CVDs such as diabetes and hypertension can occur due to increased ROS and weakened antioxidant capabilities. With ROS interfering with intracellular signaling pathways intron of vascular functions, there could be immense rapid damage to proteins,

DNA, and lipids. There has been evidence that the consumption of soybeans containing large amounts of isoflavones genistein and daidzein as glycoside conjugates or in their aglycone is associated with lower occurrences of CVD in eastern populations. Eastern diets have increased soybean intake up to $4\,\mu M$ as opposed to western diets, in which the concentrations are as low as 40 nM. The extent of isoflavone's impact on human development can be linked to as early as fetal development, in which exposure to a soy diet can reduce the vulnerability to CVD [45].

In a study involving rats, the effects of soy isoflavone deficiency versus soy isoflavone-rich diet were compared. The isoflavone-deficient rates over a span of 10–12 months led to the development of hypertension, while a balanced diet of isoflavones for only 4–6 months displayed marginal benefits in endothelial function within a significantly shorter time range. The isoflavones relaxed pre-constricted arterial rings and reduced inflammation in vessel walls [45].

As stated, the Nrf2 transcription factor provides cellular defense against oxidative stress. The mechanism involves the ingestion of soybeans to increase isoflavone content. The isoflavones activate intracellular kinase cascades to express and enhance eNOS, endothelial NO production, or ROS levels. This stimulates the modification of cysteine residues on the Keap1 to allow for the nuclear localization of Nrf2 and the subsequent binding to ARE or EprRE. The upregulation of these genes allows for the expression of antioxidant defense genes such as NQO1 or HO-1 and provides cardioprotective properties. This displays that incorporating soybeans in our daily diet could present long-term benefits for cardiovascular health [45].

CONCLUSION AND FUTURE TRENDS

Flavonoid functional foods present numerous health benefits that are continuing to be understood today. The accumulation of free radicals contributes to the development of common chronic diseases responsible for the high mortality rate throughout the world. Natural foods, including blueberry, dark chocolate, raspberry, green tea, and cabbage, are inexpensive methods of prolonging the occurrence of many chronic diseases due to their antioxidant capabilities against oxidative stress. As discussed in this chapter, an important mechanism through which flavonoids can make an impact is the activation of transcription factor Nrf2. Nrf2 has displayed optimistic results in expressing various antioxidant and anti-inflammatory genes to provide the body with an effective defense mechanism against any potential threat.

The low intake of vegetables and fruits has been linked to contributing to the overall disease burden of approximately 4.4%. Thus, the regular consumption of flavonoid-rich foods is a strongly recommended method of obtaining a proper supply of nutrients and antioxidants to reduce the risk of degenerative diseases. Eating 200–400 g of fruits and vegetables each day can fulfill the amount of nutrients we need to maintain longevity [47]. Along with major changes in lifestyle, such as exercising, consuming less alcohol and sugar, reducing smoking, and having less dairy, we can see positive changes in global life expectancy and reduced complications against fatal diseases.

REFERENCES

1. Panche AN, Diwan AD, Chandra SR. Flavonoids: An overview. *Journal of Nutritional Science*. 2016;5(47):1–15.
2. Wang TY, Li Q, Bi KS. Bioactive flavonoids in medicinal plants: Structure, activity, and biological fate. *Asian Journal of Pharmaceutical Sciences*. 2018 Jan 1;13(1):12–23.
3. de Souza Farias SA, da Costa KS, Martins JB. Analysis of conformational, structural, magnetic, and electronic properties related to antioxidant activity: Revisiting flavan, anthocyanidin, flavanone, flavonol, isoflavone, flavone, and flavan-3-ol. *Acs Omega*. 2021 Mar 24;6(13):8908–18.
4. Huang WY, Zhang HC, Liu WX, Li CY. Survey of antioxidant capacity and phenolic composition of blueberry, blackberry, and strawberry in Nanjing. *Journal of Zhejiang University Science B*. 2012 Feb;13(2):94–102.
5. National Institute of Health. *Antioxidants: In Depth*, https://www.nccih.nih.gov/health/antioxidants-in-depth. 2013 [accessed 18 December 2021].
6. Lambert SA, Jolma A, Campitelli LF, Das PK, Yin Y, Albu M, Chen X, Taipale J, Hughes TR, Weirauch MT. The human transcription factors. *Cell*. 2018 Feb 8;172(4):650–65.
7. Beyond Microgreens. *Nrf2 Activators: What They Are, and Why You Should be Eating Them!* https://beyondmicrogreens.com/blogs/microgreens-news/nrf2-activators-sulforaphane. 1 May 2021 [accessed 18 December 2021].
8. Lu MC, Zhao J, Liu YT, Liu T, Tao MM, You QD, Jiang ZY. CPUY192018, a potent inhibitor of the Keap1-Nrf2 protein-protein interaction, alleviates renal inflammation in mice by restricting oxidative stress and NF-κB activation. *Redox Biology*. 2019 Sep 1;26:101266.
9. Henry CJ. Functional foods. *European Journal of Clinical Nutrition*. 2010 Jul;64(7):657–9.
10. Arshad MS, Khalid W, Ahmad RS, Khan MK, Ahmad MH, Safdar S, Kousar S, Munir H, Shabbir U, Zafarullah M, Nadeem M. Functional foods, and human health: An overview. *Functional Foods – Phytochemicals and Health Promoting Potential*. 2021 Aug 30.
11. Musial C, Kuban-Jankowska A, Gorska-Ponikowska M. Beneficial properties of green tea catechins. *International Journal of Molecular Sciences*. 2020 Jan;21(5):1744.
12. Di Mattia CD, Sacchetti G, Mastrocola D, Serafini M. From cocoa to chocolate: The impact of processing on in vitro antioxidant activity and the effects of chocolate on antioxidant markers in vivo. *Frontiers in Immunology*. 2017 Sep 29;8:1207.
13. Gallo M, Vinci G, Graziani G, De Simone C, Ferranti P. The interaction of cocoa polyphenols with milk proteins studied by proteomic techniques. *Food Research International*. 2013 Nov 1;54(1):406–15.
14. Lippi G, Franchini M, Montagnana M, Favaloro EJ, Guidi GC, Targher G. Dark chocolate: Consumption for pleasure or therapy? *Journal of Thrombosis and Thrombolysis*. 2009 Nov;28(4):482–8.
15. Martín MA, Goya L, Ramos S. Preventive effects of cocoa and cocoa antioxidants in colon cancer. *Diseases*. 2016 Mar;4(1):6.
16. Bhakkiyalakshmi E, Sireesh D, Ramkumar KM. Redox sensitive transcription via Nrf2-Keap1 in suppression of inflammation. *Inimmunity and Inflammation in Health and Disease*. 2018 Jan 1:149–61. Academic Press.
17. Nehlig A. The neuroprotective effects of cocoa flavanol and its influence on cognitive performance. *British Journal of Clinical Pharmacology*. 2013 Mar;75(3):716–27.
18. Shah ZA, Li RC, Ahmad AS, Kensler TW, Yamamoto M, Biswal S, Doré S. The flavanol (–)-epicatechin prevents stroke damage through the Nrf2/HO1 pathway. *Journal of Cerebral Blood Flow & Metabolism*. 2010 Dec;30(12):1951–61.

19. Chacko SM, Thambi PT, Kuttan R, Nishigaki I. Beneficial effects of green tea: A literature review. *Chinese Medicine*. 2010 Dec;5(1):1–9.
20. Li J, Sapper TN, Mah E, Rudraiah S, Schill KE, Chitchumroonchokchai C, Moller MV, McDonald JD, Rohrer PR, Manautou JE, Bruno RS. Green tea extract provides extensive Nrf2-independent protection against lipid accumulation and NFκB proinflammatory responses during nonalcoholic steatohepatitis in mice fed a high-fat diet. *Molecular Nutrition & Food Research*. 2016 Apr;60(4):858–70.
21. Smith RE, Tran K, Smith CC, McDonald M, Shejwalkar P, Hara K. The role of the Nrf2/ARE antioxidant system in preventing cardiovascular diseases. *Diseases*. 2016 Dec;4(4):34.
22. Rao AV, Snyder DM. Raspberries, and human health: A review. *Journal of Agricultural and Food Chemistry*. 2010 Apr 14;58(7):3871–83.
23. Bradish CM, Perkins-Veazie P, Fernandez GE, Xie G, Jia W. Comparison of flavonoid composition of red raspberries (Rubus idaeus L.) grown in the Southern United States. *Journal of Agricultural and Food Chemistry*. 2012 Jun 13;60(23):5779–86.
24. Wood, WB. *The Nematode Caenorhabditis Elegans*. Cold Spring Harbor Laboratory Press. 1988. p. 1. ISBN 978-0-87969-433-3.
25. Song B, Zheng B, Li T, Liu RH. Raspberry extract ameliorates oxidative stress in Caenorhabditis elegans via the SKN-1/Nrf2 pathway. *Journal of Functional Foods*. 2020 Jul 1;70:103977.
26. Burton-Freeman BM, Sandhu AK, Edirisinghe I. Red raspberries, and their bioactive polyphenols: Cardiometabolic and neuronal health links. *Advances in Nutrition*. 2016 Jan;7(1):44–65.
27. Knockaert D, Van Camp J, Struijs K, Wille C, Raes K. Potential of lactic acid fermentation to produce health beneficial compounds from vegetable waste. In: *23rd International Icfmh Symposium Foodmicro 2012: Global issues in food microbiology 2012* (pp. 727–27).
28. Manchali S, Murthy KN, Patil BS. Crucial facts about health benefits of popular cruciferous vegetables. *Journal of Functional Foods*. 2012 Jan 1;4(1):94–106.
29. Uuh-Narvaez JJ, Segura-Campos MR. Cabbage (Brassica oleracea var. capitata): A food with functional properties aimed to type 2 diabetes prevention and management. *Journal of Food Science*. 2021 Nov;86(11):4775–98.
30. DeFronzo RA, Ferrannini E, Groop L, Henry RR, Herman WH, Holst JJ, Hu FB, Kahn CR, Raz I, Shulman GI, Simonson DC. Type 2 diabetes mellitus. *Nature Reviews Disease Primers*. 2015 Jul 23;1(1):1–22.
31. Kalt W, Cassidy A, Howard LR, Krikorian R, Stull AJ, Tremblay F, Zamora-Ros R. Recent research on the health benefits of blueberries and their anthocyanins. *Advances in Nutrition*. 2020 Mar 1;11(2):224–36.
32. Miller K, Feucht W, Schmid M. Bioactive compounds of strawberry and blueberry and their potential health effects based on human intervention studies: A brief overview. *Nutrients*. 2019 Jul;11(7):1510.
33. Lee SG, Kim B, Yang Y, Pham TX, Park YK, Manatou J, Koo SI, Chun OK, Lee JY. Berry anthocyanins suppress the expression and secretion of proinflammatory mediators in macrophages by inhibiting nuclear translocation of NF-κB independent of NRF2-mediated mechanism. *The Journal of Nutritional Biochemistry*. 2014 Apr 1;25(4):404–11.
34. Song Y, Huang L, Yu J. Effects of blueberry anthocyanins on retinal oxidative stress and inflammation in diabetes through Nrf2/HO-1 signaling. *Journal of Neuroimmunology*. 2016 Dec 15;301:1–6.
35. Al-Kharashi AS. Role of oxidative stress, inflammation, hypoxia, and angiogenesis in the development of diabetic retinopathy. *Saudi Journal of Ophthalmology*. 2018 Oct 1;32(4):318–23.
36. Di Lorenzo A, Bloise N, Meneghini S, Sureda A, Tenore GC, Visai L, Arciola CR, Daglia M. Effect of winemaking on the composition of red wine as a source of polyphenols for anti-infective biomaterials. *Materials*. 2016 May;9(5):316.

37. Markoski MM, Garavaglia J, Oliveira A, Olivaes J, Marcadenti A. Molecular properties of red wine compounds and cardiometabolic benefits. *Nutrition and Metabolic Insights.* 2016 Jan;9:NMI-S32909.
38. Martínez-Huélamo M, Rodríguez-Morató J, Boronat A, De la Torre R. Modulation of Nrf2 by olive oil and wine polyphenols and neuroprotection. *Antioxidants.* 2017 Dec;6(4):73.
39. Hodgson JM. Red wine flavonoids and vascular health. *Nutrition and Aging.* 2014 Jan 1;2(2–3):139–44.
40. Fernandes I, Pérez-Gregorio R, Soares S, Mateus N, De Freitas V. Wine flavonoids in health and disease prevention. *Molecules.* 2017 Feb;22(2):292.
41. Casassa LF. Flavonoid phenolics in red winemaking. Phenolic compounds – Natural sources, importance, and applications. 2017 Mar 15.
42. Basso DP, Hoshino-Bezerra AA, Sartori MM, Buitink J, Leprince O, Silva EA. Late seed maturation improves the preservation of seedling emergence during storage in soybean. *Journal of Seed Science.* 2018 Apr;40:185–92.
43. Ciampitti I, Salvagiotti F. New insights into soybean biological nitrogen fixation. *Agronomy J.* 2018;110:1185–96.
44. Rizzo G, Baroni L. Soy, soy foods and their role in vegetarian diets. *Nutrients.* 2018 Jan;10(1):43.
45. Mann GE, Bonacasa B, Ishii T, Siow RC. Targeting the redox sensitive Nrf2–Keap1 defense pathway in cardiovascular disease: Protection afforded by dietary isoflavones. *Current Opinion in Pharmacology.* 2009 Apr 1;9(2):139–45.
46. Peiretti PG, Karamać M, Janiak M, Longato E, Meineri G, Amarowicz R, Gai F. Phenolic composition, and antioxidant activities of soybean (Glycine max (L.) Merr.) plant during growth cycle. *Agronomy.* 2019 Mar;9(3):153.
47. Janabi AH, Kamboh AA, Saeed M, Xiaoyu L, BiBi J, Majeed F, Naveed M, Mughal MJ, Korejo NA, Kamboh R, Alagawany M. Flavonoid-rich foods (FRF): A promising nutraceutical approach against lifespan-shortening diseases. *Iranian Journal of Basic Medical Sciences.* 2020 Feb;23(2):140.

The Role of Nrf2 Activation and Autophagy in Aging and Neurodegenerative Diseases

12

Elizabeth Mazzio and Karam F.A. Soliman
Florida A&M University

Contents

DOI: 10.1201/9781003225225-12

THE DEFENSE SYSTEM: Keap1-Nrf2-ARE

The transcription factor Nrf2 (nuclear factor erythroid 2-related factor 2) and the Keap1-Nrf2-ARE ((Kelch-like ECH-associating protein 1)-Nrf2- (antioxidant response element)) is synonymous with a rapid and potent cellular defense mechanism against environmental oxidative toxins or those that originate from endogenous pathological or metabolic conditions. Under normal resting conditions, Nrf2 is acquiesced by being under a constant barrage of multi-ubiquitination causing rapid proteasomal degradation [1,2]. This is carried out where the absence of reactive oxygen species (ROS) (or electrophiles) on Keap1, maintains binding to cullin-based (Cul3) E3 ligase, forming the Keap1-Cul3-RBX1 (ring box protein-1)/Roc 1 E3 ligase complex, which rapidly degrades Nrf2 while interacting with the Nrf2-Neh2 domain comprising a stable Keap1-Nrf2 complex [3,4].

In contrast, in the presence of oxidants (or electrophiles), modifications occur on one or more of the 25+ cysteine residues of Keap1, causing Nrf2 to disconnect from the degradation complex, enabling freedom of movement for the full-length transcript; which houses seven functional domains, one of which include the Neh1 Cap n collar (CNC) leucine zipper [5,6]. The Nrf2 Neh1 CNC domain is responsible for dimerization and translocation to the nucleus, where Nrf2 then binds to small musculoaponeurotic fibrosarcoma proteins (sMafs), causing activation of ARE/ERE. The ARE/ERE, in turn, induces the expression of over 200 genes that augment host defense systems, including antioxidant, detoxification, anti-apoptotic, proteasomal, and ubiquitination-related, autophagy-related proteins [7]. The Nrf2/ARE defense is triggered by diverse biological threats ranging from heavy metal poisoning (e.g., Hg, Cd, Cu, Mn), hypoxia/ischemic brain injury [8–10] and mostly yields a prototypical Nfr2/ARE "signature response"; constituting upregulation of a host of sister genes simultaneously: CAT, GSH-PX, SOD, HOX-1, NQO1, GSH-R, GSH-T, TR, GCLc, GCLM, and SULFs corresponding to reduced expression of Keap1 [11–16].

Mechanistic Controls on Nrf2-ARE

While the Nrf2/Keap1 system is very complex, it can be easily simplified into two basic categories, events that suppress the system "off position" [Nrf2 degradation] or events that drive the system "on position" [Nrf2 accumulation and nuclear translocation]. The on/off switches have been studied in detail for over 30 years now and are known to involve primarily the following (a) kinase modifications that phosphorylate-specific Neh 1–7 domains on the Nrf2 transcript itself, most occurring at serine residues or (b) electrophiles/oxidants that modify Keap1 primarily occurring at cysteine residues [17].

In brief, formidable controls to sustain the pathological "off position" [*Nrf2 degradation/stability of Keap1*] involve the following enzymes/locations/modifications: (GSK-3β/location: Neh6 DSGIS (338) and DSAPGS (378) motifs/modification is mostly phosphorylation [18]), (endoplasm reticulum domain Hrd1/location: Neh4-5 on the Nrf2 [19]), (Fyn/location: Y568/modification is typically phosphorylation [20]) and (INrf2/location: Y141/modification is phosphorylation [21]). Events that control the "on" position [*Nrf2 induction/nuclear translocation/dissociation of Keap1*] (AMPK/location: serine 374, 408, and 433 on Nrf2/modification is phosphorylation [22,23]), (PKC/location: serine 40 on Nrf2, modification is phosphorylation [20]), (casein kinase 2/location: Neh4-5 on Nrf2, modification is phosphorylation [24]), (protein kinase RNA-like endoplasmic reticulum kinase (PERK)/Nrf2, modification is phosphorylation [25,26]), and (MAPK p38/location: Nrf2; Ser215, Ser408, and Ser577, modification is phosphorylation [15,27]). Controlling the enzymes responsible for these modifications can tip the Nrf2/Keap1 axis to either side.

While the Nrf2 Neh 1–7 domains are all important, particularly, Neh6 has a high controlling relevance because of its being a KEAP1-independent Nrf2 phospho degron, which is phosphorylated by glycogen synthase kinase 3 (GSK-3β), causing the formation of β-transducin repeat-containing protein (β-TrCP) CUL1 –Rbx1/Roc1 E3 ubiquitin ligase complex which rapidly degrades Nrf2 [18,28]. The discussion of GSK-3β and its upstream targets will appear through several stages in this chapter as it crosses multiple points of control suppressing the entire Nrf2/Keap1/autophagy systems.

MECHANISTIC CONTROLS ON Keap1

The second major modification that controls the "on/off positions" occur directly on Keap1, primarily at reactive cysteine (Cys) residues (thiolate switches) that sense reactive electrophiles and oxygen species prompting covalent adduct formation, followed by the release and induction of Nr2f [29]. The most important of these are housed in one of two Keap1 domains 1) the N-terminal BTB and the C-terminal DC (BTB) domains (Cys151), and an intervening region (Cys273 and Cys288) [4,30]. Cys151 is likely the most critical for modulating the E3 ubiquitin ligase activity of the Keap1-Cul3 complex causing steric stress to break the interaction upon interacting with an electrophile [31,32]. The range of molecules that react with one or more of the 25 Cys residues on

Keap1 [33,34] is very extensive, while known primary controls are believed to involve in the modification of (Cys 151, Cys 273, and Cys 288) readily with a large number of chemicals and oxidants such as (eicosapentaenoic acid and docosahexaenoic acid [35]), (artemisitene/location: Cys 151 [36]), (nitrofatty acids/location: Cys 151 [36]), (diallyl trisulfide/location: Cys 288 [37]) (15-deoxy-Δ12,14-prostaglandin J2/location: Cys 288), (prostaglandin A2, 4-hydroxynonenal, nitro-oleic fatty acid (9-OANO2), sodium arsenite/location: Cys 151, Cys 273, Cys 288), (sodium nitroprusside, CDDO-Im (Nrf2 activator)/location: Cys 151 [38]), (hydrogen peroxide/location: Cys 226, Cys 613, Cys 622, and Cys 624 [39]), (tert-butylhydroquinone (TBHQ)/location: Cys 23, Cys 151, Cys 226, and Cys 368 [40,41]), (ROS, reactive nitrogen species/location: Cys 151 [42]), (dimethyl fumarate [DMF]/location: Cys 151) [43], and (curcumin/location: Cys 151) [44]. The supposition that there is a "cysteine code hypothesis" suggests the enormity of the possibility by which each type of toxicant binds in a specific combination to Cys residues on Keap1 to trigger the dissociation and the induction of Nrf2 [38]. This code is much like a lottery ticket with vast combinatorial modifications. While research is progressing on defining these combinations, some were originally defined upon the discovery of Keap1, which came from analyzing the similarity of phase II inducers to the Nrf2 ARE detoxification genes [45,46]. Original classes of phase II molecules fell under the description of Michael reaction acceptors (e.g., rendered electrophilic by conjugation with electron-withdrawing groups) involving classes of chemicals such as alpha- and beta-unsaturated aldehydes, ketones, quinones, thioketones, sulfones, esters, nitriles, and nitro groups; these are now reflected as inducers of Nrf2/Keap1 [46,47].

Age-Related Loss of Nrf2/Keap1ARE

The age-related loss in the Nrf2/ARE occurs in diverse species, including humans [48] juxtaposed on a backdrop of increasing levels of environmental toxins and oxidants in water, air, soil, and food systems globally. The greatest vulnerability is the human brain of all the systems affected by age and a diminished Nrf2/ARE. Central nervous system (CNS) neurons are post-mitotic, and the Nrf2 cleansing system must be maintained because if it is defective, it will lead to the gradual accrual of oxidized, damaged protein aggregates, which injure the cerebral microvasculature (blood–brain barrier [BBB]), are toxic to neurons, and present the most significant risk factor for developing dementia and other CNS degenerative diseases [7,9] such as Alzheimer's disease (AD) and Parkinson's disease (PD) [15].

The age-related loss of Nrf2 defense systems in AD and PD is a controlling factor to disease severity and onset, where every study we have come across which silences Nrf2, shows exacerbating severity and early onset for all aspects of tau, amyloid, and synuclein pathologies [49,50] and a reversal afforded by overexpressed Nrf2 adenoviral gene transfers [51,52]. The age-related Nrf2 loss does not occur in a vacuum and corresponds to the direct rise in Nrf2 gene "suppressors" such as Bach1 (BTB and CNC homolog 1) c-Myc, which compete with Nrf2 for Mafs to turn off the ARE/ERE defense systems [48,53]. The rise of Nrf2 suppressors like Bach1 is equally evident in human AD and PD brain samples, corresponding to the loss of Nrf2 and mechanism uncoupling from activating modification controls like; PERK (AD) [54,55].

Overview of Nrf2-Related Autophagy

The age-related loss of Nrf2 could be one of the most critical factors in autophagy dysfunction, a relationship that is consistent throughout the literature. As co-participants in the same system, these two systems work to (a) neutralize oxidative toxins (Nrf2) and (b) remove oxidized biomass (autophagy) through proper disposing of/recycling through a lysosome-dependent process. Again, autophagy is very complex but can be simplified into two categorical process switches: ("on"/"off") with four types of autophagy defined. The most consequential kind of autophagy when it comes to Nrf2 is macrophagy (targeted removal of large proteins and organelles including damaged mitochondria), and its main "off/on" switch is the nutrient-sensitive, rapamycin-sensitive mTOR (serine-threonine kinase) complex 1 (mTORC1).

The "on" (favorable) is a process that reads like a municipal waste site protocol. In brief, the "on" switch is triggered by mTOR inhibition, which involves dephosphorylation/ then activation of ULK1/ULK2, which then, in turn, phosphorylates ATg13 and FIP200 activating the complex: ULK-Atg13- Atg101- FIP200 [56,57]. At the same time, ULK1 also phosphorylates Beclin1 (Ser 30) [58] once active, it will then incorporate into the Beclin1 complex (Beclin1, PIK3R4 (p150) - Atg14L - and the class III phosphatidylinositol 3-phosphate kinase (PI(3)K) Vps34), where Vsp34 phosphorylates phosphatidylinositol to phosphatidylinositol 3-phosphate (PtdIns(3)P) all of which initiates the bagging of trash (phagophores) for preparation for further bagging into a rugged, thick double-lined trash bag called an autophagosome positioned for an approach toward the lysosome [58–60]. PtdIns(3Ps) binds to ATG16L1 [61] and pull in the double enclosure involving Atg12-Atg5-Atg16L1 forming an E3-like complex that binds/activates Atg3, which covalently attaches LC3B-II proteins – clips (like construction bag zip ties), to the lipids on the surface of autophagosomes, enabling bag enclosure [62]. These are then loaded onto cargos with adaptor proteins (waste trucks) and receptors such as p62/sequestosome1, which self-polymerize and guide the transport of waste toward the lysosome (waste management facility) for disposal [63,64]. The autophagosomes are then fused to the lysosome requiring UVRAG (UV Radiation Resistance Associated), Rab family of small GTPases, SNARE (soluble N-ethylmaleimide-sensitive factor attachment protein receptor) the Atg17-Atg31-Atg29 complex, Atg11 proteins, and membrane tethering clip proteins [65,66]. The LC3B-II clips, formed initially via activated Atg7, are transferred to Atg3 followed by conjugation to phosphatidylethanolamine (PE) to generate processed LC3B–II.) [67]. After fusion, the waste is degraded by acid hydrolases, cathepsins and lysosomal acidic hydrolases, supplied by vacuolar-type H+-ATPases. Their building blocks are released from the vesicle through the action of permeases to be recycled. In contrast, a sustained mTOR signaling (high-nutrient state) can lead to a complete halt of autophagy, events that involve AMPK kinases that phosphorylate/deactivate ULK1/ULK2 and TSC1/2 [68].

The rate of Nrf2 controls the speed of autophagy, both of which control the clearance of AD and PD pathological aggregates [69]. Although nutrient deprivation can turn on autophagy via mTORC1 inhibition, mTORC1 inhibitors such as rapamycin and its derivatives (rapalogs) (e.g., temsirolimus) or nitazoxanide can accelerate clearance of hyperphosphorylated tau and $A\beta$, restoring the integrity of the BBB [70] and improving cognition and memory [71,72]. There is promise in the use of rapamycin/

mTOR inhibition and prevention of AD, but some are wondering why there has been no advancement toward initiating clinical trials [73].

Nrf2 SQSTM1/p62 Autophagy Age-Related Shutdown

The interdependent tether between autophagy and Nrf2 is the continual subject of advanced research that is unraveled [53,74]. They are connected by induction of Nrf2 ARE transcripts, which induce expression of genes that encode for proteins required for the 26S proteasome and autophagy (e.g., nuclear dot protein 52 (NDP52), ULK1, ATG5, and GABARAPL1 and the cargo carrier receptor p62/sequestosome1 transcripts (SQSTM1/p62) [55,75]. However, it is the SQSTM1/p62 itself, that in turn – modifies Keap1 at the (KIR) domain to degrade and release Nrf2 for nuclear translocation [15,63,76]. The "p62-Keap1-Nrf2-positive feedback loop" drives the amplification of autophagy activity in sync with greater Nrf2 induction to neutralize toxins. Furthermore, the SQSTM1/p62 also controls the off switch of mTOR by ULK1 phosphorylation/AMPK leading to autophagy induction and continual, sustained Keap1 degradation [77]. These are connected very much like a chain on a bicycle. When losses do occur, they occur in tandem. A deficiency in Nrf2/SQSTM1/p62 occurs alongside losses to collaborative partners such as calcium-binding and coiled-coil domain-containing protein 2 (CALCOCO2, NDP52), Atg7, Beclin1, and lysosomal membrane 1 (LAMP1), all corresponding to the inability to clear AD aberrant proteins from the brain [78–81]. The summation of the "off" switch being stuck is essentially an "Nrf2/autophagy shutdown". Turning back "on" the Nrf2/autophagy is the goal, and almost every study shows elevating the Nrf2/SQSTM1/p62 axis speed up degradation rates of Keap1 [82] and re-establish high-level clearance for proteinopathies (Aβ-amyloidosis, synucleinopathy tauopathy) [83,84].

AGE-RELATED Nrf2/SQSTM1/p62 SHUTDOWN AND NEURODEGENERATIVE DISEASES (ALZHEIMER'S DISEASE, PARKINSON'S DISEASE)

The Nrf2/SQSTM1/p62 loss is an all-inclusive loss involving (a) overactive mTOR (blunted autophagy) and (b) attenuated Nrf2/ARE (blunted neutralization), both pivotal in the pathogenesis of PD and AD [85].

Alzheimer's Disease

In the case of AD, the prime etiology is still not well understood, except for less than 5% of the cases to which genetic mutations are attributed to amyloid precursor protein presenilin-1 and -2 (autosomal-dominant familial AD) and apolipoprotein E-e4 (ApoE4) (autosomal recessive) [86,87]. Most cases (over 95%) are sporadic and age-related and correspond specifically to a defect in lysosomal/autophagy function, a reduction in Nrf2 and result in one of two major pathologies: (a) accumulation of inter neuronal insoluble amyloid-beta peptide (Aβ42) aggregate plagues + hippocampal neurotoxins (sAβ) and (b) accumulation of intra-neuronal neurofibrillary tangles composed of hyper-phosphorylated/acetylated tau, which polymerize into the paired helical filament aggregates [88,89]. Both these events perpetuate oxidative damage and result in striated neuropil threads causing destruction of the nucleus basalis cholinergic cortical projection, occurring in tandem with severe losses of Nrf2/SQSTM1/p62 activity [90–92].

Diseases like this related to the loss of the entire Nrf2/SQSTM1/p62 are generally associated with the onset of proteinopathies (Aβ-amyloidosis, synucleinopathy, tauopathy). Mechanistically speaking, one of the most promising avenues for boosting Nrf2 SQSTM1/p62 is gaining control over (and inhibiting) GSK-3β for the following reasons: (a) GSK-3β is highly present in resting cells, and without a trigger, it continues in its active form (dephosphorylated) being consistently elevated in AD models (e.g., APP/PS1 transgenics, 3x-Tg) and PD where it is localized to the perimeter of Lewy bodies [93,94] (b) Active GSK-3β will phosphorylate serine residues (334-338) in the Neh6 region of Nrf2 to form a structural motif recognized by SCF/β-TrCP E3 ubiquitin ligase, leading to constant Nrf2 degradation (c) alternatively suppression of GSK-3β will increase nuclear Nrf2 localization, and boost major antioxidant systems involving glutathione [95] and (d) suppression of GSK-3β is known to decrease tau hyperphosphorylation and inhibit the formation of aggregate prone Aβ 42. Some of the small molecule GSK-3β inhibitors such as pyrrolidine dithiocarbamate ammonium (PDTC), or puerarin, or PI3K/Akt activators (upstream inactivation of GSK-3β), can work to increase Nrf2 and prevent aggregates in the hippocampus of APP/PS1 mice [96]. Likewise, the use of antisense oligonucleotides for GSK-3β corresponds to the elevation of Nrf2 and reduction in tau hyperphosphorylation and alleviates disease symptoms [97]. If Nrf2/autophagy could be bolstered in the presence of a drug that prevents aggregates in the first place, this could be a powerful combination for AD prevention. As luck would have it, this too seems to be controlled by overactive GSK-3β.

Preventing the formation of aggregates (Gnt-III)

The prevention of aggregates in AD would be a valuable asset for any drug combination. First, amyloid-beta precursor protein (APP) (located in the inner plasma lipid bilayer and Golgi) is cleaved by β-secretase (β-site APP cleaving enzyme 1, BACE1 gene) at the membrane, releasing two products: a neurotoxic ectodomain (sAPPβ) + an amyloidogenic precursor protein – carboxyl-terminal fragment (CTF) CTF99 [98]. The latter product (CTF99) somehow travels through the cytosol into endosomes, where it is cleaved by γ-secretase then releasing a C-terminus of the Aβ cut at 40 amino acids (Aβ40), or 42 (Aβ42) + APP intracellular domain (AICD), the latter of which activates GSK-3β [99]. The greater the ratio of Aβ42:Aβ40, the greater the amyloid aggregation and its multimeric, diffusible Aβ deposit ridden plagues. Unfortunately, β-secretase inhibition as a drug target *is problematic* given its inherent requirement for neuronal function (axon growth, neurogenesis, synaptic plasticity), and the inhibition of γ-secretase complex *is also problematic* given its requirement in Notch signaling/embryonic lethality [100].

Inhibiting GSK-3β could bypass these problems. Not only would it heighten Nrf2/ autophagy, but it would prevent binding to and activating PS1 for rapid phosphorylation of tau [101]. Moreover, GSK-3β also appears to control O-GlcNAcylation deposits occurring on beta-amyloid (Aβ), which makes these extremely prone to forming senile plagues. These changes parallel a rise in GnT-III, also reported in APP/PS1 mice [102], and blocking GSK-3β will consistently and significantly inhibit GnT-III expression and GlcNac-coated products susceptible to aggregate, including beta-amyloid [103–105] as well as prevent full maturation of APP [106]. All in all, activating a number of kinases, including polo-like kinase2 (PLK2), can lead to the inactivation and phosphorylation of GSK-3β [107], highly sought after target drug designed to treat AD [108]. Upregulating AMPK or PI3K/Akt can also inactivate GSK-3β where the former can also activate phosphorylation of Nrf2 (location: Ser 558) and promote its nuclear accumulation [109–111].

Parkinson's Disease

PD is highly linked to autophagy failure and dysfunction of the ubiquitin-proteasome system. Deregulation of the autophagy pathways is linked to genetic mutations in PINK1 and Parkin (required for mitophagy), leucine-rich repeat kinase 2 (LRRK2), and DJ1 (ubiquitin-proteasome), to which Nrf2 dysfunction would be exacerbated [7,112]. Accumulation of proteins like α-synuclein in Lewy bodies correlates to autophagy dysfunction in the subtantia nigra (SN), which would only worsen by the extensive oxidative microenvironment circumscribing SN dopaminergic neurons. Vulnerabilities include (a) continual loss of nigral GSH [113], (b) accumulation of (Fe^{3+}) and ferrous iron (Fe^{2+}) [114], which can easily react with radical superoxide (O_2^-) and hydrogen peroxide (H_2O_2), producing a highly reactive OH radical (c) dopamine oxidation and formation of neurotoxins, dopamine quinones, tetrahydroisoquinoline alkaloids, 6-OHDA [115,116] and (d) greater MAO-B activity that generates peroxides and aldehydes [117]. The Nrf2/ SQSTM1/p62 response must be maximized to the highest level in the case of PD, in particular, given Nrf2/ARE defense genes associated with iron-induced oxidative stress and quinone detoxification along the GSH-GPX4 axis (e.g., GCLC, HMOX1, FTH, FTL, NQO1, PRDX1, GCLM, GSS, LSC7a11, GGT1, TXN, and TXNRD) [118,119].

ANTI-AGING DRUGGABLE Nrf2/SQSTM1/ p62 TARGETS: NUTRACEUTICALS

Nrf2 Activators/False Positives and Methodological Concerns

Very few Nrf2 activators are being used clinically or on the market, with DMF and RTA-408 continuing as lead candidates and interest in natural products to combat age-related vulnerabilities growing [120]. As far as natural products reported to upregulate

Nrf2 signaling [121], some issues of concern are as follows: false positives could be occurring as reported in the literature for *in vitro* studies using compounds that appear to generate a corresponding signature response (CAT, SOD, GSH-Px HO-1, NQO1, etc.) but occurring only as a result of auto-oxidative, pro-oxidant properties (e.g., gallic acid (-)-gallocatechin gallate, gallols, quinones), instability issues or compounds that could contribute to electrophilic artifacts [122–131]. Some Nrf2 activators, when tested *in vitro*, are reversible by adding antioxidants, as in the case of thymoquinone and curcumin, suggesting some type of radical generation or compound instability [132–134]. Moreover, Nrf2 activators such as EGCG, when tested *in vitro,* can reportedly worsen heavy metal toxicity, explained by the authors as interfering auto-oxidation or (Fe(3+)) interactions [131]. Furthermore, many Nrf2 activation studies use immortal cancer cell line models, which are by nature in direct contradiction concerning aging (senescence) versus cancer (immortality), which are inverted through the entire Nrf2 p62/SQSTM1 axis [135,136]. Cancer cells maintain high activity level of Nrf2/p62/SQSTM1, which bestow resistance to oxidative chemotherapy drugs, radiation, the immune system, and forcibly drive oncogenic beta-catenin signaling [137] and mesenchymal-epithelial plasticity [138–141]. Lastly, and most interesting, when working *in vitro,* particularly with polyphenolics containing a phenol ring such as phloretin, phloridzin, naringenin, apigenin, curcumin, resveratrol, isoliquiritigenin, are pro-oxidant properties and generation of polyphenolic phenoxyl radicals, which can oxidize cellular GSH and also interact with metals such as Fe^{3+}, Fe^{2+}, the ramification of which needs further investigation, as this actually could be a defining attribute, rather than an artifact [142–144].

Normalization of Nrf2 p62/SQSTM1 Axis: Effective Nutraceuticals in Animal Models

There is no question that natural products can activate Nrf2 as demonstrated in hundreds if not thousands of studies employing diverse models ranging from zebrafish [145,146] primary cells backed by corresponding transgenic animal models [147] and structure-based molecular analysis [148]. Across these studies, reported effects are set forth as a chemical or drug that "upregulates the Nrf2 p62/SQSTM1 axis" parallel to "attenuated biological injury". Similarly, age-related losses in Nrf2 p62/SQSTM1 have been substantiated in hundreds of studies showing greater vulnerability to oxidative toxicological injury [74,149,150]. The data regarding this topic are overwhelming, so we provide a brief theme throughout the literature by the system, by the model of injury and protective Nrf2-activating compounds.

AD – Model of injury transgenic (amyloid precursor protein APP/presenilin 1 PS1 double transgenic mice, 3x-Tg (APP Swedish, MAPT P301L, and PSEN1 M146V), Abeta1-42 intrahippocampal injection, scopolamine, and galactose induced: (**Nrf2** ↑/ pterostilbene [151], fasudil [152], pinoresinol diglucoside [153], rhynchophylline [154], vitamin D [155], polysaccharide of *Taxus chinensis* [156], lithium chloride [157], acetyl-11-keto-beta-boswellic acid [158], syringing [159], curcumin analogs [160], astragalus polysaccharide [161], coniferaldehyde [162], ginsenoside compound K [163], caffeic acid phenethyl ester derivative from honeybee (FA-97) [164], *Amanita caesarea* polysaccharides [165], artemether [166], resveratrol [167], hesperetin [168], sulforaphane [169], hesperidin [170], puerarin [96], orientin [171], carnosinic acid [172], hydrogen sulfide (H2S) [173], kavalactone [174], linalool [175], anthocyanins extracted from Korean black beans [176], and niacinamide [177]).

PD – Model of injury: Heat shock factor 1/MPTP (*Andrographis paniculata* leaf/ andrographolide [178], Brucein D (BD) from *Brucea javanica* [179], Danshensu [180], astragaloside IV [181], and sulforaphane) [182].

Liver – Model of injury – acetaminophen, alcohol, concanavalin A, hepatic sinus with monocrotaline, toosendanin-induced high-fat diet and non–alcoholic steatohepatitis:(**Nrf2** ↑/ protected by Ginsenoside Rg1 [183], Baicalein, baicalin [184], chlorogenic acid [185], (-)-epicatechin [186], essential oils from eucalyptol and Artemisia vulgaris L [187], querce-tin [188], H_2S donor GYY4137 [189], green tea [190], physalin B [191], Bixon [192], *Veronica ciliata* Fisch [193], melatonin [194], nicotinic acid [195], vine tea polyphenol [196], carveol [197], myricetin [198], resveratrol [199], *Schisandra chinensis* polysaccharides [200], sul-foraphane [201], tetrahydrocurcumin, and octahydrocurcumin [202], nicotinamide, glycyr-rhetinic acid, magnesium isoglycyrrhizinate [203–205], and curcumin [206]).

Atherosclerosis – Model of injury tert-butyl hydroperoxide or calcification: (**Nrf2** ↑/ protected by acacetin [207], z-ligustilide [208], rosmarinic acid [209]).

Dementia/cognition and brain – Model of injury (specific)/scopolamine/(**Nrf2** ↑/ walnut peptide YVLLPSPK [210], and ginsenoside compound K [163]), methamphet-amine/(**Nrf2** ↑/resveratrol [211]), bisphenol A/(**Nrf2** ↑/alpha-lipoic acid [212]), phenycy-clidine-induced schizophrenia/(**Nrf2** ↑/*Andrographis paniculate*) [207], BBB-sepsis/ (**Nrf2** ↑/GYY4137, synthetic compound of hydrogen sulfide (H2S) [213], blast injury to the brain/(**Nrf2** ↑/resveratrol) [214], hypoxia/(**Nrf2** ↑/echinacoside) [215], traumatic brain injury/(**Nrf2** ↑/melatonin [216]), galactose toxicity/(**Nrf2** ↑/sesamol) [217], brain injury/(**Nrf2** ↑/ginger and turmeric [218]).

Intestinal – Model of injury – Mycotoxin deoxynivalenol (DON): (**Nrf2** ↑/ L-carnosine [219] and lycopene [220]).

Diabetes – Model of injury – high-fat diet/streptozotocin: (**Nrf2** ↑/protected by *Salvia officinalis, Panax ginseng, Trigonella foenum*-graeceum, and *Cinnamomum zey-lanicum* [221], hinokinin [222], and scutellarin [223]).

Cardiac – Model of injury – ischemia/reperfusion, isoproterenol, arsenic trioxide, diabetic cardiomyopathy: (**Nrf2** ↑/protected by dioscin [224], hesperidin [225], penta-methyl quercetin [226], baicalin [227], salvia miltiorrhiza [228], and mangiferin [229]).

Lung – Model of injury – methicillin-resistant *Staphylococcus aureus*, PM2.5, sep-sis, particle injury and pulmonary fibrosis: (**Nrf2** ↑/protected by itaconate (4-OI) [230], melatonin [231], sinomenine [232], vitamin D [233], *Salvia miltiorrhiza* [234], and tan-shinone IIA from *Salvia miltiorrhiza* [235]).

These are just a few examples that represent thousands of studies in all types of models of injury while monitoring the Nrf2/ARE/Keap1/p62 axis.

Data Interpretation Concerns

Even with appropriate models, there is a major issue regarding the study of nutraceuti-cals and Nrf2 induction and its interpretation of biological consequences. Many natu-ral compounds can activate PI3K/Akt/PKC/ERK/p38MAPK/AMPK/NF-κB [7,121], which activates Nrf2, its release from Keap1 [15] to turn on ARE genes [27]. All these natural inhibitors (including negative controls on GSKβ) are all pathways of a highly complex nature involved with diverse pathological intertwining events. This makes it very difficult to suggest that protective effects are entirely a result of the Nrf2/ARE/ autophagy axis. More importantly, the Nrf2-inducing compounds themselves (e.g., melatonin, tocotrienols, mangiferin, curcumin, epigallocatechin gallate, schisandra B resveratrol, silybin, sulforaphane, genistein, phenethyl isothiocyanate, naringenin, honokiol, quercetin, sulforaphane, triptolide, allicin, berberine, piperlongumine, fisetin, 18α-glycyrrhetinic acid, chitosan oligosaccharide and phloretin [236,237] or even the drugs (oltipraz, rosiglitazone, dimethyl fumarate) [85,238,239] have a plethora of other biological targets some of which act as antioxidants/pro-oxidants, anti-inflammatories, making it impossible to tie efficacy of upregulation of Nrf2, which is of equal signaling complexity on a finite pathological endpoint [15,134,238].

CONCLUSION

This is a fascinating area of research but will require accuracy in reporting to propel this field rapidly. This field of study, due to its very nature (electrophilic/oxidative adduct formation), is open to false positives in vitro, and contradictions may present themselves with the use of immortal cell lines that contain an inverted Nrf2 p62/SQSTM1 axis. Moreover, the mechanism by which this axis would be controlled (drug or nutraceutical-wise) is subject to multi-kinase balances, which are highly complex and interwoven, making it difficult to determine if an alleviation of a pathological endpoint indicator is a direct result of the Nrf2 system alone. However, all together, these studies suggest a need to develop more specific Nrf2/autophagy inducers, which can pass the BBB and prevent or delay CNS degenerative diseases such as AD or PD. Lastly, nature has inherently bestowed upon us medicines that, in their natural forms, are being orally ingested by millions (if not billions) across the globe, seeking to alleviate age-related conditions. These nutraceuticals (in their raw forms) should be wholly assessed for efficacy in established models, rather than individual compounds, which become non-applicable if not sold OTC or by prescription.

REFERENCES

1. Furukawa M and Xiong Y. BTB protein Keap1 targets antioxidant transcription factor Nrf2 for ubiquitination by the Cullin 3-Roc1 ligase. *Mol Cell Biol* 2005; 25: 162–171. DOI: 10.1128/MCB.25.1.162-171.2005.
2. McMahon M, Itoh K, Yamamoto M, et al. Keap1-dependent proteasomal degradation of transcription factor Nrf2 contributes to the negative regulation of antioxidant response element-driven gene expression. *J Biol Chem* 2003; 278: 21592–21600. DOI: 10.1074/jbc. M300931200.

3. Kaspar JW and Jaiswal AK. An autoregulatory loop between Nrf2 and Cul3-Rbx1 controls their cellular abundance. *J Biol Chem* 2010; 285: 21349–21358. DOI: 10.1074/jbc.M110.121863.
4. Kobayashi A, Kang MI, Okawa H, et al. Oxidative stress sensor Keap1 functions as an adaptor for Cul3-based E3 ligase to regulate proteasomal degradation of Nrf2. *Mol Cell Biol* 2004; 24: 7130–7139. DOI: 10.1128/MCB.24.16.7130-7139.2004.
5. Hong F, Sekhar KR, Freeman ML, et al. Specific patterns of electrophile adduction trigger Keap1 ubiquitination and Nrf2 activation. *J Biol Chem* 2005; 280: 31768–31775. DOI: 10.1074/jbc.M503346200.
6. Zipper LM and Mulcahy RT. The Keap1 BTB/POZ dimerization function is required to sequester Nrf2 in the cytoplasm. *J Biol Chem* 2002; 277: 36544–36552. DOI: 10.1074/jbc. M206530200.
7. Yang T and Zhang F. Targeting transcription factor Nrf2 (nuclear factor erythroid 2-related factor 2) for the intervention of vascular cognitive impairment and dementia. *Arterioscler Thromb Vasc Biol* 2021; 41: 97–116. DOI: 10.1161/ATVBAHA.120.314804.
8. Buha A, Baralic K, Djukic-Cosic D, et al. The role of toxic metals and metalloids in Nrf2 signaling. *Antioxidants (Basel)* 2021; 10. DOI: 10.3390/antiox10050630.
9. Farina M, Vieira LE, Buttari B, et al. The Nrf2 pathway in ischemic stroke: A review. *Molecules* 2021; 26. DOI: 10.3390/molecules26165001.
10. Alam J, Wicks C, Stewart D, et al. Mechanism of heme oxygenase-1 gene activation by cadmium in MCF-7 mammary epithelial cells. Role of p38 kinase and Nrf2 transcription factor. *J Biol Chem* 2000; 275: 27694–27702. DOI: 10.1074/jbc.M004729200.
11. Zhong CC, Zhao T, Hogstrand C, et al. Copper (Cu) induced changes of lipid metabolism through oxidative stress-mediated autophagy and Nrf2/PPARgamma pathways. *J Nutr Biochem* 2021: 108883. DOI: 10.1016/j.jnutbio.2021.108883.
12. Shang X, Yu P, Yin Y, et al. Effect of selenium-rich Bacillus subtilis against mercury-induced intestinal damage repair and oxidative stress in common carp. *Comp Biochem Physiol C Toxicol Pharmacol* 2021; 239: 108851. DOI: 10.1016/j.cbpc.2020.108851.
13. Ramadan SS, Almeer RS, Alkahtani S, et al. Ziziphus spina-christi leaf extract attenuates mercuric chloride-induced liver injury in male rats via inhibition of oxidative damage. *Environ Sci Pollut Res Int* 2021; 28: 17482–17494. DOI: 10.1007/s11356-020-12160-6.
14. Ni M, Li X, Yin Z, et al. Comparative study on the response of rat primary astrocytes and microglia to methylmercury toxicity. *Glia* 2011; 59: 810–820. DOI: 10.1002/glia.21153.
15. Yu C and Xiao JH. The Keap1-Nrf2 system: A mediator between oxidative stress and aging. *Oxid Med Cell Longev* 2021; 2021: 6635460. DOI: 10.1155/2021/6635460.
16. Fao L, Mota SI and Rego AC. Shaping the Nrf2-ARE-related pathways in Alzheimer's and Parkinson's diseases. *Ageing Res Rev* 2019; 54: 100942. DOI: 10.1016/j.arr.2019.100942.
17. Villavicencio Tejo F and Quintanilla RA. Contribution of the Nrf2 pathway on oxidative damage and mitochondrial failure in Parkinson and Alzheimer's disease. *Antioxidants (Basel)* 2021; 10. DOI: 10.3390/antiox10071069.
18. Chowdhry S, Zhang Y, McMahon M, et al. Nrf2 is controlled by two distinct beta-TrCP recognition motifs in its Neh6 domain, one of which can be modulated by GSK-3 activity. *Oncogene* 2013; 32: 3765–3781. DOI: 10.1038/onc.2012.388.
19. Wu T, Zhao F, Gao B, et al. Hrd1 suppresses Nrf2-mediated cellular protection during liver cirrhosis. *Genes Dev* 2014; 28: 708–722. DOI: 10.1101/gad.238246.114.
20. Niture SK, Khatri R and Jaiswal AK. Regulation of Nrf2-an update. *Free Radic Biol Med* 2014; 66: 36–44. DOI: 10.1016/j.freeradbiomed.2013.02.008.
21. Jain AK, Mahajan S and Jaiswal AK. Phosphorylation and dephosphorylation of tyrosine 141 regulate stability and degradation of INrf2: A novel mechanism in Nrf2 activation. *J Biol Chem* 2008; 283: 17712–17720. DOI: 10.1074/jbc.M709854200.
22. Sharma A, Anand SK, Singh N, et al. Berbamine induced AMPK activation regulates mTOR/SREBP-1c axis and Nrf2/ARE pathway to allay lipid accumulation and oxidative stress in steatotic HepG2 cells. *Eur J Pharmacol* 2020; 882: 173244. DOI: 10.1016/j. ejphar.2020.173244.

23. Matzinger M, Fischhuber K, Poloske D, et al. AMPK leads to phosphorylation of the tran-scription factor Nrf2, tuning transactivation of selected target genes. *Redox Biol* 2020; 29: 101393. DOI: 10.1016/j.redox.2019.101393.
24. Apopa PL, He X and Ma Q. Phosphorylation of Nrf2 in the transcription activation domain by casein kinase 2 (CK2) is critical for the nuclear translocation and transcription activa-tion function of Nrf2 in IMR-32 neuroblastoma cells. *J Biochem Mol Toxicol* 2008; 22: 63–76. DOI: 10.1002/jbt.20212.
25. Cullinan SB and Diehl JA. PERK-dependent activation of Nrf2 contributes to redox homeostasis and cell survival following endoplasmic reticulum stress. *J Biol Chem* 2004; 279: 20108–20117. DOI: 10.1074/jbc.M314219200.
26. Aydin Y, Chedid M, Chava S, et al. Activation of PERK-Nrf2 oncogenic signaling pro-motes Mdm2-mediated Rb degradation in persistently infected HCV culture. *Sci Rep* 2017; 7: 9223. DOI: 10.1038/s41598-017-10087-6.
27. Zipper LM and Mulcahy RT. Inhibition of ERK and p38 MAP kinases inhibits binding of Nrf2 and induction of GCS genes. *Biochem Biophys Res Commun* 2000; 278: 484–492. DOI: 10.1006/bbrc.2000.3830.
28. Rada P, Rojo AI, Chowdhry S, et al. SCF/{beta}-TrCP promotes glycogen synthase kinase 3-dependent degradation of the Nrf2 transcription factor in a Keap1-independent manner. *Mol Cell Biol* 2011; 31: 1121–1133. DOI: 10.1128/MCB.01204-10.
29. Antelmann H and Helmann JD. Thiol-based redox switches and gene regulation. *Antioxid Redox Signal* 2011; 14: 1049–1063. DOI: 10.1089/ars.2010.3400.
30. Sekhar KR, Rachakonda G and Freeman ML. Cysteine-based regulation of the CUL3 adaptor protein Keap1. *Toxicol Appl Pharmacol* 2010; 244: 21–26. DOI: 10.1016/j.taap.2009.06.016.
31. Eggler AL, Small E, Hannink M, et al. Cul3-mediated Nrf2 ubiquitination and antioxidant response element (ARE) activation are dependent on the partial molar volume at position 151 of Keap1. *Biochem J* 2009; 422: 171–180. DOI: 10.1042/BJ20090471.
32. Zhang DD, Lo SC, Sun Z, et al. Ubiquitination of Keap1, a BTB-Kelch substrate adaptor protein for Cul3, targets Keap1 for degradation by a proteasome-independent pathway. *J Biol Chem* 2005; 280: 30091–30099. DOI: 10.1074/jbc.M501279200.
33. He X and Ma Q. NRF2 cysteine residues are critical for oxidant/electrophile-sensing, Kelch-like ECH-associated protein-1-dependent ubiquitination-proteasomal degrada-tion, and transcription activation. *Mol Pharmacol* 2009; 76: 1265–1278. DOI: 10.1124/mol.109.058453.
34. Wakabayashi N, Dinkova-Kostova AT, Holtzclaw WD, et al. Protection against electro-phile and oxidant stress by induction of the phase 2 response: Fate of cysteines of the Keap1 sensor modified by inducers. *Proc Natl Acad Sci U S A* 2004; 101: 2040–2045. DOI: 10.1073/pnas.0307301101.
35. Gao L, Wang J, Sekhar KR, et al. Novel n-3 fatty acid oxidation products activate Nrf2 by destabilizing the association between Keap1 and Cullin3. *J Biol Chem* 2007; 282: 2529–2537. DOI: 10.1074/jbc.M607622200.
36. Kansanen E, Bonacci G, Schopfer FJ, et al. Electrophilic nitro-fatty acids activate NRF2 by a KEAP1 cysteine 151-independent mechanism. *J Biol Chem* 2011; 286: 14019–14027. DOI: 10.1074/jbc.M110.190710.
37. Kim S, Lee HG, Park SA, et al. Keap1 cysteine 288 as a potential target for diallyl trisulfide-induced Nrf2 activation. *PLoS One* 2014; 9: e85984. DOI: 10.1371/journal.pone.0085984.
38. Saito R, Suzuki T, Hiramoto K, et al. Characterizations of three major cysteine sensors of Keap1 in stress response. *Mol Cell Biol* 2016; 36: 271–284. DOI: 10.1128/MCB.00868-15.
39. Suzuki T, Muramatsu A, Saito R, et al. Molecular mechanism of cellular oxidative stress sensing by Keap1. *Cell Rep* 2019; 28: 746–758 e744. DOI: 10.1016/j.celrep.2019.06.047.
40. Abiko Y, Miura T, Phuc BH, et al. Participation of covalent modification of Keap1 in the activation of Nrf2 by tert-butylbenzoquinone, an electrophilic metabolite of butylated hydroxyanisole. *Toxicol Appl Pharmacol* 2011; 255: 32–39. DOI: 10.1016/j.taap.2011.05.013.

41. Yamamoto M, Kensler TW and Motohashi H. The KEAP1-NRF2 system: A thiol-based sensor-effector apparatus for maintaining redox homeostasis. *Physiol Rev* 2018; 98: 1169–1203. DOI: 10.1152/physrev.00023.2017.

42. Fourquet S, Guerois R, Biard D, et al. Activation of NRF2 by nitrosative agents and H2O2 involves KEAP1 disulfide formation. *J Biol Chem* 2010; 285: 8463–8471. DOI: 10.1074/jbc.M109.051714.

43. Sauerland M, Mertes R, Morozzi C, et al. Kinetic assessment of Michael addition reactions of alpha, beta-unsaturated carbonyl compounds to amino acid and protein thiols. *Free Radic Biol Med* 2021; 169: 1–11. DOI: 10.1016/j.freeradbiomed.2021.03.040.

44. Shin JW, Chun KS, Kim DH, et al. Curcumin induces stabilization of Nrf2 protein through Keap1 cysteine modification. *Biochem Pharmacol* 2020; 173: 113820. DOI: 10.1016/j.bcp.2020.113820.

45. Itoh K, Wakabayashi N, Katoh Y, et al. Keap1 represses nuclear activation of antioxidant responsive elements by Nrf2 through binding to the amino-terminal Neh2 domain. *Genes Dev* 1999; 13: 76–86. DOI: 10.1101/gad.13.1.76.

46. Dinkova-Kostova AT, Holtzclaw WD, Cole RN, et al. Direct evidence that sulfhydryl groups of Keap1 are the sensors regulating induction of phase 2 enzymes that protect against carcinogens and oxidants. *Proc Natl Acad Sci U S A* 2002; 99: 11908–11913. DOI: 10.1073/pnas.172398899.

47. Talalay P. Mechanisms of induction of enzymes that protect against chemical carcinogenesis. *Adv Enzyme Regul* 1989; 28: 237–250. DOI: 10.1016/0065-2571(89)90074-5.

48. Davies KJA and Forman HJ. Does Bach1 & c-Myc dependent redox dysregulation of Nrf2 & adaptive homeostasis decrease cancer risk in aging? *Free Radic Biol Med* 2019; 134: 708–714. DOI: 10.1016/j.freeradbiomed.2019.01.028.

49. Ren P, Chen J, Li B, et al. Nrf2 ablation promotes Alzheimer's disease-like pathology in APP/PS1 transgenic mice: The role of neuroinflammation and oxidative stress. *Oxid Med Cell Longev* 2020; 2020: 3050971. DOI: 10.1155/2020/3050971.

50. Rojo AI, Pajares M, Rada P, et al. NRF2 deficiency replicates transcriptomic changes in Alzheimer's patients and worsens APP and TAU pathology. *Redox Biol* 2017; 13: 444–451. DOI: 10.1016/j.redox.2017.07.006.

51. Kanninen K, Malm TM, Jyrkkanen HK, et al. Nuclear factor erythroid 2-related factor 2 protects against beta-amyloid. *Mol Cell Neurosci* 2008; 39: 302–313. DOI: 10.1016/j.mcn.2008.07.010.

52. Kanninen K, Heikkinen R, Malm T, et al. Intrahippocampal injection of a lentiviral vector expressing Nrf2 improves spatial learning in a mouse model of Alzheimer's disease. *Proc Natl Acad Sci U S A* 2009; 106: 16505–16510. DOI: 10.1073/pnas.0908397106.

53. Pajares M, Jimenez-Moreno N, Garcia-Yague AJ, et al. Transcription factor NFE2L2/NRF2 is a regulator of macroautophagy genes. *Autophagy* 2016; 12: 1902–1916. DOI: 10.1080/15548627.2016.1208889.

54. Lanzillotta C, Zuliani I, Tramutola A, et al. Chronic PERK induction promotes Alzheimer-like neuropathology in down syndrome: Insights for therapeutic intervention. *Prog Neurobiol* 2021; 196: 101892. DOI: 10.1016/j.pneurobio.2020.101892.

55. Ahuja M, Ammal Kaidery N, Attucks OC, et al. Bach1 derepression is neuroprotective in a mouse model of Parkinson's disease. *Proc Natl Acad Sci U S A* 2021; 118. DOI: 10.1073/pnas.2111643118.

56. Hosokawa N, Hara T, Kaizuka T, et al. Nutrient-dependent mTORC1 association with the ULK1-Atg13-FIP200 complex required for autophagy. *Mol Biol Cell* 2009; 20: 1981–1991. DOI: 10.1091/mbc.E08-12-1248.

57. Alers S, Loffler AS, Paasch F, et al. Atg13 and FIP200 act independently of Ulk1 and Ulk2 in autophagy induction. *Autophagy* 2011; 7: 1423–1433. DOI: 10.4161/auto.7.12.18027.

58. Park JM, Seo M, Jung CH, et al. ULK1 phosphorylates Ser30 of BECN1 in association with ATG14 to stimulate autophagy induction. *Autophagy* 2018; 14: 584–597. DOI: 10.1080/15548627.2017.1422851.

59. Hong Z, Pedersen NM, Wang L, et al. PtdIns3P controls mTORC1 signaling through lyso-somal positioning. *J Cell Biol* 2017; 216: 4217–4233. DOI: 10.1083/jcb.201611073.
60. Gallagher LE, Williamson LE, and Chan EY. Advances in autophagy regulatory mecha-nisms. *Cells* 2016; 5. DOI: 10.3390/cells5020024.
61. Dooley HC, Wilson MI and Tooze SA. WIPI2B link PtdIns3P to LC3 lipidation through binding ATG16L1. *Autophagy* 2015; 11: 190–191. DOI: 10.1080/15548627.2014.996029.
62. Fujita N, Itoh T, Omori H, et al. The Atg16L complex specifies the site of LC3 lipidation for membrane biogenesis in autophagy. *Mol Biol Cell* 2008; 19: 2092–2100. DOI: 10.1091/mbc.E07-12-1257.
63. Kageyama S, Gudmundsson SR, Sou YS, et al. p62/SQSTM1-droplet serves as a platform for autophagosome formation and antioxidative stress response. *Nat Commun* 2021; 12: 16. DOI: 10.1038/s41467-020-20185-1.
64. Itakura E and Mizushima N. p62 Targeting to the autophagosome formation site requires self-oligomerization but not LC3 binding. *J Cell Biol* 2011; 192: 17–27. DOI: 10.1083/jcb.201009067.
65. Liu X and Klionsky DJ. The Atg17-Atg31-Atg29 complex and Atg11 regulate autophago-some-vacuole fusion. *Autophagy* 2016; 12: 894–895. DOI: 10.1080/15548627.2016.1162364.
66. Liang C, Sir D, Lee S, et al. Beyond autophagy: The role of UVRAG in membrane traffick-ing. *Autophagy* 2008; 4: 817–820. DOI: 10.4161/auto.6496.
67. Frudd K, Burgoyne T, and Burgoyne JR. Oxidation of Atg3 and Atg7 mediates inhibition of autophagy. *Nat Commun* 2018; 9: 95. DOI: 10.1038/s41467-017-02352-z.
68. Chan EY. mTORC1 phosphorylates the ULK1-mAtg13-FIP200 autophagy regulatory complex. *Sci Signal* 2009; 2: pe51. DOI: 10.1126/scisignal.284pe51.
69. Kuang H, Tan CY, Tian HZ, et al. Exploring the bi-directional relationship between autoph-agy and Alzheimer's disease. *CNS Neurosci Ther* 2020; 26: 155–166. DOI: 10.1111/cns.13216.
70. Van Skike CE, Jahrling JB, Olson AB, et al. Inhibition of mTOR protects the blood-brain barrier in models of Alzheimer's disease and vascular cognitive impairment. *Am J Physiol Heart Circ Physiol* 2018; 314: H693–H703. DOI: 10.1152/ajpheart.00570.2017.
71. Jiang T, Yu JT, Zhu XC, et al. Temsirolimus promotes autophagic clearance of amyloid-beta and provides protective effects in cellular and animal models of Alzheimer's disease. *Pharmacol Res* 2014; 81: 54–63. DOI: 10.1016/j.phrs.2014.02.008.
72. Li X, Lu J, Xu Y, et al. Discovery of nitazoxanide-based derivatives as autophagy activa-tors for the treatment of Alzheimer's disease. *Acta Pharm Sin B* 2020; 10: 646–666. DOI: 10.1016/j.apsb.2019.07.006.
73. Kaeberlein M and Galvan V. Rapamycin and Alzheimer's disease: Time for a clinical trial? *Sci Transl Med* 2019; 11. DOI: 10.1126/scitranslmed.aar4289.
74. Kopacz A, Kloska D, Targosz-Korecka M, et al. Keap1 governs ageing-induced pro-tein aggregation in endothelial cells. *Redox Biol* 2020; 34: 101572. DOI: 10.1016/j.redox.2020.101572.
75. Komatsu M, Kageyama S and Ichimura Y. p62/SQSTM1/A170: Physiology and pathology. *Pharmacol Res* 2012; 66: 457–462. DOI: 10.1016/j.phrs.2012.07.004.
76. Lau A, Wang XJ, Zhao F, et al. A noncanonical mechanism of Nrf2 activation by autophagy deficiency: Direct interaction between Keap1 and p62. *Mol Cell Biol* 2010; 30: 3275–3285. DOI: 10.1128/MCB.00248-10.
77. Lee DH, Park JS, Lee YS, et al. SQSTM1/p62 activates NFE2L2/NRF2 via ULK1-mediated autophagic KEAP1 degradation and protects mouse liver from lipotoxicity. *Autophagy* 2020; 16: 1949–1973. DOI: 10.1080/15548627.2020.1712108.
78. Jo C, Gundemir S, Pritchard S, et al. Nrf2 reduces levels of phosphorylated tau protein by inducing autophagy adaptor protein NDP52. *Nat Commun* 2014; 5: 3496. DOI: 10.1038/ncomms4496.
79. Carvalho C, Santos MS, Oliveira CR, et al. Alzheimer's disease and type 2 diabetes-related alterations in brain mitochondria, autophagy, and synaptic markers. *Biochim Biophys Acta* 2015; 1852: 1665–1675. DOI: 10.1016/j.bbadis.2015.05.001.

80. Guo C, Zhang Y, Nie Q, et al. SQSTM1/ p62 oligomerization contributes to Abeta-induced inhibition of Nrf2 signaling. *Neurobiol Aging* 2021; 98: 10–20. DOI: 10.1016/j.neurobiolaging.2020.05.018.

81. Salminen A, Kaarniranta K, Kauppinen A, et al. Impaired autophagy and APP processing in Alzheimer's disease: The potential role of Beclin 1 interactome. *Prog Neurobiol* 2013; 106–107: 33–54. DOI: 10.1016/j.pneurobio.2013.06.002.

82. Knatko EV, Tatham MH, Zhang Y, et al. Downregulation of Keap1 confers features of a fasted metabolic state. *iScience* 2020; 23: 101638. DOI: 10.1016/j.isci.2020.101638.

83. Zhao X, Shi Y, Zhang D, et al. Autophagy inducer activates Nrf2-ARE pathway to attenuate aberrant alveolarization in neonatal rats with bronchopulmonary dysplasia. *Life Sci* 2020; 252: 117662. DOI: 10.1016/j.lfs.2020.117662.

84. Salminen A, Kaarniranta K, Haapasalo A, et al. Emerging role of p62/sequestosome-1 in the pathogenesis of Alzheimer's disease. *Prog Neurobiol* 2012; 96: 87–95. DOI: 10.1016/j.pneurobio.2011.11.005.

85. Yuan H, Xu Y, Luo Y, et al. Role of Nrf2 in cell senescence regulation. *Mol Cell Biochem* 2021; 476: 247–259. DOI: 10.1007/s11010-020-03901-9.

86. Van Cauwenberghe C, Van Broeckhoven C and Sleegers K. The genetic landscape of Alzheimer disease: Clinical implications and perspectives. *Genet Med* 2016; 18: 421–430. DOI: 10.1038/gim.2015.117.

87. Cacace R, Sleegers K and Van Broeckhoven C. Molecular genetics of early-onset Alzheimer's disease revisited. *Alzheimer's Dement* 2016; 12: 733–748. DOI: 10.1016/j.jalz.2016.01.012.

88. Ruben GC, Iqbal K, Wisniewski HM, et al. Alzheimer neurofibrillary tangles contain 2.1 nm filaments structurally identical to the microtubule-associated protein tau: A high-resolution transmission electron microscope study of tangles and senile plaque core amyloid. *Brain Res* 1993; 602: 164–179. DOI: 10.1016/0006-8993(92)91092-s.

89. Joshi G, Gan KA, Johnson DA, et al. Increased Alzheimer's disease-like pathology in the APP/ PS1DeltaE9 mouse model lacking Nrf2 through modulation of autophagy. *Neurobiol Aging* 2015; 36: 664–679. DOI: 10.1016/j.neurobiolaging.2014.09.004.

90. Murphy GM, Jr., Greenberg BD, Ellis WG, et al. Alzheimer's disease. Beta-amyloid precursor protein expression in the nucleus basalis of Meynert. *Am J Pathol* 1992; 141: 357–361.

91. Xu Y, Zhang S, and Zheng H. The cargo receptor SQSTM1 ameliorates neurofibrillary tangle pathology and spreads through selective targeting of pathological MAPT (microtubule-associated protein tau). *Autophagy* 2019; 15: 583–598. DOI: 10.1080/15548627.2018.1532258.

92. Tian Y, Wang W, Xu L, et al. Activation of Nrf2/ARE pathway alleviates the cognitive deficits in PS1V97L-Tg mouse model of Alzheimer's disease through modulation of oxidative stress. *J Neurosci Res* 2019; 97: 492–505. DOI: 10.1002/jnr.24357.

93. Nagao M and Hayashi H. Glycogen synthase kinase-3beta is associated with Parkinson's disease. *Neurosci Lett* 2009; 449: 103–107. DOI: 10.1016/j.neulet.2008.10.104.

94. Li DW, Liu ZQ, Chen W, et al. Association of glycogen synthase kinase-3beta with Parkinson's disease (review). *Mol Med Rep* 2014; 9: 2043–2050. DOI: 10.3892/mmr.2014.2080.

95. Cuadrado A. Structural and functional characterization of Nrf2 degradation by glycogen synthase kinase 3/beta-TrCP. *Free Radic Biol Med* 2015; 88: 147–157. DOI: 10.1016/j.freeradbiomed.2015.04.029.

96. Zhou Y, Xie N, Li L, et al. Puerarin alleviates cognitive impairment and oxidative stress in APP/PS1 transgenic mice. *Int J Neuropsychopharmacol* 2014; 17: 635–644. DOI: 10.1017/S146114571300148X.

97. Farr SA, Ripley JL, Sultana R, et al. Antisense oligonucleotide against GSK-3beta in brain of SAMP8 mice improves learning and memory and decreases oxidative stress: Involvement of transcription factor Nrf2 and implications for Alzheimer disease. *Free Radic Biol Med* 2014; 67: 387–395. DOI: 10.1016/j.freeradbiomed.2013.11.014.

98. Yan R, Han P, Miao H, et al. The transmembrane domain of the Alzheimer's beta-secretase (BACE1) determines its late Golgi localization and access to beta-amyloid precursor protein (APP) substrate. *J Biol Chem* 2001; 276: 36788–36796. DOI: 10.1074/jbc.M104350200.

99. Ryan KA and Pimplikar SW. Activation of GSK-3 and phosphorylation of CRMP2 in transgenic mice expressing APP intracellular domain. *J Cell Biol* 2005; 171: 327–335. DOI: 10.1083/jcb.200505078.

100. Ng HL, Quail E, Cruickshank MN, et al. To be, or notch to be: Mediating cell fate from embryogenesis to lymphopoiesis. *Biomolecules* 2021; 11. DOI: 10.3390/biom11060849.

101. Takashima A, Murayama M, Murayama O, et al. Presenilin 1 associate with glycogen synthase kinase-3beta and its substrate tau. *Proc Natl Acad Sci U S A* 1998; 95: 9637–9641. DOI: 10.1073/pnas.95.16.9637.

102. Wang Y, Chen S, Xu Z, et al. GLP-1 receptor agonists downregulate aberrant GnT-III expression in Alzheimer's disease models through the Akt/GSK-3beta/beta-catenin signaling. *Neuropharmacology* 2018; 131: 190–199. DOI: 10.1016/j.neuropharm.2017.11.048.

103. Xu Q, Akama R, Isaji T, et al. Wnt/beta-catenin signaling down-regulates N-acetylglucosaminyltransferase III expression: the implications of two mutually exclusive pathways for regulation. *J Biol Chem* 2011; 286: 4310–4318. DOI: 10.1074/jbc.M110.182576.

104. Akasaka-Manya K, Manya H, Sakurai Y, et al. Protective effect of N-glycan bisecting GlcNAc residues on beta-amyloid production in Alzheimer's disease. *Glycobiology* 2010; 20: 99–106. DOI: 10.1093/glycob/cwp152.

105. Fiala M, Mahanian M, Rosenthal M, et al. MGAT3 mRNA: A biomarker for prognosis and therapy of Alzheimer's disease by vitamin D and curcuminoids. *J Alzheimers Dis* 2011; 25: 135–144. DOI: 10.3233/JAD-2011-101950.

106. Aplin AE, Jacobsen JS, Anderton BH, et al. Effect of increased glycogen synthase kinase-3 activity upon the maturation of the amyloid precursor protein in transfected cells. *Neuroreport* 1997; 8: 639–643. DOI: 10.1097/00001756-199702100-00012.

107. Fan Y, Wang J, He N, et al. PLK2 protects retinal ganglion cells from oxidative stress by potentiating Nrf2 signaling via GSK-3beta. *J Biochem Mol Toxicol* 2021; 35: e22815. DOI: 10.1002/jbt.22815.

108. Ma QL, Lim GP, Harris-White ME, et al. Antibodies against beta-amyloid reduce Abeta oligomers, glycogen synthase kinase-3beta activation and tau phosphorylation in vivo and in vitro. *J Neurosci Res* 2006; 83: 374–384. DOI: 10.1002/jnr.20734.

109. Ren J, Liu T, Han Y, et al. GSK-3beta inhibits autophagy and enhances radiosensitivity in non-small cell lung cancer. *Diagn Pathol* 2018; 13: 33. DOI: 10.1186/s13000-018-0708-x.

110.   Sun A, Li C, Chen R, et al. GSK-3beta controls autophagy by modulating the LKB1-AMPK pathway in prostate cancer cells. *Prostate* 2016; 76: 172–183. 2015/10/07. DOI: 10.1002/pros.23106.

111. Park SY, Choi YW and Park G. Nrf2-mediated neuroprotection against oxygen-glucose deprivation/reperfusion injury by emodin via AMPK-dependent inhibition of GSK-3beta. *J Pharm Pharmacol* 2018; 70: 525–535. DOI: 10.1111/jphp.12885.

112. Gumeni S, Papanagnou ED, Manola MS, et al. Nrf2 activation induces mitophagy and reverses Parkin/Pink1 knock down-mediated neuronal and muscle degeneration phenotypes. *Cell Death Dis* 2021; 12: 671. DOI: 10.1038/s41419-021-03952-w.

113. Zeevalk GD, Manzino L, Sonsalla PK, et al. Characterization of intracellular elevation of glutathione (GSH) with glutathione monoethyl ester and GSH in brain and neuronal cultures: Relevance to Parkinson's disease. *Exp Neurol* 2007; 203: 512–520. DOI: 10.1016/j.expneurol.2006.09.004.

114. Riederer P, Monoranu C, Strobel S, et al. Iron as the concert master in the pathogenic orchestra playing in sporadic Parkinson's disease. *J Neural Transm (Vienna)* 2021; 128: 1577–1598. DOI: 10.1007/s00702-021-02414-z.

115. Monzani E, Nicolis S, Dell'Acqua S, et al. Dopamine, oxidative stress and protein-quinone modifications in Parkinson's and other neurodegenerative diseases. *Angew Chem Int Ed Engl* 2019; 58: 6512–6527. DOI: 10.1002/anie.201811122.

116. Parga JA, Rodriguez-Perez AI, Garcia-Garrote M, et al. NRF2 activation and downstream effects: Focus on Parkinson's disease and brain angiotensin. *Antioxidants (Basel)* 2021; 10. DOI: 10.3390/antiox10111649.

117. Goldstein DS. The catecholaldehyde hypothesis: Where MAO fits in. *J Neural Transm (Vienna)* 2020; 127: 169–177. DOI: 10.1007/s00702-019-02106-9.

118. Song S, Gao Y, Sheng Y, et al. Targeting NRF2 to suppress ferroptosis in brain injury. *Histol Histopathol* 2021; 36: 383–397. DOI: 10.14670/HH-18-286.

119. Okada K, Warabi E, Sugimoto H, et al. Nrf2 inhibits hepatic iron accumulation and counteracts oxidative stress-induced liver injury in nutritional steatohepatitis. *J Gastroenterol* 2012; 47: 924–935. DOI: 10.1007/s00535-012-0552-9.

120. Ma B, Lucas B, Capacci A, et al. Design, synthesis and identification of novel, orally bioavailable non-covalent Nrf2 activators. *Bioorg Med Chem Lett* 2020; 30: 126852. DOI: 10.1016/j.bmcl.2019.126852.

121. Zgorzynska E, Dziedzic B and Walczewska A. An overview of the Nrf2/ARE pathway and its role in neurodegenerative diseases. *Int J Mol Sci* 2021; 22. DOI: 10.3390/ijms22179592.

122. Sang S, Hou Z, Lambert JD, et al. Redox properties of tea polyphenols and related biological activities. *Antioxid Redox Signal* 2005; 7: 1704–1714. DOI: 10.1089/ars.2005.7.1704.

123. Totsune H. [Production of active oxygen by autooxidation; quinone antineoplastic agents]. *Tanpakushitsu Kakusan Koso* 1988; 33: 2781–2789.

124. Ouyang J, Zhu K, Liu Z, et al. Prooxidant effects of epigallocatechin-3-gallate in health benefits and potential adverse effect. *Oxid Med Cell Longev* 2020; 2020: 9723686. DOI: 10.1155/2020/9723686.

125. Munoz-Munoz JL, Garcia-Molina F, Molina-Alarcon M, et al. Kinetic characterization of the enzymatic and chemical oxidation of the catechins in green tea. *J Agric Food Chem* 2008; 56: 9215–9224. DOI: 10.1021/jf8012162.

126. Canada AT, Giannella E, Nguyen TD, et al. The production of reactive oxygen species by dietary flavonols. *Free Radic Biol Med* 1990; 9: 441–449. DOI: 10.1016/0891-5849(90)90022-b.

127. Wu QQ, Liang YF, Ma SB, et al. Stability and stabilization of (-)-gallocatechin gallate under various experimental conditions and analyses of its epimerization, auto-oxidation, and degradation by LC-MS. *J Sci Food Agric* 2019; 99: 5984–5993. DOI: 10.1002/jsfa.9873.

128. Perron NR, Wang HC, Deguire SN, et al. Kinetics of iron oxidation upon polyphenol binding. *Dalton Trans* 2010; 39: 9982–9987. DOI: 10.1039/c0dt00752h.

129. Halliwell B. Dietary polyphenols: Good, bad, or indifferent for your health? *Cardiovasc Res* 2007; 73: 341–347. DOI: 10.1016/j.cardiores.2006.10.004.

130. Tedesco I, Spagnuolo C, Russo GL, et al. The pro-oxidant activity of red wine polyphenols induces an adaptive antioxidant response in human erythrocytes. *Antioxidants (Basel)* 2021; 10. DOI: 10.3390/antiox10050800.

131. Zwolak I. Epigallocatechin gallate for management of heavy metal-induced oxidative stress: Mechanisms of action, efficacy, and concerns. *Int J Mol Sci* 2021; 22. DOI: 10.3390/ijms22084027.

132. Kundu J, Kim DH, Kundu JK, et al. Thymoquinone induces heme oxygenase-1 expression in HaCaT cells via Nrf2/ARE activation: Akt and AMPKalpha as upstream targets. *Food Chem Toxicol* 2014; 65: 18–26. DOI: 10.1016/j.fct.2013.12.015.

133. McNally SJ, Harrison EM, Ross JA, et al. Curcumin induces heme oxygenase 1 through generation of reactive oxygen species, p38 activation and phosphatase inhibition. *Int J Mol Med* 2007; 19: 165–172.

134. Jayasuriya R, Dhamodharan U, Ali D, et al. Targeting Nrf2/Keap1 signaling pathway by bioactive natural agents: Possible therapeutic strategy to combat liver disease. *Phytomedicine* 2021; 92: 153755. DOI: 10.1016/j.phymed.2021.153755.

135. Jiang G, Liang X, Huang Y, et al. p62 promotes proliferation, apoptosisresistance and invasion of prostate cancer cells through the Keap1/Nrf2/ARE axis. *Oncol Rep* 2020; 43: 1547–1557. DOI: 10.3892/or.2020.7527.

136. Yang H, Ni HM and Ding WX. The double-edged sword of MTOR in autophagy deficiency induced-liver injury and tumorigenesis. *Autophagy* 2019; 15: 1671–1673. DOI: 10.1080/15548627.2019.1634445.

137. Savall M, Senni N, Lagoutte I, et al. Cooperation between the NRF2 pathway and oncogenic beta-catenin during HCC tumorigenesis. *Hepatol Commun* 2021; 5: 1490–1506. DOI: 10.1002/hep4.1746.

138. Martinez VD, Vucic EA, Thu KL, et al. Disruption of KEAP1/CUL3/RBX1 E3-ubiquitin ligase complex components by multiple genetic mechanisms: Association with poor prognosis in head and neck cancer. *Head Neck* 2015; 37: 727–734. DOI: 10.1002/hed.23663.

139. Li T, Jiang D and Wu K. p62 promotes bladder cancer cell growth by activating KEAP1/NRF2-dependent antioxidative response. *Cancer Sci* 2020; 111: 1156–1164. DOI: 10.1111/cas.14321.

140. Tan CT, Chang HC, Zhou Q, et al. MOAP-1-mediated dissociation of p62/SQSTM1 bodies releases Keap1 and suppresses Nrf2 signaling. *EMBO Rep* 2021; 22: e50854. DOI: 10.15252/embr.202050854.

141. Kamble D, Mahajan M, Dhat R, et al. Keap1-Nrf2 pathway regulates ALDH and contributes to radioresistance in breast cancer stem cells. *Cells* 2021; 10. DOI: 10.3390/cells10010083.

142. Xing J, Chen X and Zhong D. Stability of baicalin in biological fluids in vitro. *J Pharm Biomed Anal* 2005; 39: 593–600. DOI: 10.1016/j.jpba.2005.03.034.

143. Chan TS, Galati G, Pannala AS, et al. Simultaneous detection of the antioxidant and prooxidant activity of dietary polyphenolics in a peroxidase system. *Free Radic Res* 2003; 37: 787–794. DOI: 10.1080/1071576031000094899.

144. Galati G, Chan T, Wu B, et al. Glutathione-dependent generation of reactive oxygen species by the peroxidase-catalyzed redox cycling of flavonoids. *Chem Res Toxicol* 1999; 12: 521–525. DOI: 10.1021/tx980271b.

145. Zhao X, Gong L, Wang C, et al. Quercetin mitigates ethanol-induced hepatic steatosis in zebrafish via P2X7R-mediated PI3K/ Keap1/Nrf2 signaling pathway. *J Ethnopharmacol* 2021; 268: 113569. DOI: 10.1016/j.jep.2020.113569.

146. Nguyen VT, Bian L, Tamaoki J, et al. Generation and characterization of keap1a- and keap1b-knockout zebrafish. *Redox Biol* 2020; 36: 101667. DOI: 10.1016/j.redox.2020.101667.

147. Xu XX, Zheng G, Tang SK, et al. Theaflavin protects chondrocytes against apoptosis and senescence via regulating Nrf2 and ameliorates murine osteoarthritis. *Food Funct* 2021; 12: 1590–1602. DOI: 10.1039/d0fo02038a.

148. Zhang L, Xu L, Chen H, et al. Structure-based molecular hybridization design of Keap1-Nrf2 inhibitors as novel protective agents of acute lung injury. *Eur J Med Chem* 2021; 222: 113599. DOI: 10.1016/j.ejmech.2021.113599.

149. Cordaro M, D'Amico R, Morabito R, et al. Physiological and biochemical changes in NRF2 pathway in aged animals subjected to brain injury. *Cell Physiol Biochem* 2021; 55: 160–179. DOI: 10.33594/000000353.

150. Oishi T, Matsumaru D, Ota N, et al. Activation of the NRF2 pathway in Keap1-knockdown mice attenuates progression of age-related hearing loss. *NPJ Aging Mech Dis* 2020; 6: 14. DOI: 10.1038/s41514-020-00053-4.

151. Xu J, Liu J, Li Q, et al. Pterostilbene alleviates Abeta1-42-induced cognitive dysfunction via inhibition of oxidative stress by activating Nrf2 signaling pathway. *Mol Nutr Food Res* 2021; 65: e2000711. DOI: 10.1002/mnfr.202000711.

152. Wei W, Wang Y, Zhang J, et al. Fasudil ameliorates cognitive deficits, oxidative stress and neuronal apoptosis via inhibiting ROCK/MAPK and activating Nrf2 signalling pathways in APP/PS1 mice. *Folia Neuropathol* 2021; 59: 32–49. DOI: 10.5114/fn.2021.105130.

153. Lei S, Wu S, Wang G, et al. Pinoresinol diglucoside attenuates neuroinflammation, apoptosis and oxidative stress in a mice model with Alzheimer's disease. *Neuroreport* 2021; 32: 259–267. DOI: 10.1097/WNR.0000000000001583.

154. Jiang P, Chen L, Xu J, et al. Neuroprotective effects of rhynchophylline against Abeta1-42-induced oxidative stress, neurodegeneration, and memory impairment via Nrf2-ARE activation. *Neurochem Res* 2021; 46: 2439–2450. DOI: 10.1007/s11064-021-03343-9.

155. Ali A, Shah SA, Zaman N, et al. Vitamin D exerts neuroprotection via SIRT1/nrf-2/ NF-kB signaling pathways against D-galactose-induced memory impairment in adult mice. *Neurochem Int* 2021; 142: 104893. DOI: 10.1016/j.neuint.2020.104893.

156. Zhang S, Li L, Hu J, et al. Polysaccharide of Taxus chinensis var. mairei Cheng et L.K.Fu attenuates neurotoxicity and cognitive dysfunction in mice with Alzheimer's disease. *Pharm Biol* 2020; 58: 959–968. DOI: 10.1080/13880209.2020.1817102.

157. Xiang J, Cao K, Dong YT, et al. Lithium chloride reduced the level of oxidative stress in brains and serums of APP/PS1 double transgenic mice via the regulation of GSK3beta/Nrf2/ HO-1 pathway. *Int J Neurosci* 2020; 130: 564–573. DOI: 10.1080/00207454.2019.1688808.

158. Wei C, Fan J, Sun X, et al. Acetyl-11-keto-beta-boswellic acid ameliorates cognitive deficits and reduces amyloid-beta levels in APPswe/PS1dE9 mice through antioxidant and anti-inflammatory pathways. *Free Radic Biol Med* 2020; 150: 96–108. DOI: 10.1016/j. freeradbiomed.2020.02.022.

159. Wang CY, Zhang Q, Xun Z, et al. Increases of iASPP-Keap1 interaction mediated by syringin enhance synaptic plasticity and rescue cognitive impairments via stabilizing Nrf2 in Alzheimer's models. *Redox Biol* 2020; 36: 101672. DOI: 10.1016/j.redox.2020.101672.

160. Su IJ, Chang HY, Wang HC, et al. A curcumin analog exhibits multiple biologic effects on the pathogenesis of Alzheimer's disease and improves behavior, inflammation, and beta-amyloid accumulation in a mouse model. *Int J Mol Sci* 2020; 21. DOI: 10.3390/ ijms21155459.

161. Qin X, Hua J, Lin SJ, et al. Astragalus polysaccharide alleviates cognitive impairment and beta-amyloid accumulation in APP/PS1 mice via Nrf2 pathway. *Biochem Biophys Res Commun* 2020; 531: 431–437. DOI: 10.1016/j.bbrc.2020.07.122.

162. Dong Y, Stewart T, Bai L, et al. Coniferaldehyde attenuates Alzheimer's pathology via activation of Nrf2 and its targets. *Theranostics* 2020; 10: 179–200. DOI: 10.7150/thno.36722.

163. Yang Q, Lin J, Zhang H, et al. Ginsenoside compound K regulates amyloid-beta via the Nrf2/Keap1 signaling pathway in mice with scopolamine hydrobromide-induced memory impairments. *J Mol Neurosci* 2019; 67: 62–71. DOI: 10.1007/s12031-018-1210-3.

164. Wan T, Wang Z, Luo Y, et al. FA-97, a new synthetic caffeic acid phenethyl ester derivative, protects against oxidative stress-mediated neuronal cell apoptosis and scopolamine-induced cognitive impairment by activating Nrf2/HO-1 signaling. *Oxid Med Cell Longev* 2019; 2019: 8239642. DOI: 10.1155/2019/8239642.

165. Li Z, Chen X, Zhang Y, et al. Protective roles of Amanita caesarea polysaccharides against Alzheimer's disease via Nrf2 pathway. *Int J Biol Macromol* 2019; 121: 29–37. DOI: 10.1016/j.ijbiomac.2018.09.216.

166. Li S, Zhao X, Lazarovici P, et al. Artemether activation of AMPK/GSK3beta(ser9)/ Nrf2 signaling confers neuroprotection towards beta-Amyloid-Induced neurotoxicity in 3xTg Alzheimer's mouse model. *Oxid Med Cell Longev* 2019; 2019: 1862437. DOI: 10.1155/2019/1862437.

167. Kong D, Yan Y, He XY, et al. Effects of resveratrol on the mechanisms of antioxidants and estrogen in Alzheimer's disease. *Biomed Res Int* 2019; 2019: 8983752. DOI: 10.1155/2019/8983752.

168. Ikram M, Muhammad T, Rehman SU, et al. Hesperetin confers neuroprotection by regulating Nrf2/TLR4/NF-kappaB signaling in an abeta mouse model. *Mol Neurobiol* 2019; 56: 6293–6309. DOI: 10.1007/s12035-019-1512-7.

169. Pu D, Zhao Y, Chen J, et al. Protective effects of sulforaphane on cognitive impairments and AD-like lesions in diabetic mice are associated with the upregulation of Nrf2 transcription activity. *Neuroscience* 2018; 381: 35–45. DOI: 10.1016/j.neuroscience.2018.04.017.

170. Hong Y and An Z. Hesperidin attenuate learning and memory deficits in APP/PS1 mice through activation of Akt/Nrf2 signaling and inhibition of RAGE/NF-kappaB signaling. *Arch Pharm Res* 2018; 41: 655–663. DOI: 10.1007/s12272-015-0662-z.

171. Yu L, Wang S, Chen X, et al. Orientin alleviates cognitive deficits and oxidative stress in Abeta1-42-induced mouse model of Alzheimer's disease. *Life Sci* 2015; 121: 104–109. DOI: 10.1016/j.lfs.2014.11.021.

172. Lipton SA, Rezaie T, Nutter A, et al. Therapeutic advantage of pro-electrophilic drugs to activate the Nrf2/ARE pathway in Alzheimer's disease models. *Cell Death Dis* 2016; 7: e2499. DOI: 10.1038/cddis.2016.389.

173. Liu Y, Deng Y, Liu H, et al. Hydrogen sulfide ameliorates learning memory impairment in APP/PS1 transgenic mice: A novel mechanism mediated by the activation of Nrf2. *Pharmacol Biochem Behav* 2016; 150–151: 207–216. DOI: 10.1016/j.pbb.2016.11.002.

174. Fragoulis A, Siegl S, Fendt M, et al. Oral administration of methysticin improves cognitive deficits in a mouse model of Alzheimer's disease. *Redox Biol* 2017; 12: 843–853. DOI: 10.1016/j.redox.2017.04.024.

175. Xu P, Wang K, Lu C, et al. Protective effects of linalool against amyloid beta-induced cognitive deficits and damages in mice. *Life Sci* 2017; 174: 21–27. DOI: 10.1016/j.lfs.2017.02.010.

176. Ali T, Kim T, Rehman SU, et al. Natural dietary supplementation of anthocyanins via PI3K/Akt/Nrf2/HO-1 pathways mitigate oxidative stress, neurodegeneration, and memory impairment in a mouse model of Alzheimer's disease. *Mol Neurobiol* 2018; 55: 6076–6093. DOI: 10.1007/s12035-017-0798-6.

177. Ghosh D, LeVault KR, and Brewer GJ. Dual-energy precursor and nuclear erythroid-related factor 2 activator treatment additively improve redox glutathione levels and neuron survival in aging and Alzheimer mouse neurons upstream of reactive oxygen species. *Neurobiol Aging* 2014; 35: 179–190. DOI: 10.1016/j.neurobiolaging.2013.06.023.

178. Dutta N, Ghosh S, Nelson VK, et al. Andrographolide upregulates protein quality control mechanisms in cell and mouse through upregulation of mTORC1 function. *Biochim Biophys Acta Gen Subj* 2021; 1865: 129885. DOI: 10.1016/j.bbagen.2021.129885.

179. Yang Y, Kong F, Ding Q, et al. Bruceine D elevates Nrf2 activation to restrain Parkinson's disease in mice through suppressing oxidative stress and inflammatory response. *Biochem Biophys Res Commun* 2020; 526: 1013–1020. DOI: 10.1016/j.bbrc.2020.03.097.

180. Wang T, Li C, Han B, et al. Neuroprotective effects of Danshensu on rotenone-induced Parkinson's disease models in vitro and in vivo. *BMC Complement Med Ther* 2020; 20: 20. DOI: 10.1186/s12906-019-2738-7.

181. Yang C, Mo Y, Xu E, et al. Astragaloside IV ameliorates motor deficits and dopaminergic neuron degeneration via inhibiting neuroinflammation and oxidative stress in a Parkinson's disease mouse model. *Int Immunopharmacol* 2019; 75: 105651. DOI: 10.1016/j.intimp.2019.05.036.

182. Zhou Q, Chen B, Wang X, et al. Sulforaphane protects against rotenone-induced neurotoxicity in vivo: Involvement of the mTOR, Nrf2, and autophagy pathways. *Sci Rep* 2016; 6: 32206. DOI: 10.1038/srep32206.

183. Ning C, Gao X, Wang C, et al. Ginsenoside Rg1 protects against acetaminophen-induced liver injury via activating Nrf2 signaling pathway in vivo and in vitro. *Regul Toxicol Pharmacol* 2018; 98: 58–68. DOI: 10.1016/j.yrtph.2018.07.012.

184. Shi L, Hao Z, Zhang S, et al. Baicalein and baicalin alleviate acetaminophen-induced liver injury by activating Nrf2 antioxidative pathway: The involvement of ERK1/2 and PKC. *Biochem Pharmacol* 2018; 150: 9–23. DOI: 10.1016/j.bcp.2018.01.026.

185. Wei M, Zheng Z, Shi L, et al. Natural polyphenol chlorogenic acid protects against acetaminophen-induced hepatotoxicity by activating ERK/Nrf2 antioxidative pathway. *Toxicol Sci* 2018; 162: 99–112. DOI: 10.1093/toxsci/kfx230.
186. Huang Z, Jing X, Sheng Y, et al. (-)-Epicatechin attenuates hepatic sinusoidal obstruction syndrome by inhibiting liver oxidative and inflammatory injury. *Redox Biol* 2019; 22: 101117. DOI: 10.1016/j.redox.2019.101117.
187. Jiang Z, Guo X, Zhang K, et al. The essential oils and eucalyptol from Artemisia vulgaris L. prevent acetaminophen-induced liver injury by activating Nrf2-Keap1 and enhancing APAP clearance through non-toxic metabolic pathway. *Front Pharmacol* 2019; 10: 782. DOI: 10.3389/fphar.2019.00782.
188. Jin Y, Huang ZL, Li L, et al. Quercetin attenuates toosendanin-induced hepatotoxicity through inducing the Nrf2/GCL/GSH antioxidant signaling pathway. *Acta Pharmacol Sin* 2019; 40: 75–85. DOI: 10.1038/s41401-018-0024-8.
189. Zhao S, Song T, Gu Y, et al. Hydrogen sulfide alleviates liver injury through the S-sulfhydrated-kelch-like ECH-associated protein 1/nuclear erythroid 2-related factor 2/low-density lipoprotein receptor-related protein 1 pathway. *Hepatology* 2021; 73: 282–302. DOI: 10.1002/hep.31247.
190. Zhang YP, Yang XQ, Yu DK, et al. Nrf2 signalling pathway and autophagy impact on the preventive effect of green tea extract against alcohol-induced liver injury. *J Pharm Pharmacol* 2021; 73: 986–995. DOI: 10.1093/jpp/rgab027.
191. Zhang MH, Li J, Zhu XY, et al. Physalin B ameliorates non-alcoholic steatohepatitis by stimulating autophagy and NRF2 activation mediated improvement in oxidative stress. *Free Radic Biol Med* 2021; 164: 1–12. DOI: 10.1016/j.freeradbiomed.2020.12.020.
192. Tao S, Yang Y, Li J, et al. Bixin attenuates high-fat diet-caused liver steatosis and inflammatory injury through Nrf2/PPARalpha signals. *Oxid Med Cell Longev* 2021; 2021: 6610124. DOI: 10.1155/2021/6610124.
193. Lu Q, Shu Y, Wang L, et al. The protective effect of Veronica ciliata Fisch. Extracts on relieving oxidative stress-induced liver injury via activating AMPK/p62/Nrf2 pathway. *J Ethnopharmacol* 2021; 270: 113775. DOI: 10.1016/j.jep.2021.113775.
194. Joshi A, Upadhyay KK, Vohra A, et al. Melatonin induces Nrf2-HO-1 reprogramming and corrections in hepatic core clock oscillations in non-alcoholic fatty liver disease. *FASEB J* 2021; 35: e21803. DOI: 10.1096/fj.202002556RRR.
195. Hu D, Zhang L, Jiang R, et al. Nicotinic acid against acetaminophen-induced hepatotoxicity via Sirt1/Nrf2 antioxidative pathway in mice. *J Nutr Sci Vitaminol (Tokyo)* 2021; 67: 145–152. DOI: 10.3177/jnsv.67.145.
196. Xie K, He X, Chen K, et al. Ameliorative effects and molecular mechanisms of vine tea on western diet-induced NAFLD. *Food Funct* 2020; 11: 5976–5991. DOI: 10.1039/d0fo00795a.
197. Rahman ZU, Al Kury LT, Alattar A, et al. Carveol a naturally-derived potent and emerging Nrf2 activator protects against acetaminophen-induced hepatotoxicity. *Front Pharmacol* 2020; 11: 621538. DOI: 10.3389/fphar.2020.621538.
198. Lv H, An B, Yu Q, et al. The hepatoprotective effect of myricetin against lipopolysaccharide and D-galactosamine-induced fulminant hepatitis. *Int J Biol Macromol* 2020; 155: 1092–1104. DOI: 10.1016/j.ijbiomac.2019.11.075.
199. Hosseini H, Teimouri M, Shabani M, et al. Resveratrol alleviates non-alcoholic fatty liver disease through epigenetic modification of the Nrf2 signaling pathway. *Int J Biochem Cell Biol* 2020; 119: 105667. DOI: 10.1016/j.biocel.2019.105667.
200. Shan Y, Jiang B, Yu J, et al. Protective effect of schisandra chinensis polysaccharides against the immunological liver injury in mice based on Nrf2/ARE and TLR4/NF-kappaB signaling pathway. *J Med Food* 2019; 22: 885–895. DOI: 10.1089/jmf.2018.4377.
201. Panda H, Keleku-Lukwete N, Kuga A, et al. Dietary supplementation with sulforaphane attenuates liver damage and heme overload in a sickle cell disease murine model. *Exp Hematol* 2019; 77: 51–60 e51. DOI: 10.1016/j.exphem.2019.08.001.

202. Luo DD, Chen JF, Liu JJ, et al. Tetrahydrocurcumin and octahydrocurcumin, the primary and final hydrogenated metabolites of curcumin, possess superior hepatic-protective effect against acetaminophen-induced liver injury: Role of CYP2E1 and Keap1-Nrf2 pathway. *Food Chem Toxicol* 2019; 123: 349–362. DOI: 10.1016/j.fct.2018.11.012.
203. Xu J, Zhang L, Jiang R, et al. Nicotinamide improves NAD(+) levels to protect against acetaminophen-induced acute liver injury in mice. *Hum Exp Toxicol* 2021; 40: 1938–1946. DOI: 10.1177/09603271211014573.
204. Yan M, Guo L, Yang Y, et al. Glycyrrhetinic acid protects alpha-naphthylisothiocyanate-induced cholestasis through regulating transporters, inflammation and apoptosis. *Front Pharmacol* 2021; 12: 701240. DOI: 10.3389/fphar.2021.701240.
205. Liu M, Zheng B, Liu P, et al. Exploration of the hepatoprotective effect and mechanism of magnesium isoglycyrrhizinate in mice with arsenic trioxideinduced acute liver injury. *Mol Med Rep* 2021; 23. DOI: 10.3892/mmr.2021.12077.
206. Wang X, Chang X, Zhan H, et al. Curcumin and Baicalin ameliorate ethanol-induced liver oxidative damage via the Nrf2/HO-1 pathway. *J Food Biochem* 2020: e13425. DOI: 10.1111/jfbc.13425.
207. Wang X, Liu J, Dai Z, et al. Andrographolide improves PCP-induced schizophrenia-like behaviors through blocking the interaction between NRF2 and KEAP1. *J Pharmacol Sci* 2021; 147: 9–17. DOI: 10.1016/j.jphs.2021.05.007.
208. Zhu Y, Zhang Y, Huang X, et al. Z-Ligustilide protects vascular endothelial cells from oxidative stress and rescues high-fat diet-induced atherosclerosis by activating multiple NRF2 downstream genes. *Atherosclerosis* 2019; 284: 110–120. DOI: 10.1016/j.atherosclerosis.2019.02.010.
209. Ji R, Sun H, Peng J, et al. Rosmarinic acid exerts an antagonistic effect on vascular calcification by regulating the Nrf2 signalling pathway. *Free Radic Res* 2019; 53: 187–197. DOI: 10.1080/10715762.2018.1558447.
210. Zhao F, Liu C, Fang L, et al. Walnut-derived peptide activates PINK1 via the NRF2/KEAP1/HO-1 pathway, promotes mitophagy, and alleviates learning and memory impairments in a mice model. *J Agric Food Chem* 2021; 69: 2758–2772. DOI: 10.1021/acs.jafc.0c07546.
211. Zeng Q, Xiong Q, Zhou M, et al. Resveratrol attenuates methamphetamine-induced memory impairment via inhibition of oxidative stress and apoptosis in mice. *J Food Biochem* 2021; 45: e13622. DOI: 10.1111/jfbc.13622.
212. Wu D, Liu H, Liu Y, et al. Protective effect of alpha-lipoic acid on bisphenol A-induced learning and memory impairment in developing mice: nNOS and keap1/Nrf2 pathway. *Food Chem Toxicol* 2021; 154: 112307. DOI: 10.1016/j.fct.2021.112307.
213. Cui W, Chen J, Yu F, et al. GYY4137 protected the integrity of the blood-brain barrier via activation of the Nrf2/ARE pathway in mice with sepsis. *FASEB J* 2021; 35: e21710. DOI: 10.1096/fj.202100074R.
214. Cong P, Wang T, Tong C, et al. Resveratrol ameliorates thoracic blast exposure-induced inflammation, endoplasmic reticulum stress, and apoptosis in the brain through the Nrf2/Keap1 and NF-kappaB signaling pathway. *Injury* 2021; 52: 2795–2802. DOI: 10.1016/j.injury.2021.08.019.
215. Zheng H, Su Y, Sun Y, et al. Echinacoside alleviates hypobaric hypoxia-induced memory impairment in C57 mice. *Phytother Res* 2019; 33: 1150–1160. DOI: 10.1002/ptr.6310.
216. Wang J, Jiang C, Zhang K, et al. Melatonin receptor activation provides cerebral protection after traumatic brain injury by mitigating oxidative stress and inflammation via the Nrf2 signaling pathway. *Free Radic Biol Med* 2019; 131: 345–355. DOI: 10.1016/j.freeradbiomed.2018.12.014.
217. Ren B, Yuan T, Diao Z, et al. Protective effects of sesamol on systemic oxidative stress-induced cognitive impairments via regulation of Nrf2/Keap1 pathway. *Food Funct* 2018; 9: 5912–5924. DOI: 10.1039/c8fo01436a.

218. Zarei M, Uppin V, Acharya P, et al. Ginger, and turmeric lipid-solubles attenuate heated oil-induced oxidative stress in the brain via the upregulation of NRF2 and improve cognitive function in rats. *Metab Brain Dis* 2021; 36: 225–238. DOI: 10.1007/s11011-020-00642-y.
219. Zhou JY, Lin HL, Qin YC, et al. l-Carnosine protects against deoxynivalenol-induced oxidative stress in intestinal stem cells by regulating the Keap1/Nrf2 signaling pathway. *Mol Nutr Food Res* 2021; 65: e2100406. DOI: 10.1002/mnfr.202100406.
220. Rajput SA, Liang SJ, Wang XQ, et al. Lycopene protects intestinal epithelium from deoxynivalenol-induced oxidative damage via regulating Keap1/Nrf2 signaling. *Antioxidants (Basel)* 2021; 10. DOI: 10.3390/antiox10091493.
221. Rahimi G, Heydari S, Rahimi B, et al. A combination of herbal compound (SPTC) along with exercise or metformin more efficiently alleviated diabetic complications through down-regulation of stress oxidative pathway upon activating Nrf2-Keap1 axis in AGE rich diet-induced type 2 diabetic mice. *Nutr Metab (Lond)* 2021; 18: 14. DOI: 10.1186/s12986-021-00543-6.
222. Lu Q, Zheng R, Zhu P, et al. Hinokinin alleviates high-fat diet/streptozotocin-induced cardiac injury in mice through modulation in oxidative stress, inflammation, and apoptosis. *Biomed Pharmacother* 2021; 137: 111361. DOI: 10.1016/j.biopha.2021.111361.
223. Huo Y, Mijiti A, Cai R, et al. Scutellarin alleviates type 2 diabetes (HFD/low dose STZ)-induced cardiac injury through modulation of oxidative stress, inflammation, apoptosis, and fibrosis in mice. *Hum Exp Toxicol* 2021; 40: S460–S474. DOI: 10.1177/09603271211045948.
224. Li R, Qi Y, Yuan Q, et al. Protective effects of dioscin against isoproterenol-induced cardiac hypertrophy via adjusting PKCepsilon/ERK-mediated oxidative stress. *Eur J Pharmacol* 2021; 907: 174277. DOI: 10.1016/j.ejphar.2021.174277.
225. Jia Y, Li J, Liu P, et al. Based on activation of p62-Keap1-Nrf2 pathway, hesperidin protects arsenic-trioxide-induced cardiotoxicity in mice. *Front Pharmacol* 2021; 12: 758670. DOI: 10.3389/fphar.2021.758670.
226. Du J, He W, Zhang C, et al. Pentamethylquercetin attenuates cardiac remodeling via activation of the sestrins/Keap1/Nrf2 pathway in MSG-induced obese mice. *Biomed Res Int* 2020; 2020: 3243906. DOI: 10.1155/2020/3243906.
227. Li R, Liu Y, Shan YG, et al. Bailcalin protects against diabetic cardiomyopathy through Keap1/Nrf2/AMPK-mediated antioxidative and lipid-lowering effects. *Oxid Med Cell Longev* 2019; 2019: 3206542. DOI: 10.1155/2019/3206542.
228. Zeng H, Wang L, Zhang J, et al. Activated PKB/GSK-3beta synergizes with PKC-delta signaling in attenuating myocardial ischemia/reperfusion injury via potentiation of NRF2 activity: Therapeutic efficacy of dihydrotanshinone-I. *Acta Pharm Sin B* 2021; 11: 71–88. DOI: 10.1016/j.apsb.2020.09.006.
229. Song J, Meng Y, Wang M, et al. Mangiferin activates Nrf2 to attenuate cardiac fibrosis via redistributing glutaminolysis-derived glutamate. *Pharmacol Res* 2020; 157: 104845. DOI: 10.1016/j.phrs.2020.104845.
230. Liu G, Wu Y, Jin S, et al. Itaconate ameliorates methicillin-resistant Staphylococcus aureus-induced acute lung injury through the Nrf2/ARE pathway. *Ann Transl Med* 2021; 9: 712. DOI: 10.21037/atm-21-1448.
231. Guohua F, Tieyuan Z, Xinping M, et al. Melatonin protects against PM2.5-induced lung injury by inhibiting ferroptosis of lung epithelial cells in an Nrf2-dependent manner. *Ecotoxicol Environ Saf* 2021; 223: 112588. DOI: 10.1016/j.ecoenv.2021.112588.
232. Wang W, Yang X, Chen Q, et al. Sinomenine attenuates septic-associated lung injury through the Nrf2-Keap1 and autophagy. *J Pharm Pharmacol* 2020; 72: 259–270. DOI: 10.1111/jphp.13202.
233. Tao S, Zhang H, Xue L, et al. Vitamin D protects against particles-caused lung injury through induction of autophagy in an Nrf2-dependent manner. *Environ Toxicol* 2019; 34: 594–609. DOI: 10.1002/tox.22726.

234. Peng LY, An L, Sun NY, et al. Salvia miltiorrhiza restrains reactive oxygen species-associated pulmonary fibrosis via targeting Nrf2-Nox4 redox balance. *Am J Chin Med* 2019; 47: 1113–1131. DOI: 10.1142/S0192415X19500575.
235. An L, Peng LY, Sun NY, et al. Tanshinone IIA activates nuclear factor-erythroid 2-related factor 2 to restrain pulmonary fibrosis via regulation of redox homeostasis and glutaminolysis. *Antioxid Redox Signal* 2019; 30: 1831–1848. DOI: 10.1089/ars.2018.7569.
236. Malavolta M, Bracci M, Santarelli L, et al. Inducers of senescence, toxic compounds, and senolytics: The multiple faces of Nrf2-activating phytochemicals in cancer adjuvant therapy. *Mediators Inflamm* 2018; 2018: 4159013. DOI: 10.1155/2018/4159013.
237. Yamagata K. Dietary docosahexaenoic acid inhibits neurodegeneration and prevents stroke. *J Neurosci Res* 2021; 99: 561–572. DOI: 10.1002/jnr.24728.
238. Zhao F, Ci X, Man X, et al. Food-derived pharmacological modulators of the Nrf2/ARE pathway: Their role in the treatment of diseases. *Molecules* 2021; 26. DOI: 10.3390/molecules26041016.
239. Zhou YQ, Mei W, Tian XB, et al. The therapeutic potential of Nrf2 inducers in chronic pain: Evidence from preclinical studies. *Pharmacol Ther* 2021; 225: 107846. DOI: 10.1016/j.pharmthera.2021.107846.

Index

Note: **Bold** page numbers refer to tables; *italic* page numbers refer to figures.

For Product Safety Concerns and Information please contact our EU
representative GPSR@taylorandfrancis.com
Taylor & Francis Verlag GmbH, Kaufingerstraße 24, 80331 München, Germany